TAKE YOUR PEDIATRICIAN WITH YOU

A JOHNS HOPKINS PRESS

HEALTH BOOK

Take Your Pediatrician with You

Keeping Your Child Healthy at Home and on the Road

Dr. Christopher S. Ryder

THE JOHNS HOPKINS UNIVERSITY PRESS
Baltimore

Note to the Reader: This book is not intended to take the place of the advice of your child's doctor at home or to take the place of medical advice and treatment while you and your child are traveling. All travelers should visit a travel clinic or travel physician before traveling to lesser-developed countries or tropical countries. This book is not intended to take the place of a visit to a health provider.

Drug Dosage: The author and publisher have made reasonable efforts to determine that the selection and dosage of drugs discussed in this text conform to the practices of the general medical community. The medications described do not necessarily have specific approval by the U.S. Food and Drug Administration for use in the diseases and dosages for which they are recommended. In view of ongoing research, changes in governmental regulations, and the constant flow of information relating to drug therapy and drug reactions, the reader is urged to check the package insert of each drug for any change in indications and dosage and for warnings and precautions. This is particularly important when the recommended agent is a new and/or infrequently used drug.

© 2004, 2007 by Christopher S. Ryder
All rights reserved. Published 2007
Printed in the United States of America on acid-free paper
9 8 7 6 5 4 3 2 1

An earlier version was published in 2004 as *Handbook for Pediatric Health Problems at Home and on the Road*

The Johns Hopkins University Press
2715 North Charles Street
Baltimore, Maryland 21218-4363
www.press.jhu.edu

Library of Congress Cataloging-in-Publication Data

Ryder, Christopher S., 1947–
   Take your pediatrician with you : keeping your child healthy at home and on the road /
Christopher S. Ryder.
      p. cm.
   Rev. ed. of: Handbook for pediatric health problems at home and on the road. © 2004.
   Includes index.
   ISBN-13: 978-0-8018-8601-0 (pbk. : alk. paper)
   ISBN-10: 0-8018-8601-5 (pbk. : alk. paper)
   1. Pediatric emergencies—Handbooks, manuals, etc. 2. Travel—Health aspects—
Handbooks, manuals, etc. 3. Children—Travel—Handbooks, manuals, etc. I. Ryder,
Christopher S., 1947–   Handbook for pediatric health problems at home and on the road.
II. Title.
   RJ370.R94 2007
   618.92'0025—dc22   2006023120

A catalog record for this book is available from the British Library.

To my best friend and wife, Alixe,

the perfect traveling companion,

and to my son, David.

Thank you both for all your love, patience, support,

and understanding during the writing of this book.

And to Nelson Mandela,

who enabled all South Africans to "Walk Tall."

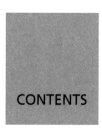

CONTENTS

PART ONE

Traveling with Children

PART TWO

Common Childhood Illnesses

PART THREE

Summer Woes

PART FOUR

Accidents, Injuries, and Emergencies

PART FIVE

A Medical Kit for Children   569

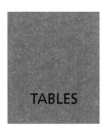

TABLES

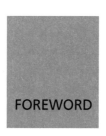

FOREWORD

As the world becomes more accessible in our age of the Internet, cruise ships, jets, and cars, more families are traveling with children. But the joy of a vacation may be ruined by faulty planning, lack of knowledge of the destination, visa requirements, endemic disease, and cultural differences.

Christopher Ryder, M.D., an outstanding pediatrician and a parent with a young son, has traveled extensively. He has personally experienced the joys and trials of traveling with his family, and he describes these "encounters of travel kind" in this book.

The book succeeds admirably, providing state-of-the-art information in a comprehensive and easy-to-understand manner. It deals with the preparation for travel and how this differs if one has children in tow, and the prevention and treatment of common illnesses and accidents experienced by traveling families. Travel-related medical and nonmedical problems are discussed.

Although Dr. Ryder originally intended this book just for travelers, it will be an invaluable resource for expectant parents, parents planning a foreign adoption, and all families with children.

The earlier version of this book, entitled *Handbook for Pediatric Health Problems at Home and on the Road,* proved to be very popular, and this newer version has added valuable information on the prevention of another increasingly important mosquito-borne illness (dengue fever) and guidelines on the prevention of that all-important emerging infection avian (bird) flu. Other new topics include a discussion of many common childhood diseases such as croup, bronchiolitis, and roseola, as well as important pointers relating to traveling teenagers. For those of you venturing not only to the water's edge but into the water, this new version has added an excellent review on the prevention and management of stings and other injuries caused by marine animals.

I believe this book should be required reading for all pediatric and family practice residents in training, not only for the outstanding travel advice it contains but also for the insight it offers into common childhood illnesses. As a professional colleague, I highly recommend this all-encompassing book for families both at home and on the road, medical personnel, and travel clinics. This aptly named book allows you to "take your pediatrician with you."

—B. K. Varma, M.D.
Chairman, Department of Pediatrics
Pinnacle Health Hospitals
Harrisburg, Pennsylvania
Clinical Professor of Pediatrics
Pennsylvania State University of Medicine
Hershey, Pennsylvania

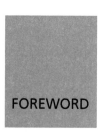

FOREWORD

If you have children, you need this book! Comprehensive and easy to use, it will inform, empower, and encourage you. The author of this book, Dr. Christopher Ryder, is one of the best pediatricians I have ever known, with more than 25 years of experience caring for children and their families. His incredible depth and breadth of knowledge allowed him to write this most comprehensive, well-researched, and practical book. It should be used not only during travel with children but in everyday life as well.

This edition of the book has a greatly expanded travel section that now includes chapters on traveling with adolescents, how to deal with headaches, and some common mosquito-borne diseases. Dr. Ryder has also added some very valuable information on common childhood infections, like RSV, croup, and hand, foot, and mouth disease, among others. His chapter on bringing home your internationally adopted child is excellent. It walks you through the whole process starting with pre-adoption medical preparations for parents. It lists illnesses that are common in international adoptees and gives very specific recommendations on what to bring with you on your trip.

If you have this book, you can feel very comfortable that you are prepared to deal with any medical issue that may face you or your child both at home and on the road.

—*Boris Skurkovich, M.D.*
Clinical Associate Professor of Pediatrics
Brown Medical School
Director, International Adoption Clinic
Hasbro Children's Hospital
Providence, Rhode Island

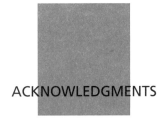

ACKNOWLEDGMENTS

I would like to give special thanks to my editor, Grace Carino, who did a wonderful job of making this book more readable. Her suggestions and insights I gratefully acknowledge. I would also like to thank Jacqueline Wehmueller and her staff for guiding me through the writing and publishing process and always being so helpful and optimistic.

Thanks are due to Dr. Richard Levine for his suggestions on the section on traveling with adolescents and to Dr. Boris Skurkovich for sharing his knowledge on international adoption.

An earlier edition of this book was published with the title *Handbook for Pediatric Problems at Home and on the Road.* I am indebted to Steve Pedersen and Barb Moore for their help and encouragement with this edition. Neither of them ever seemed to lose faith in me or in the success of the book. Alice Duncan gave me some valuable early pointers in making this earlier edition more lucid. I would also like to thank the editing staff at Bookmasters for their help with the previous edition.

Thanks to all the children, their parents, and my colleagues for all they have taught me over the years.

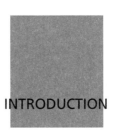

INTRODUCTION

Soon after completing my medical training I left South Africa and visited England for the first time. The sense of freedom and independence I experienced was exhilarating, and I can remember as though it were yesterday the excitement I felt as I explored London. I would rise early and jog along the often damp pavements, marveling at the sights and sounds of that great city as it woke to greet a new day.

Other European countries followed England, and even after I returned to South Africa, the generous vacations I enjoyed allowed me to continue to travel. I then went to the Middle East and worked in Bahrain for three years before settling in the United States.

Although those month-long annual vacations are but a dream, my wife and I still use our free time to indulge ourselves and to share with our son the adventures that travel offers. Together we have traveled through much of Europe, parts of Africa, Asia, and America.

Some years ago, friends of ours were taking their six-year-old child to China for three months and asked us what they should take with them so they would be prepared to treat minor illnesses while away. We suggested they buy a first aid kit. They arrived on our doorstep, bulging shopping bags in hand, and together we unpacked a variety of drugstore first aid and medical kits on our dining room table. As we checked the contents of the various kits, it became obvious that most of them contained a collection of Band-Aids and bandages and medications suitable only for adults. Not one of these kits was suitable for a family traveling with a child. In fact, none of the medications contained in any of these kits could even be *swallowed* by a young child! This was the inspiration for the creation of a child-friendly travel kit.

My wife and I then started to assemble some basic items that we knew we would use when traveling with our child. As the kit evolved, it became obvious that this was something that every family could use both at home and while on vacation. Many families rely on their pediatrician or family doctor for advice when faced with the common ailments of childhood. When they are away from home, however, they can't always reach their doctor, so I wrote a book to accompany the kit. In addition to instructions for assembling a medical kit for children, this book covers many of the more common childhood illnesses and problems that a parent might encounter both at home and while traveling, as well as travel advice and prevention and treatment of travel-related illnesses.

I recognize that a parent's level of stress is higher away from home and away from familiar surroundings and familiar and trusted health care. I always urge parents to use common sense and parental intuition. Whenever a parent is in doubt, however, he or she should seek experienced medical help. Guidelines are given throughout this book about when to seek expert medical help and how to locate physicians abroad, including physicians who speak English.

THE BOOK IS DIVIDED INTO FIVE PARTS. Part One suggests how parents can prepare to travel with children in the United States and abroad. It covers common problems such as earaches while flying, jet lag, and motion sickness as well as less common and more serious diseases such as malaria and altitude sickness. It also includes a section on traveling with children who have chronic diseases such as asthma and diabetes. Part of my job as a pediatrician involves taking care of children who have been adopted from foreign countries, so I have included a chapter on traveling to fetch the foreign adoptee.

By far the majority of the calls I receive from anxious parents who are traveling with their children are not about exotic travel diseases but about the relatively minor and common illnesses children also get at home. This is why Part Two, on common childhood symptoms and illnesses, became such an important part of the book. This section includes most of the common sicknesses that children get as they grow up, such as fevers, coughs and colds, strep throat, constipation, vomiting, and diarrhea.

Part Three discusses common summer ailments because summer is when most families travel, and that is also the season when certain diseases and accidents are more likely to occur. The most important topic covered here is the prevention of sunburn. Other topics include the prevention of insect and tick bites, West Nile fever, Lyme disease, and poison ivy rashes.

Although this book discusses exotic diseases such as malaria, the most likely reason your child will land in the hospital while traveling in the United States or abroad is an accident. Accidents are one of the most common causes of death in childhood in the United States, and motor vehicle accidents are the leading cause of death while traveling. Part Four, on accidents, injuries, and emergencies, discusses how to prevent more common accidents as well as extremely rare events such as lightning strikes.

Part Five describes the items you will want to include in a medical kit for your children. The contents listed could also be the basis for a family or adult medical and travel kit.

You will see that I go into detail on how to manage the very common childhood problems that occur at home and while traveling, such as travelers' diarrhea, diarrhea and dehydration, and fevers. While most families who use this book will have ready access to medical care, others may be in a remote location and will need to cope with these problems entirely on their own. This book contains information intended to help get these families safely through these illnesses, which many times may relate to one another. For example, you may have a child who develops a cold that brings with it a sore throat. Therefore I group together chapters on connected ailments and their symptoms. This book, however, does not contain an exhaustive list of all the problems your children are likely to develop. References are provided for parents who want more detailed information and suggestions for additional reading.

This book primarily applies to children and childhood diseases, but much of the information it contains is also applicable to adults. Topics such as preparing for travel abroad, travelers' diarrhea, selecting safe food and water, malaria prevention, motion sickness, cruise ships, altitude sickness, jet lag, preventing insect stings and bites, and many others apply to both children and adults. One topic, "economy class syndrome"/traveler's thrombosis (blood clot), which is discussed in Part One, applies only to adults. I thought it was important to include this topic because children seldom travel alone, and if the adults fall ill, the children will certainly be affected.

This book contains many important warnings. But travel should be fun and educational, and the cautions in this book are meant to help you and your family have more fun and education and fewer illnesses, accidents, and emergencies—or, if medical problems do come up, to limit their impact on your child's health and your travels. Understanding and learning the reasons for various precautions will help you and your children follow them. The better prepared you are, the less likely you are to need medical care while away from home.

PART ONE

Traveling with Children

1

Planning, Packing, and Pacing

Anyone who has children will acknowledge that they change one's life! You'll want to remember this when making your travel plans.

Traveling with children poses unique challenges and requires much more planning than traveling without them. The stresses of travel escalate when you have a child in tow, but so do the fun and enjoyment. You will probably have more laughs—and more tears. Through the eyes of your child you will see the world in a very different way.

Travel often brings families closer together. Think back to your childhood. Some of your happiest and most vivid memories may be those of the vacations you spent with your parents and siblings. These memories become even more precious once your parents are no longer living. At the end of the day, the rewards of traveling with children are worth the extra hassles, the extra effort, and the added stresses.

SOME POINTS TO CONSIDER WHEN PLANNING YOUR TRAVELS

The Ages of Your Children

Newborn to Three Months

Home is the best place to be with a newborn. Traveling exposes all of us to infections. If an infant gets an infection and a fever in the first three months of life, immediate medical attention will be required. For this reason, it is better to wait until your baby is a little older before venturing far from home.

Four to Twelve Months

This may be a relatively easy time to travel. You have become used to your baby, and the days of colic should be behind you.

You are in charge, which is not always the case when your child is older! Your baby has limited mobility, and if you have a comfortable baby carrier, you may not need a stroller.

Your baby may be breast-fed (the healthiest, easiest, cheapest, and most convenient method) or formula fed. If you use formula, a source of safe water is essential. If you are unsure of the safety of the water supply, it may be easier to boil water once a day and store it in clean, sealed feeding bottles. (It is necessary only to bring the water to a boil to kill organisms, but for an extra margin of safety you can allow the water to boil for one minute.) Just before feeding, add the powdered formula. It is not necessary to reheat the formula. Discard any unused formula.

Bottles and nipples must be kept clean and can be steril-

ized by soaking in boiling water or in water to which a sterilizing tablet has been added. Ready-to-use formula is convenient but bulky and heavy. This may be a good choice if you
are planning a short trip.

Once your baby is eating solids, take along a supply of
cereal and other baby foods. The foods you are familiar with
may not be available in other countries.

Babies and toddlers require a lot of paraphernalia. Baby
carriers, car seats, strollers, portable cribs, diapers—the list
seems endless. Take what you need, and do not economize
when safety is involved. Taking along an infant car seat is essential, unless you are sure you will have one at your destination. Even then, slipups can happen, and the promised seat
may not be available. Also, in many countries infant car seats
are not readily available or may not be in good condition or
be the right size for your child.

One to Four Years

This is probably the most challenging time to travel with
children. They are usually more demanding and easily frus-
trated, and they may be prone to temper tantrums. They are
active and striving for independence on the one hand and yet
totally reliant on their parents on the other. Their attention
span is usually short, and they need to be entertained. (Have
you ever been seated next to someone else's two-year-old on
a long bus or plane ride?)

- Children of this age require a more diverse diet, and it
  is more difficult to provide safe food and water for them

when traveling in developing countries. Always carry a supply of snacks, small boxes of juice, and plenty of wet wipes.

- Everything they lay their hands on is usually put straight into their mouth, and you will have trouble keeping their hands clean.
- Until your child is potty trained, you will need a supply of diapers. Disposable diapers usually make life easier but may not be readily available in developing countries. Always have a change of clothing easily accessible. Although one assumes life becomes easier once your child is toilet trained, this is not always the case. Young children need to "go now" and often have fixed ideas about where they will go, especially for a bowel movement. At times one longs for the diaper days!
- The equipment list you made for your infant is often even longer for your toddler. Toys that can be linked together make an adult's life a lot easier because less time is spent trying to retrieve or hunt for that "essential" toy beneath the aircraft seat or behind the bus seat.

Five Years and Older

As your children grow older, involve them in the planning of your trip. Let them help you research the places you intend to visit. Collect maps and brochures, visit the library or the bookstore, and search the Web for information.

If you are traveling to another country, prepare your children for differences in culture and living conditions.

Children of this age should carry their own backpacks.

Let them have some responsibility for what they choose to carry, but supervise them as they choose. You may end up carrying the backpack if it is too heavy. (Don't forget to include teddy.)

Your Vacation Location: Deciding Where to Go

Vacations that seem exotic and romantic when reading tourist brochures may be the exact opposite if you travel with children. Especially when traveling with young children, it may be sensible to stick to one of your tried-and-true vacation destinations where there will be few surprises. The more exotic and off the beaten path the location, the greater the preparation and the greater the potential for disaster.

When planning your vacation, ask yourself what you expect from your vacation.

- Do you want to spend most of the time together as a family or do you feel you need time apart from your children?
- Do you want to stay in one location or do you want more variety?
- Is the purpose of your vacation relaxation or are you seeking stimulation and activity? Are you looking for a combination of these?
- Do you enjoy camping or does a luxury hotel have a greater appeal? What does your budget allow?
- Are you more comfortable revisiting a favorite and familiar place or do you want to try something completely different?

- Do you want to stay in your own country or are you ready for foreign travel?

Decide what is right for you and your family. Know your own limits. With the right attitude and realistic expectations, your vacation will be a success.

For Your Reference

These family-friendly and kid-friendly Internet sites can help you plan your trip:

1. www.familytravelforum.com
2. www.travelforkids.com

PACKING FOR YOUR TRIP

Travel with as little luggage as possible, but remember to take along a favorite toy or blanket that will comfort your children and make them feel more secure.

When packing, you need to choose carefully not only what things are packed but also where things are packed. On plane and bus journeys, keep a supply of snacks and a change of diapers and clothing easily available. Sunscreen, insect repellent, and medications should be easily accessible but in a safe place away from your toddler's inquisitive hands.

If traveling to a tropical or very warm country, you will want to take cotton clothes, which are by far the coolest. Although you may be tempted to pack just a T-shirt and shorts for your young children, it is wise to take long pants and long-sleeved shirts as well to help protect against sunburn and insect bites. One-piece sleep suits and special infant sleeping bags will help protect infants and young children from insect bites at night.

Take comfortable, broken-in shoes. Include an extra pair of shoes in case one pair gets wet. It is often unsafe to walk barefoot in developing countries because of the potential not only for injuries from glass or other sharp objects but also for parasitic infections.

Take a hat to protect your child from the sun. If traveling to a cold location, you will need something to keep his head warm. A baby can lose a lot of heat from his head. In cold climates, it is a good idea to dress your child in layers and have spare gloves and extra tights to keep her warm.

MAKING YOUR JOURNEY MORE ENJOYABLE

All of us are happier if not confined to a car or airplane or bus seat for long periods. If you are traveling by car, stop frequently to give children a chance to exercise and use a restroom. It is better to arrive late but safely and smiling.

Take along toys, crayons, music, playing cards, and other diversions to entertain your children as you journey.

Older children can use guidebooks and tourist bureau pamphlets to alert the family about upcoming places of interest. They can also follow along on a map and use a marker to trace the journey.

Games like "I Spy" help pass the time and keep children aware of their surroundings.

Encourage children to walk while waiting in an airport. They need to burn up as much energy as possible.

Use the restroom just before boarding the plane. You may have to wait an hour or more after boarding before being permitted to leave your seat; also, there are a limited number of toilets on the plane. The toilets are cramped, and changing an infant or helping a toddler "go to the bathroom" in airplane toilets is not easy.

CHOOSING YOUR ACCOMMODATIONS

Consider safety and the ages of your children when choosing a place to stay.

Make sure children are welcome. It certainly is not relaxing to constantly ask your child to be quiet or to worry that a priceless piece of furniture might be damaged.

Consider upgrading your hotel accommodation to provide greater comfort for tired parents and children.

A beach or a swimming pool is a treat, but remember that children need constant supervision around water.

Children need time to feel at home in a hotel room. Allow time and space for them to settle in.

Many vacation resorts have "kid clubs" that offer supervised activities. This allows the adults to spend time together while giving children the opportunity to make new friends. Such an arrangement is especially important if you are traveling with just one child.

PLANNING YOUR ITINERARY

When traveling with children, less is often more, so do not plan to do too much. Allow time for unstructured play. Visiting the park to throw a Frisbee around may be the highlight of the day.

When we visited Disney World with our four-year-old, we all enjoyed ourselves more when we spent the afternoons at the hotel pool. By evening we were well rested and ready to return to the park to enjoy the fireworks.

Plan your days so that there is something of interest for each of your children.

Try to maintain your child's routine as much as possible. Plan excursions around your child's normal nap time, for example.

Museums, cathedrals, and other educational and historical attractions may not hold a child's attention for long, but most children will discover *something* that interests them.

Looking for lions in various shapes and forms kept our child alert and interested for hours when we spent an afternoon in St. Mark's Square in Venice. In Rome, our son found the antics of the cats on the grounds of the Coliseum infinitely more fascinating and entertaining than the ruins.

At times it may be sensible to let one parent have fun with the kids while the other parent pursues more intellectual or strenuous activities.

Be flexible.

Memories of having fun feeding flocks of pigeons, tossing coins into a fountain, or racing up the Spanish steps are more valuable than being able to say "I went to every Disney attraction" or "I saw every cathedral in Paris!"

2

Staying Safe, Staying Healthy, and Preventing Accidents

Although this chapter was primarily intended for international travelers, you will see that much of it applies to those who never leave the shores of the continental United States. If you watch the evening news or read your local newspaper, you will realize that you do not have to visit Beirut, Baghdad, or Johannesburg to be mugged or conned—it can happen in your own backyard!

If traveling to lesser-developed countries, you should visit a travel clinic to learn more about the risks pertaining to those countries. Topics such as malaria and other serious diseases are covered elsewhere in this book.

Accident prevention is just as important while traveling as it is at home—perhaps even more so, as you and your family are in unfamiliar surroundings.

STAYING TOGETHER AND OTHER
GENERAL SAFETY MEASURES

We worry about our child getting lost at home. While traveling, the worry may be even greater. Ground rules for safety need to be established before departing and should be reinforced frequently.

- Dress your children in bright clothes so that they are easily visible.
- Pin a whistle on the jacket of young children so that they can signal if they become separated from you.
- Decide on a meeting place in each location should you become separated.
- Young children should carry on their person a card listing their name, parents' names, and contact numbers. This information should not be visible but should be carried in a safe pocket.
- Children should carry on their person a card listing the name and address of their hotel or motel. It is a good idea for parents to do this also, especially when in a foreign country.
- Parents should carry with them a recent photograph of their child.
- During wilderness travel, children should be taught to hug the nearest tree if they become lost.
- Teach children not to go anywhere with strangers.
- Teach children to identify the police, security guards, and similar authorities. These are the people they can ask for help.

- Travel inconspicuously. Do not wear expensive jewelry and watches. Do not flash money around. Teach your children to do the same.
- Keep valuables and travel documents in your room safe or your hotel safe.

Also keep in mind these other important aspects of personal safety when traveling abroad:

- Avoid countries that are known to have drug-related violence or significant drug problems.
- Never purchase, transport, or use illegal drugs. Teach your children not to carry packages for strangers.
- Travel in groups, especially at night.
- Don't go out alone on beaches at night, and never sleep on the beach.
- Camp only in designated campsites.
- If you intend to travel to locations where there is a possibility of political turmoil, it is an excellent idea to research the country of destination thoroughly and learn what measures you can take to safeguard yourself and your family.

For Your Reference

Here are some excellent sources for information on travel safety:

1. *The Safe Travel Book,* by Peter Savage (1998).
2. *Travel Safely at Home and Abroad,* by Raymond W.

Worring, Whitney S. Hibbard, and Samantha Schroeder (1996).

3. Shorelands, a travel health information company. Phone: (800) 433-5256. Web site: www.tripprep.com/index.html.

4. U.S. State Department Travel Warnings and Consular Information Sheets. Phone: (202) 647-5225 or (888) 407-4747. If outside the United States, call (317) 472-2328. Fax: (202) 747-3000. Bureau of Consular Affairs home page: www.travel.state.gov.

5. U.S. Department of State. Phone: (202) 647-4000; ask to be connected to the desk covering your destination country.

KEEPING YOUR FAMILY HEALTHY

Exposure to the Elements

Children are far more susceptible to extremes in temperature than adults are, and special care should be taken in unusually hot or cold climates.

Hot Climates

Precautions should be taken in hot climates to avoid sunburn, dehydration, and heat-related syndromes.

- Increase fluid intake to maintain hydration.
- Wear appropriate clothing, including a hat with a wide brim.

- Use sunscreen.
(See Chapter 57.)

Cold Climates

Hypothermia (a drop in body temperature) can occur in cold weather. Children lose heat very easily. Heat loss is aggravated by windy conditions and also by excessive perspiration in rainproof and windproof clothing. Hypothermia, however, can also occur in warmer temperatures and even in places that have a hot climate year-round, especially if a person is wearing damp or wet clothing.

- Change children's clothing as soon as it is wet.
- Dress appropriately. Dress in layers.
- Young children, especially infants, may lose a large amount of heat from their head. A warm hat is essential.
(See Chapter 58.)

Infectious Disease

Throughout this book mention is made of avoiding infectious diseases. Chapter 3 has a large section devoted to proper immunizations, especially if traveling abroad. Hand washing is stressed repeatedly, and Chapter 17 goes into great detail on how to avoid acquiring an emerging infectious disease such as SARS or Avian flu.

Help, in the form of child-care providers, gardeners, and cooks, is often quite easy to come by and relatively cheap in developing countries. Tuberculosis is one of the scourges of these countries and can be easily spread to children who often spend a lot of time around these helpers. Be aware of this, especially if you will be staying in a lesser-developed country for an extended period.

Animal Bites

Caution children about petting and playing with stray dogs and cats and other animals. They might not be as tolerant as the family pet back home and may carry rabies. Rabies is especially common in parts of the Far East, Asia, and Africa (see Chapters 55 and 56). It is a good general rule to tell your children never to approach or pet unknown animals, even if they appear friendly. Watch, take photos, but don't touch.

PREVENTING ACCIDENTS

Accidents are the leading cause of death among travelers under the age of 55. Motor vehicle accidents top the list, followed by drowning. People tend to exaggerate and worry about such unlikely dangers as airplane accidents and terrorism and to minimize the far more common dangers of motor vehicle accidents and drowning, both of which are preventable. As some pilots tell passengers upon landing, "The safest part of your journey is now over and the dangerous part is about to begin!"

Motor Vehicle Accidents

Several precautions can be taken to help prevent motor vehicle accidents:

- Always use seat belts. If renting a car, reserve a vehicle that has them. In many countries seat belts are not standard equipment on cars. Extra time and effort may be needed to locate a car with seat belts.
- Children younger than four years of age need a car seat. Reserve one when booking a rental car or take your own.
- Older children may need a booster seat (see Chapter 46).
- Rent the largest car you can afford, but also take into consideration the roads you will be driving on. Some narrow lanes may not accommodate large vehicles.
- Familiarize yourself with your rental vehicle. Get used to the controls. Don't just head out onto a busy highway. Drive around the parking lot a few times first.
- Avoid driving when you are fatigued. If you have just had a long flight, rest for a night or day before getting behind the wheel of an unfamiliar vehicle. When renting a camper, you should be aware that some companies require a person to wait 24 hours before driving it if that person has arrived on an international flight.
- Drive slowly. Roads may contain potholes and often are poorly signposted. Local children may be playing on the roads. Animals may stray onto the road. Take extra care if you are traveling in a country where people drive on the other side of the road.

- Avoid traveling at night, especially in rural areas and especially if you are unsure of the way.
- Do not drink and drive.
- Do not sleep in your car or RV on the roadside at night.
- Be very careful when stopping at view sites. In many countries these are prime targets for hijackers, pickpockets, and thieves. While you are admiring the scenery, someone else may be admiring your valuables!
- Avoid traveling in open vehicles and in the back of trucks.
- Avoid overcrowded vehicles.
- Carrying children on motorbikes is especially dangerous. Don't do this! In fact, it is better to avoid scooters and mopeds completely, despite their obvious attraction. Scooter accidents and injuries are common, even in quiet resort locations. Don't be the sucker who keeps the local orthopedic surgeon in business!
- If you are traveling by taxi or have hired a driver, do not be afraid to ask your driver to slow down and drive more cautiously. Although some drivers may appear very nonchalant and confident, their appearance may be misleading. Motor vehicle accidents occur with far greater frequency in developing countries where poor roads, poor vehicle maintenance, and poor traffic law enforcement are common. You may need to offer the driver a financial incentive to drive more slowly.
- Insist upon safe behavior on sidewalks and when crossing roads. Traffic may be approaching from a direction you are not expecting.

Remember, vehicle accidents are the number one cause of death while on vacation or traveling.

Hotel Safety

Americans may be surprised when they realize that safety standards in many countries are not equivalent to those in the United States. This may be true even in good hotels in many Western countries. Hotels may not have smoke alarms and may have balconies that are not adequately protected and windows that do not lock. Many windows open completely, even on very high floors where a fall may mean certain death.

When we traveled to Paris with our five-year-old son, we were shown to our room on the seventh floor of the hotel and immediately marveled at the spectacular view, which was seen through our floor-to-ceiling windows. We were somewhat alarmed when we realized that the window had no lock and there was no outside balcony or railing. It would have been quite easy for either an adult or a child to have opened the window and toppled out!

Here are steps you can take to keep you and your family safer in your hotel:

- Locate fire exits. Be able to locate them in the dark. Check that they can be opened from the inside and that they are not blocked off.

- Check new living and play areas from a safety point of view. Pay particular attention to windows, balconies, electrical outlets, and electrical cords.
- Do not allow children to play on balconies.
- Never sit on the balcony railing! Many tragic deaths have occurred when vacationers have fallen to their death from balconies.
- In the bathroom, beware of hot water temperatures. In many hotels, the hot water temperature is close to boiling! Severe burns can result.

Swimming

Drowning is the second most common cause of death while traveling.

Swimming in unknown waters carries not only the risk of drowning but also the risk of acquiring waterborne diseases. These may enter the body directly through the skin or by swallowing water. Children tend to swallow much more water than adults while swimming and so are more prone to waterborne diseases.

Many swimming areas have dangerous currents, and frequently there is no lifeguard on duty. Deserted beaches are often deserted for a reason. They may have dangerous cross-currents or backwashes or generally be unsafe for swimming. Find out from local people where it is safe to swim. Teach your children water safety.

Alcohol and swimming do not mix. You cannot supervise your children adequately if you have been drinking.

A vacation is often the time when people try new water sports. Get adequate instruction. When snorkeling or scuba diving, always have a partner close by.

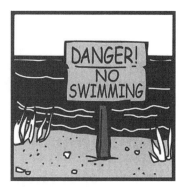

Many tropical waters contain a variety of poisonous fish, and dangerous or even fatal stings may result. It is a good idea to wear rubber shoes or sandals when swimming in tropical waters. Ask the locals what the local hazards are (see Chapter 41).

In certain countries, sharks may be a problem. Rivers in Africa contain not only many disease-causing parasites but also crocodiles and hippos! Hippopotamuses are responsible for many deaths in Africa.

Walking and Hiking

When walking and hiking, it is wise to wear closed shoes, not only to avoid bites from snakes but also to protect yourself from insect stings, sand fleas, and parasitic diseases such as hookworm. If walking in snake- or tick-infested areas, it is a good idea to wear boots and long pants (see Chapter 39).

Wear comfortable shoes or boots. Whether you sprain an ankle on the cobblestone streets of Florence or on the Appalachian Trail, the end result will be very similar. Your vacation will be spoiled (see Chapter 45).

3

Traveling with Children Outside the United States

Traveling, especially abroad, is an enriching experience for both adults and children. Visiting foreign countries is one of the most important educational experiences a child can have, and it encourages all of us to become more tolerant of foreign customs and cultures.

Traveling with children is a lot more work and more stressful than traveling without them, but it can also be a lot more fun. Barriers erected by race and language often fall away in the company of children. Children are less inhibited than adults and often help break the ice. In many countries, when you travel with a child, local people open their hearts and homes to you and your family.

Traveling abroad can be as safe as staying at home if you are sensible about your choice of destination, make proper preparations, and take precautions. Remote and primitive destinations are just not suitable for young children, particularly if you are traveling on a shoestring budget.

If you are planning to travel to remote and dangerous places, seek medical advice and information beforehand about the hazards and dangers that you are likely to encounter there.

When you are considering the risks of travel, some important differences between children and adults should be kept in mind.

- Children, especially preschool children, may not be fully immunized and are therefore prone to certain infectious diseases such as measles, polio, and chicken pox.
- Travelers' diarrhea is usually only an inconvenience to adults, but young children may rapidly become dehydrated and require urgent medical attention.
- Children are more susceptible to extremes in environmental temperature. They more easily develop heat stroke and hypothermia.
- Children are more likely to get sunburned.
- Children are risk takers and often have poor judgment. They are more prone to accidents, drowning, animal bites, and poisoning.
- Illnesses such as malaria and tuberculosis tend to be more common and more severe in children. Rabies occurs more commonly in children.

Although most infectious illnesses that you acquire while traveling abroad cause symptoms early on, the symptoms of some illnesses (such as tuberculosis, malaria, and some causes of diarrhea) may not appear until weeks or even months after you return.

Despite warnings about dreaded diseases, these fortunately are rare. Don't forget about motor vehicle accidents. They pose the greatest risk of death and serious medical problems during travel.

When traveling outside the United States, it is especially important to be honest with yourself about the level of discomfort and hardship you are willing to tolerate:

- Do you feel very insecure when you can't understand the local language?
- Do you feel that everyone should be able to speak English?
- Are you easily upset by uncertainty and unexpected delays and changes in your schedule?
- Does your anxiety level increase when you don't have access to medical care?
- Does unfamiliar food put you off?
- Do you need a hot shower every day?
- Does the absence of clean toilet facilities upset you?

Don't underestimate the psychological stress caused by lack of sleep, minor ailments (such as diarrhea, constipation, and skin rashes), unfamiliar food, lack of clean toilet facilities, and the inability to understand foreign languages.

It is vital to keep your sense of humor and not to overextend yourself.

Attitude is everything when you travel, especially when you travel with children. Minor mishaps may open doors to unexpected adventures and opportunities.

A family we met when we were hopelessly lost in Hong Kong showed us parts of the city the guidebooks would never have told us about!

PREPARING FOR INTERNATIONAL TRAVEL

Preparing for travel is essential, especially with young children. Knowledge and preparation are the keys to a successful and medically uneventful trip. The extent of preparation depends not only on which country you visit but also on the specific location within the country. Are you traveling to large cities or to rural areas, to cool, dry areas or to humid, tropical areas? The length and purpose of the journey will also influence your preparation.

Learning more about the country you intend to visit, including its health problems, is wise. Involve older children and teenagers in this research. It can be fun as well as educational.

Traveling to developing countries that lack clean water and disease-control programs requires specific preventative measures to avoid illnesses. Many of these measures are covered in this book. Additional sources for obtaining information on travel-related medical issues are listed below.

Preparation is especially important if you plan to travel to countries with radically different cultures. You should prepare your children for different lifestyles and different standards of living. It may come as quite a shock to you and your children to witness the extent of poverty and disease in many developing countries.

When traveling to remote, primitive, or undeveloped areas, it is especially important to have backup and evacuation plans. If you are traveling to remote locations, it would certainly be worthwhile for the adult and adolescent members of your party to take a first aid course before traveling.

 For Your Reference

The following sources provide information on medical issues related to foreign travel:

1. The Centers for Disease Control and Prevention (CDC). Phone: (888) 232-3228. Fax: (888) 232-3299. Web site: www.cdc.gov/travel. The CDC publishes an excellent book, *Health Information for International Travel,* which can be purchased in hard-copy form and is also available on the Internet. This book is updated every two years.

2. *International Travel Health Guide,* by Stuart R. Rose and Jay S. Keystone, is *the best* of the travel health guides, and it is updated frequently. It is recommended for the serious international traveler and contains a wealth of information on all aspects of travel. It can be purchased by calling (800) 872-8633 or at the Web

site www.travmed.com. The 13th edition was published in 2006.

3. *Travellers' Health: How to Stay Healthy Abroad,* by Dr. Richard Dawood, 4th ed. (2002). An extremely comprehensive guide to travel and living abroad. Excellent!

4. American Society of Tropical Medicine and Hygiene (ASTMH). Phone: (847) 480-9592. Web site: www.astmh.org. This society publishes a very useful booklet entitled "Health Hints for the Tropics."

5. International Society of Travel Medicine (ISTM), P.O. Box 871089, Stone Mountain, GA 30087. Phone: (770) 736-7060. Fax: (770) 736-6732. Web site: www.istm.org.

6. Shorelands, Inc., 10625 West North Avenue, Milwaukee, WI 53226. Phone: (800) 433-5256. Web site: www.tripprep.com. This is an excellent Web site with a wealth of information. It is highly recommended.

7. MD Travel Health. www.mdtravelhealth.com.

8. Travel Medicine Inc. www.travmed.com.

9. *Travelling Well,* by Dr. Deborah Mills, 12th ed. (2005).

10. If you plan to travel to exotic, lesser-developed countries or undertake more serious adventure or wilderness travel, two pocket-sized books are highly recommended. One is *Pocket Doctor: A Passport to Healthy Travel,* by Dr. Stephen Bezruchka, which contains a lot of commonsense advice and sensitive sentiments regarding the environment and respect for other peo-

ples. The other is *A Comprehensive Guide to Wilderness and Travel Medicine,* by Eric A. Weiss, M.D., which has a wealth of practical advice for handling medical emergencies in places where medical care is not readily available.

GETTING A PRE-TRAVEL MEDICAL CONSULTATION

A pre-travel consultation with a family physician or at a travel clinic is recommended for *everyone* who plans an extended stay in a developing or tropical country. Ideally, this visit should take place 6 to 10 weeks before departure to allow sufficient time for the special vaccinations recommended for some countries. However, even if you've left this part of your travel planning to the last minute, a visit just prior to your departure is still worthwhile.

Note: Your own physician or your child's pediatrician may not be familiar with the latest health recommendations for travel to countries outside the United States. For this reason, it's a good idea to consult a specialist in travel medicine or an infectious disease physician if you intend to travel to developing, tropical, or subtropical countries.

Some travel clinics have limited expertise in dealing with children, so if your child has any chronic diseases or special needs, you should also visit your child's pediatrician to discuss these.

The cost of consulting a travel clinic and getting the immunizations that you and your child may require is not insignificant and may not be covered by your medical insurance. However, this will be money well spent because the consequences of diseases such as malaria and hepatitis can result in serious long-term health problems. Consulting a travel medical specialist will also help you to avoid accidents and to make wise choices regarding safe food and water, and a specialist can guide you on the many complex issues that you may encounter. The travel clinic will also advise you about medications you should take with you to prevent and treat travelers' diarrhea, malaria, motion sickness, acute mountain sickness, and other travel-related illnesses.

If you intend to spend some time in a country that has a significant risk of tuberculosis, all members of your family should have a tuberculin skin test prior to departure. This test should be repeated when you return.

 For Your Reference

Most teaching hospitals and many community hospitals have travel clinics. The following Web sites can also help you locate a travel medicine clinic in your area:

1. International Society of Travel Medicine (ISTM). www.istm.org.
2. American Society of Tropical Medicine and Hygiene (ASTMH). www.astmh.org/clinics/clinindex.html.
3. Shoreland's Travel Health Online. www.tripprep.com.
4. Travel Medicine, Inc. www.travmed.com.
5. MD Travel Health. www.travelhealth.com.

HOW YOUNG IS TOO YOUNG TO TRAVEL?

It is unwise to travel to developing countries with infants who are younger than six months of age. Their primary immunization series is not complete, and it is more difficult to prevent and treat insectborne illnesses such as malaria in this age group.

In addition, many immunizations recommended for travel cannot be given to children younger than two years of age. The immunization against typhoid is one example.

It is also important to remember that diarrheal illness tends to be more severe in infants and young children and is more likely to lead to dehydration.

The younger the child, the harder it is to assess the degree of illness. Children younger than three years of age cannot pinpoint exactly where their pain is or explain their symptoms well. Diagnosis is often difficult, and young children may become very ill very quickly.

Some authorities hold the more conservative view that it is preferable not to travel to developing countries with children younger than age three because of the risk of travelers' diarrhea, tuberculosis, and malaria. This may be solid advice if you intend to travel to a country that has a drug-resistant type of malaria (chloroquine-resistant falciparum malaria).

IMMUNIZATIONS

Recommending appropriate vaccinations for travel, especially to lesser-developed countries, is extremely complex. For this reason we advise you to consult a travel clinic or travel medicine physician or infectious disease physician to ensure you receive accurate information and the correct immunizations.

Many of these vaccinations are expensive, and their cost may not be covered by your medical insurance. An experienced travel clinic physician can help you evaluate the cost-benefit ratio and advise you as to which are the most important immunizations to receive.

Remember that immunizations against infectious diseases are one of the most important medical advances made, and they may *save you and your child from serious illness and even death*. There are no cures for many of the illnesses that immunization prevents. Antibiotics are not effective against measles, hepatitis, rabies, yellow fever, and many other vaccine-preventable diseases.

Note: The pre-travel medical consultation (discussed earlier) is also a good time for adults to update their routine immunizations.

Immunizations fall into three categories: routine, recommended, and required. These immunizations frequently change categories. For example, recommended immunizations often become routine, and some recommended vaccines may be required immunizations for entry into certain countries.

Routine Immunizations

These are the immunizations most children routinely receive during infancy and childhood, and most adults should receive as part of their normal preventive health care. Make sure your child's routine immunizations are up to date because many of the diseases that these immunizations protect against are still prevalent in other parts of the world. These routine immunizations may be even more important than the travel immunizations discussed later in this section. *Do not* skip these routine immunizations if you plan extensive travels outside the United States with your child, especially to developing countries.

The routine preventive immunization schedule varies from country to country, and even in the United States it is frequently updated and changed.

Immunization schedules can be modified and accelerated if a family is traveling to a foreign country, especially a developing country. For example, your child's first measles immunization may be given as early as six months of age and repeated at one year of age.

DTaP

Diphtheria, tetanus, and pertussis (whooping cough) vaccines are usually combined into one vaccine known as the DTaP. The DTaP may also be combined with other vaccines in the same shot.

Once the primary DTaP vaccination series is complete, tetanus-diphtheria (Td) boosters should be given every 10 years. In certain circumstances—for example, after getting a contaminated wound—an additional dose of Td may be required to prevent tetanus. Because you cannot guarantee that your child will not get a contaminated wound while you are traveling, a Td (tetanus) booster may be recommended every five years. Newer tetanus-diphtheria-pertussis (Tdap) boosters also give added protection against whooping cough (pertussis). These are preferable to the older Td immunization, as immunity to whooping cough wanes fairly rapidly. Whooping cough remains a significant illness at all ages, even in the United States.

Diphtheria boosters are recommended for all travelers to countries where the risk of diphtheria is high, such as the Russian Federation, Ukraine, and Tajikistan and for long-term visits (more than four weeks) to Africa, Asia, and South America. Again, the Tdap is the preferred immunization.

Polio Vaccine

In the United States, this vaccine is given as an injectable vaccine known as the IPV. In many countries, the oral polio vaccine (OPV) is still used. A one-time booster of IPV is recommended for travelers to developing countries. Recently, there has been a resurgence of polio in central and North Africa, particularly in Nigeria. Wild polio still occurs in other lesser-developed areas including the Middle East and Asia.

Measles-Mumps-Rubella (MMR) Vaccine

Measles is still common in many developing countries and is a common cause of childhood death in these countries. Measles may cause a severe life-threatening illness, even in well-nourished, otherwise healthy children. Some people, especially those born before 1957 in the United States, and between 1970 and 1990 in Canada, may not have immunity against measles. Their immunity to measles should be checked prior to travel to developing countries, or alternatively a repeat dose of the measles vaccine administered.

Hemophilus *Type B (HIB) Vaccine*

This vaccine prevents illnesses due to the *Hemophilus* type B bacterium. This bacterium was a common cause of pneumonia and meningitis in the United States. These illnesses are still common in many countries.

Hepatitis B (Hep B) vaccine

For details, see the next section ("Recommended Immunizations"). The hepatitis B vaccine became a routine immunization only in the past 15 years. For this reason many older adolescents and adults may not have received this immunization.

Varicella (Chicken Pox) Vaccine

Although usually a mild infection, chicken pox can occasionally cause severe disease, even death. Nonimmune adolescents and adults are particularly likely to get a more severe form of chicken pox. Again, this vaccine was only recently introduced as a routine immunization, and so many people may not have immunity against this disease. All susceptible individuals should receive this vaccine prior to their travels.

Pneumococcal Vaccine

The bacterium *Streptococcus pneumoniae* is the most important bacterial cause of ear infections (otitis media) and sinusitis in most parts of the world, including the United States. It may also cause pneumonia, severe bloodstream infections (septicemia), and bacterial meningitis. This immunization is definitely worth getting, even in the United States.

A conjugate vaccine (Prevnar) was recently introduced as a routine immunization for children in the first five years of life. A polysaccharide vaccine (Pneumovax) has been available for many years and may be administered to certain high-risk persons who are older than two years of age.

Meningococcal Vaccine

This vaccine was originally recommended in the United States only for adolescents entering college, for military recruits, and for people traveling to certain countries. However, in 2005 the recommendations were expanded to cover children 11 years of age and older.

A new conjugate vaccine (Menactra) has recently been introduced in the United States. This vaccine gives longer-lasting immunity than the older polysaccharide vaccine (Menomune). There is no vaccine that is effective for prevention of meningococcal disease caused by the serogroup B meningococcus.

Although the meningococcal vaccine appears here as a *routine* immunization, it is also a *recommended* immunization for travel to specific high-risk areas and a *required* immunization for travel to Saudi Arabia.

NEW COMBINATIONS OF THE ROUTINE VACCINATIONS discussed above become available almost every year. The bottom line is that your child needs to be protected against diphtheria, tetanus, whooping cough (pertussis), polio, measles, mumps, rubella, *Hemophilus* type B disease, hepatitis B, chicken pox (varicella), and pneumococcal disease. Protection against meningococcal disease is recommended for specific age groups and populations.

Recommended Immunizations

Some of these immunizations are often recommended even if you do not intend to travel.

Hepatitis A Vaccine

Hepatitis A is the most common vaccine-preventable disease that affects travelers. This is an extremely important vaccine, especially for adults. It can be given to children at one year of age. Children younger than one year of age can be given immune globulin to prevent hepatitis A.

Although travelers frequently worry about acquiring cholera or typhoid, they are far more likely to acquire hepatitis A. Hepatitis A can cause severe liver disease and even death in adults, especially in the older population. It's not unusual for children to acquire hepatitis A and not show any signs of significant illness; however, they can pass hepatitis A on to their parents or grandparents, who may become seriously ill. *Do not* forgo receiving this very effective vaccination.

Hepatitis A is now a *routine* immunization in many parts of the United States.

Hepatitis B Vaccine

This vaccination is recommended for everyone. Not all children and adults will have received the hepatitis B vaccine as part of their routine immunization series in childhood. Hepatitis B is a preventable disease that can lead to severe liver disease later in life, including cirrhosis of the liver and liver cancer.

Individuals who have received neither the hepatitis B nor the hepatitis A vaccine can be given a combination vaccine (Twinrix).

Typhoid Vaccine

Typhoid fever is a hazard in some developing countries. The typhoid vaccine may be given orally or as an injection. Children older than six years of age and adults may receive the oral vaccine. Children from two to six years of age should receive the injectable vaccine.

Typhoid immunization is especially important for VFRs (see Chapter 4), as their risk of acquiring typhoid is particularly high, and for people who intend to visit developing countries where poor sanitation is a problem. This vaccine does *not* give total immunity, and so safe food and water precautions are still *essential*.

Influenza Vaccine

This vaccine is recommended if you are traveling over the winter months, especially if your child has a chronic disease such as asthma or heart disease. Different countries, however, have outbreaks of influenza at different times of the year. In the Southern Hemisphere the flu season is between April and September. Travelers should consider getting this vaccine at their travel destination, as the antigenic compo-

nents of the vaccine differ in the Southern Hemisphere.
Outbreaks may occur year-round in the tropics.

If your child has not had a flu shot before, he or she may
need two shots at least a month apart.

The influenza vaccine is recommended for most children
and adults, even if not traveling.

Other Vaccines

Other vaccines that fall into the group of recommended vaccines include those against Japanese encephalitis, rabies, meningococcal disease, plague, and tickborne encephalitis. In many parts of the world, especially Southeast Asia, rabies poses a significant risk, particularly to children. Rabies vaccine is recommended for children who will be spending many months in an area where rabies is prevalent. The meningococcal vaccine is recommended for travel to the meningitis belt in sub-Saharan Africa.

Required Immunizations

A vaccination that falls into this category is one that is required for entry into certain countries. If you have not had the immunization(s) required by the country you are traveling to, you will be denied entry to that country.

Yellow Fever Vaccine

Yellow fever vaccine is required by some countries as a condition of entry. At present this is the only vaccine *officially* required. However, see the comments for meningococcal disease and cholera just below. Yellow fever is a viral infection that may be fatal and is transmitted by the bite of infected *Aedes aegypti* mosquitoes (see Chapter 16).

The yellow fever vaccine can be given only in designated yellow fever vaccination centers. Proof of yellow fever immunization should be recorded on the International Certificate of Vaccination (also known as the Yellow Card). If you do not have this card, you may be denied entry into certain countries. If you are unable to receive this vaccination for medical reasons, you should obtain a waiver from the destination country's embassy or consulate before your departure. To see which countries require a Yellow Card, visit www.cdc .gov/travel/yelfever.htm.

Cholera Vaccine

The cholera vaccine is not "officially" required for entry into any country, but it may be a good idea to get the cholera vaccine (if possible) or get an exemption letter from the destination country's embassy or consulate to avoid problems with entry to that country. Alternatively, a notation of vaccine contraindication stamped on an official-looking document with an official stamp may be sufficient to satisfy local immigration authorities. These comments apply mainly to Saudi Arabia and more specifically when going on the Hajj.

At present no cholera vaccine is available in the United States. Many countries, including Canada and some European countries, offer a fairly effective oral cholera vaccine. One of these vaccines, Dukoral, also provides some immunity against the most common cause of travelers' diarrhea, enterotoxigenic *E. coli*. Some travel experts recommend trying to get this vaccine to certain high-risk travelers and relief and health care workers who intend to work in refugee camps and other high-risk environments. Getting the cholera vaccine does *not* mean you can ignore observing safe food and water precautions.

Meningococcal Vaccine

This is also not officially a required immunization, but it may be needed for entry into Saudi Arabia during the Hajj. Getting this vaccine is definitely worthwhile.

DENTAL CHECKUP

A visit to your dentist is a good idea if you are planning a long stay in a developing country or if you are having any dental problems prior to your departure. Arrange this visit well in advance to allow sufficient time to get all necessary dental work done. Good dental care may be hard to find in lesser-developed countries. Sterility might not be maintained for dental procedures, thus increasing the risk of acquiring severe infections such as HIV infection, hepatitis B, and hepatitis C.

- Many children with congenital heart defects require antibiotic prophylaxis when they receive dental treatment. These children should take along a supply of an appropriate antibiotic.
- If you are likely to need dental care or are planning a

long stay in a developing country, you should take with you a supply of sterile syringes and needles or even consider purchasing a dental kit from an appropriate commercial source—for example, Travel Medicine Inc. (800-TRAV-MED) or Chinook Medical Gear (800-766-1365). Discuss this possibility with your dentist.

EYEGLASSES

The following suggestions will be helpful for family members who wear eyeglasses or contact lenses:

- If you or your child wears contact lenses or eyeglasses, take a spare pair with you.
- Keep a copy of eyeglass and contact lens prescriptions with you.
- It is a good idea for contact lens wearers to take along a pair of eyeglasses as well in case they develop an eye infection, such as conjunctivitis (pink eye). If this happens, it is important not to wear contact lenses until the infection has cleared.
- It is also a good idea to ask your physician or eye doctor for a prescription for antibacterial eyedrops to take with you.

DOCUMENTS, PASSPORTS, VISAS

Photocopies should be made of all important travel documents. You should carry a copy, file one at home, and leave one or two sets with people you can trust as emergency contacts. Copies should not be left in luggage, which can be lost or stolen.

Carry tickets, passports, and travelers checks on your person while traveling. At your destination, it may be wiser to leave passports and plane tickets in the hotel safe. Travelers should assume that pickpockets are everywhere.

Passports

Each family member must have his or her own passport. Check the expiration date to make sure all the passports are valid for the duration of the trip. Many countries require that a passport be valid for an additional four to six months beyond the expected duration of the trip.

Just a few days before we were leaving for South Africa, my wife discovered that our son's passport had expired. This discovery was a life-shortening experience for her! Our family relies on her organizational skills for tickets, passports, and visas. A desperate phone call to our travel agent produced the name of a company that would expedite passport renewals. The next few hours were spent writing large checks, and soon the passport, a handful of forms, and new photographs were on their way to the company, which was on the other side of the country. The precious passport was returned just 30 minutes before we left for the airport. No FedEx van has ever received a greater welcome at our home. What a tribute to American efficiency!

Allow six to eight weeks when applying for a new passport or renewing an old one. Specialized passport services are able to obtain passports on much shorter notice but at far greater cost. One such service is American Passport Express: (800) 841-6778 or www.americanpassport.com.

Visas

You and your children will need a visa to visit some countries. A visa is obtained from the embassy or consulate of the country you intend to visit. It allows you to enter the country and stay for a specified time. If you are visiting a number of countries, it may take some time to get all the required visas, so allow adequate time for this processing. Double check any information you are given about visas.

Check with your travel agent or contact the embassies of the countries you intend to visit or write to Passport Services, U.S. Department of State, Washington, DC 20524. Another source for obtaining information about visa requirements is the Web site of the Bureau of Consular Affairs: www.travel .state.gov.

My wife travels on a South African passport and was told she did not need a visa to visit Italy. En route to Rome we had a stopover in Brussels. It was here that the "fun" began. The customs official said, "You have a small problem. You do not have a visa for Belgium." My wife explained that we were en route to Rome and did not intend to leave the Brussels airport. The official's face tightened, and he announced that we now had a "big" problem! "Where is the visa for Italy?" he asked. We were escorted to a holding room to await an interview with a senior immigration official. He courteously stated that my wife should not have been allowed to board the plane in the United States without a visa for Italy. He said she would have to return to the United States on the next flight out of Brussels. Our son and I would be permitted to continue to Italy!

Our seven-year-old was devastated by the thought that "Mummy" might have to go home. Big tears trickled down from under his "Harry Potter" glasses and he said, "But Mum, it's your birthday." We saw the immigration officer's eyes glance down at my wife's passport, and his expression softened for just a second. "Return to the waiting room and I will see what I can do."

The next hour was spent in the company of two men traveling with forged passports and a suspected drug dealer who was in handcuffs. This was enough to impress upon us the seriousness of my wife's predicament.

Finally we were summoned back into the interview room, and my wife was handed her passport, which now sported two new visas, one for Belgium and one for Italy. Also in the passport was a note that read, "Happy Birthday, from the Belgian immigration authorities."

Custody Papers

Single parents should carry copies of custody papers in case questions arise when crossing international borders with a child, especially when the child has a different last name. Some countries require a certified letter from the other parent giving his or her consent for the child to cross borders.

PERSONAL MEDICAL INFORMATION AND MEDICATIONS

If anyone in your family has a complex medical illness, photocopies of the relevant medical records should be carried with you. These records should include a complete list of medications with their correct pharmacological names because the trade names of the medications vary from country to country. Take copies of all prescriptions with you. It is also a good idea to take along a letter from your child's doctor listing medications she is on and their dosage. Such a letter is essential if you are carrying syringes and needles.

Medicines should be carried in their original containers.

Keep medications with you in your carry-on luggage. Medicines should *not* be left with your checked luggage, which may be separated from you for prolonged periods or be lost.

Emergency medications such as epinephrine kits (Epipen), asthma medications, seizure medications, and diabetic medications (insulin, glucagon, and syringes) should *always* be easily accessible.

It is a good idea to take along extra medications in case of unscheduled delays.

Do not forget to take along your medical kit.

TRAVEL INSURANCE

It is often stated that if you can't afford travel insurance you can't afford to travel! This point of view may be somewhat extreme, and it would deprive many people of the excitement and advantages of travel. Think carefully about your need for travel insurance. Be sensible, taking into account your travel destination and the medical facilities located there, as well as the individual health needs of everyone in your travel party. If anyone in your party has a chronic disease such as asthma or diabetes or is elderly, make sure you get adequate health insurance. This also applies if you intend to take part in dangerous activities such as extreme sports.

As is mentioned elsewhere in this book, prevention is always better than cure. This begins with getting the correct immunizations for *all* the people traveling, adults included. Your travel clinic or physician will also guide you on malaria prophylaxis (if indicated), ways to avoid insect and tick bites, prevention and treatment of travelers' diarrhea, and general safety measures (see Chapter 2). Remember to pack your medical kit and to update the medications in it. Don't forget to take along adequate amounts of all your and your child's regular (routine) medications. Consider purchasing a cell phone plan that enables you to make international calls. This will make getting hold of your physician back home and your medical insurance company a lot easier.

Types of Travel Insurance

There are many types of insurance related to travel. These include travel health (medical) insurance, medical evacuation insurance, trip cancellation and trip interruption insurance, and lost baggage insurance.

Medical Insurance

The first step is to determine whether the medical insurance you have back home in the United States will cover medical expenses incurred while outside the country. Check the fine print in your health insurance policy, and phone your insurance company and confirm what services will be covered. Get this in writing. Even if your regular health insurance back home covers expenses while traveling, there are often many bridges you have to cross:

- Most medical insurances require preauthorization if you want to receive care from "out-of-plan" or out-of-state institutions or providers.
- Exclusions, restrictions, and deductibles frequently apply.
- The health care provider, clinic, or hospital that you are visiting may not accept this insurance and will often insist on payment up front.

There are many types of travel medical insurance. The best type is medical insurance *with assistance,* which means that your insurance plan guarantees you assistance from "home" with sorting out complex and not so complex medical issues. This includes locating English-speaking physicians when abroad, providing you with an interpreter to help you converse with health care providers, helping you find adequate medical facilities, and helping you decide whether you need to come home and whether you require medical evacuation. If anyone in your travel party becomes seriously ill, such an insurance policy is worth its weight in gold! Get it if you think you might need it and can afford it.

Your travel agent may be able to help you locate good travel medical insurance. The Internet is a good source for this as well.

For Your Reference

Well-known companies to help you find travel medical insurance include the following:

1. Travel Assistance International, 9200 Keystone Crossing, Suite 300, Indianapolis, IN 46240. Phone: (800) 821-2828.
2. TravMed-Medex, Box 10623, Baltimore, MD 21285. Phone: (800) 732-5309.
3. International SOS Assistance Inc., 3600 Horizon Boulevard, Suite 300, Trevose, PA 19053. Web site: www.internationalsos.com.
4. Worldwide Assistance Services, Inc., 1133 15th Street, NW, Suite 400, Washington, DC 20005. Phone:

(877) 238-1234 or (202) 331-1609. Web site: www
.worldwideassistance.com.

Evacuation Insurance

Evacuation insurance may not be covered in your travel medical insurance, although many of the medical insurance with
assistance plans described above offer it. Evacuation insurance should definitely be considered for travelers with specialized medical problems or when planning dangerous activities or when visiting especially remote and dangerous
parts of the world. Injuries sustained during motor vehicle
accidents are the most common reason travelers require
medical evacuation.

 For Your Reference

Many of the companies listed above provide evacuation insurance. Other companies include the following:

1. US Air Ambulance. Phone: (800) 633-5384.
2. American Air Ambulance. Phone: (800) 863-0312.
3. Medjet Assist. Phone: (800) 963-3538.

FINDING HEALTH CARE WHILE TRAVELING

Again, long before you depart on your travels, consider the
preventive measures outlined above. If you follow these, you
are less likely to need medical care.

Before traveling, especially to lesser-developed countries and out-of-the-way places, stop and think what you would do if someone in your family or party becomes ill or disabled while traveling. If you have a well-thought-out plan and appropriate phone numbers and addresses, you are less likely to panic and will be better able to cope with the situation. Keep these phone numbers and addresses easily accessible. If you have a mobile phone with you on which you can make international calls, your job just got easier! If you have your medical kit with you and this book, you will be able to take care of most minor (and some not so minor!) medical problems in children and will know when you need to find medical help. Consider purchasing a medical phrase book or dictionary in the language of your destination country.

Many people born and brought up in the United States are inclined to think that the United States is the only country in the world capable of providing good medical care. This is simply not true. The standard of medical care in many countries may be just as high as that in the United States. This applies particularly to the countries of Western Europe, Canada, Australia, New Zealand, many Asian countries, and the Republic of South Africa.

The medical facilities in some countries may appear less modern and sophisticated than in the United States and often don't meet the same hygiene and cleanliness standards. However, the physician taking care of you may have far greater expertise in tropical diseases such as malaria and typhoid than your physician back home. It is natural to feel insecure in a strange environment, and the following are some suggestions for obtaining medical care when traveling.

Before you go any further, try to assess the severity and urgency of the problem: chest pain in adults, major injuries with bleeding, or broken bones need urgent care. Try to get to the nearest hospital immediately. If the problem is not so severe or urgent, work through the list below:

- Local contacts. Ask yourself if you know anyone locally (for example, a member of the expatriate community) who can recommend a good physician.
- Hotels and resorts. If you are staying in a hotel or resort, the hotel staff may be able to recommend a doctor who may even visit you in your room. Some large hotels and resorts have a physician "in house." Alternatively, they may be able to refer you to a reputable clinic or hospital in the vicinity.
- Embassy or consulate. The United States embassy or consulate (and many other embassies) will often be able to recommend local physicians, clinics, hospitals, and other medical care.
- Do you have medical insurance with assistance as discussed above? Contact your insurance carrier. These companies offer a wide variety of services to their members including physician-backed assistance. Most of these companies offer 24-hour access to coordinators who can help locate physicians overseas.
- Are you a member of IAMAT? The International As-

sociation of Medical Assistance to Travelers (IAMAT) is established throughout the world. Members can call and be referred to a local physician who speaks the traveler's native language. To access the service, the traveler must be a member of IAMAT. The address is 417 Center Street, Lewiston, NY 14092, and the phone number is (716) 754-4883. Contact IAMAT before you travel and consider joining this organization. There is no charge to join IAMAT, but a donation will be gratefully acknowledged. This organization will provide you with a booklet of recommended physicians in different countries as well as other useful information for your travels.

- Personal Physicians Worldwide. This organization provides truly excellent service but is very expensive. If you plan extensive travels and a member of your family has a medical problem, and you can afford these services, consider joining this organization. Address: 815 Connecticut Avenue NW, Washington, DC 20006. Phone: (888) 657-8114. Web site: www.personalphysicians.com.
- Credit card cardholder assistance. Some credit card companies provide medical help hotlines to their card holders. Check this before you set out on your travels.
- MedicAlert Travel Plus program. If you are a member of this program, this organization will help you locate medical care while abroad (see Chapter 5).

Remember, to prevent is better than to cure. For travelers, this is particularly important. Most of the diseases and medical problems that people encounter abroad can be prevented.

The farther afield you travel and the more remote and primitive the location, the more important it is to be well prepared.

As mentioned earlier, if traveling to remote locations, it will certainly be a good idea for the adult and adolescent members of your party to take a first aid course before traveling.

Checklist for International Travel (especially to lesser-developed countries)

1. Medical checkup
   - Immunizations
   - Prescriptions for travelers' diarrhea
   - Prescriptions for malaria prophylaxis (if necessary)
2. Dental checkup
3. Documents
   - Passports/Green Cards (with copies)
   - Visas (with copies)
   - Custody papers
   - Medical record summary (if indicated)
   - Copy of itinerary with addresses (also leave one with contact back home)
4. Insurance
   - Medical
   - Evacuation
   - Trip cancellation, trip interruption, lost baggage
5. Details for locating health care abroad (addresses, phone numbers, IAMAT card)
6. Mobile phone with international calling capability
7. Bookings/reservations
   - Lists with contact phone numbers and addresses

Continued

Checklist for International Travel (especially to lesser-developed countries) *continued*

8. Financial
   - Credit cards (with theft insurance and numbers to report stolen card)
   - Travelers checks (with numbers in a separate location)
9. Other
   - Airline tickets
   - Driver's license
   - Extra passport photos
   - International certificate of vaccination (Yellow Card)
   - Student ID card, AAA card, AARP card, etc.
   - Medical phrase book or dictionary
10. Medical kit
    - Check and restock. Include insect repellents, alcohol hand sanitizer, OTC meds for travelers' diarrhea, etc.
11. Routine medications
12. Other important phone numbers
    - Family and friends
    - Family practitioner, pediatrician, etc.

POST-TRAVEL PHYSICAL

A post-travel physical with your child's doctor is a good idea if your child has been ill while away, has diarrhea lasting longer than 10 days or diarrhea that recurs, or develops an unexplained fever. Remind your child's doctor that you have traveled recently and tell him or her where you have been. This is especially important if you have traveled to areas where malaria is prevalent. Insist on blood tests to exclude malaria and have these tests repeated if your child remains ill. Most people who acquire malaria on their travels do not develop symptoms until they have returned home.

If you have traveled to an area with a high prevalence of tuberculosis, a tuberculin skin test should be done 12 weeks after returning home.

If you or your child develops unusual symptoms after traveling, especially to tropical or developing countries, visit your doctor immediately. If the symptoms persist, *insist* on a referral to an infectious disease specialist or a physician who specializes in travel-related illnesses.

Some travel medicine experts recommend that you consult a physician if you have spent an extended time away in a tropical or lesser-developed country even if you have no symptoms. Many diseases do not produce any symptoms for years but can be detected by specific screening tests. Examples of these are tuberculosis (mentioned above), hepatitis, and schistosomiasis (bilharzia). Some of these diseases may be spread to other people without your even being aware that you or your child has the disease.

IN SUMMARY

Despite the hazards discussed above, traveling abroad can be safe if you are sensible and take appropriate precautions and preventive measures. Do not let these hazards deter you from foreign travel, as the positive aspects of travel usually outweigh the negative ones.

Remember that most travelers return home quite safely without having had any serious illnesses. Remember, also, that most travel illnesses and accidents can be prevented.

You should take the following items to your travel clinic appointment:

- A list of your travel destinations.
- The vaccine records of all the travelers.
- A summary of the medical history of each of the travelers, including allergies and a list of the medications each traveler is taking.

4

Advice for Visiting Friends and Relatives

VFR is the term applied to immigrants and their children who return to their country of origin to visit friends and relatives. It applies particularly to immigrants to very developed countries (such as the United States, Canada, Western Europe, Australia, and New Zealand) returning to lesser-developed countries in Asia, Africa, and South America.

In 2002, 10 percent of the U.S. population was foreign-born. If you add the children of this 10 percent of the population, the combined numbers amounted to 20 percent of the U.S. population. This group of people account for 40 percent of all overseas journeys made by U.S. citizens.

Why single out this group? VFRs are far more likely to suffer from travel-related disease than other travelers. These illnesses include travelers' diarrhea, fish-toxin poisoning, typhoid, hepatitis A, malaria, tuberculosis, dengue fever, and respiratory tract infections, including influenza. Typhoid is a particularly common infection that VFRs get. VFRs are also more likely to be involved in accidents, especially motor vehicle accidents. Animal bites and poisonings by venom are also more common. Why is this? There are many reasons, some of which are listed here:

- VFRs are less likely to receive travel counseling prior to departure. They are less likely to have the appropriate immunizations, both routine and travel. VFRs feel they know the country they are visiting and assume they have immunity against many of the diseases that occur there.
- They tend to assume greater risks while traveling, especially with regard to transportation, food and water consumption, and accommodations.
- They are more likely to stay in rural and remote villages without sophisticated accommodations or facilities. They may sleep on the floor and in crowded rooms.
- They tend to stay longer and mix more with the local population.

If you are a VFR, you need to take extra precautions when traveling to lesser-developed countries.

 What to Do before You Go

- Visit a travel clinic or travel physician before your departure. Try to make this visit some months before your journey to allow sufficient time for immunizations. You may not be up to date on your routine immunizations. A tetanus booster is often required. Travel immunizations, such as those against typhoid, may also be necessary. Children may need rabies immunizations. Just because you were born in the country, do not think you will be more immune to the local diseases. The exact opposite is true.

- Purchase or make up a travel medical kit. This should include an alcohol-based hand sanitizer lotion or spray, as well as a good insect repellent. If traveling to an area where malaria and other insectborne diseases are prevalent, read the chapters in this book on malaria, other insectborne diseases, and prevention of insect bites. If malaria is present in the area you intend to visit, and especially if you are traveling to rural areas, consider purchasing mosquito bed nets. This is particularly important for young children.
- Check your health insurance. Consider purchasing additional health insurance.

What to Do while You Are Traveling

- Avoid traveling in unsafe vehicles.
- Pay attention to safe food and water precautions.
- Wash your hands frequently.
- Use insect repellents appropriately. Pay attention to other insect precautions.

- Be cautious around animals. This is especially important for children. Clean all wounds well. Rabies is a major problem in many developing countries.
- Wash your hands.

 ### *What to Do once You Return*

If anyone in your family becomes ill after you return home, seek medical care early. Inform your health care provider of your recent travels so that she or he will be aware of the need to check for more unusual diseases, such as malaria and typhoid.

5

Traveling with Children Who Have Chronic Illnesses and Special Needs

Traveling with children who have chronic illnesses or special needs poses added challenges and requires additional preparation. Do not plan a too hectic or strenuous schedule. Think your travel plans through carefully. Minor alterations in your itinerary may make the trip more suitable for the person with an underlying disease. Reliable medical care may not be available in remote areas, and parents need to be certain that they are capable of handling their child's illness on their own. If not, it may be prudent to select a different travel destination.

If you have a child with a chronic illness or other medical problem, it is especially important to visit a travel clinic or travel physician before your travels. It is essential that your child's immunizations are up to date and that you are adequately prepared to prevent such travel-related illnesses as travelers' diarrhea and malaria.

It is also important to visit the physician who is taking care of your child's chronic illness so that you are sure the underlying condition is under optimal control. Adjustments to medication are usually best made weeks in advance, rather than on the day of departure. Make sure you have a *written* disease management plan so that you know how to adjust medication if the need arises.

Wear a MedicAlert bracelet. Consider joining the Medic-Alert Travel Plus program. Its services include helping you locate a physician when you are out of the United States, helping with medical evacuation, and numerous other benefits. MedicAlert can be contacted by phone at (888) 633-4298; from outside the United States call (209) 669-2450. Web site: www.medicalert.org.

Anyone with a chronic disease who travels internationally should definitely have good travel and evacuation insurance.

Know how to locate medical care in your destination country and how to contact your physician back home.

Carry medication with you in your carry-on baggage. This medication needs to be in the original containers with the pharmacy labels. Bring extra medication in case of unscheduled delays, spoilage, or loss. Also carry backup prescriptions for additional medication. These scripts should have the correct pharmacological names of the drugs, as the trade names often vary from country to country. Discuss with your physician the need for additional medication to treat complications of the underlying disease, and also discuss the advisability of taking along an antibiotic to treat infections. Get specific guidelines for using these medications.

Many airports have upgraded their security measures because of the increase in the threat of terrorism. Consequently it is very important to check with the Federal Aviation Administration (FAA) and your airline if your child uses any medical equipment that you will need to take on board the aircraft. Do this several days before your departure date so that you have enough time to get any necessary letters, prescriptions, and other paperwork from your child's doctor to document the reasons your child needs to carry these items on board.

 For Your Reference

The following Web sites provide additional information on traveling with disabilities:

1. www.access-able.com
2. www.miusa.org
3. www.mossresourcenet.org/travel.htm

The U.S. Department of Transportation has a toll-free hotline for disabled travelers requiring assistance. This service covers travel within the United States and abroad, on U.S. and foreign airlines. It will give real-time advice to travelers who need help. The phone number is (800) 778-4838.

CHILDREN WITH ASTHMA

If your child has very unstable asthma and is prone to severe attacks, it is unwise to travel to countries with limited medical facilities. In fact, it is not sensible to travel anywhere until asthma is under good control.

While your child is on vacation, his asthma may act up as he is exposed to a variety of "asthma triggers," which include the following:

- Molds, which are very common in hot and humid environments and especially at seaside resorts. Many people appear to have well-controlled asthma until they open up their seaside cottage at the beginning of summer and are met with a barrage of mold spores.
- Upper respiratory infections picked up while traveling and being in confined spaces with many other people.
- Exposure to irritants such as cigarette smoke. This is common in buses, aircraft, trains, and public places in many countries.
- The excitement and the anxiety that often go with travel.
- Forgetting to take medication because of the disruption in your child's usual routine.

Often a combination of triggers results in the worsening of your child's asthma.

Discuss with your child's doctor whether your child's asthma medication needs to be increased before and during your trip. This applies particularly to the "controller" (preventer) medications such as inhaled corticosteroids. Make sure you take along enough medication, especially sufficient "rescue" medication such as albuterol or other short-acting bronchodilators and a course of oral steroids. All of this should be discussed with your doctor prior to travel. You should have with you a written asthma action plan outlining the steps to be taken in the event your child has an asthma attack or her asthma symptoms increase.

It is always better to err on the side of being overcautious and to overtreat rather than undertreat asthma, especially while away on vacation or in unfamiliar surroundings.

Early signs that asthma may be getting out of control are a cough late at night (10 p.m. to 2 a.m.) and a cough with exercise. If your child needs to use his "rescue" inhaler more often than usual, this suggests that the asthma is worsening. A person with well-controlled asthma should not need to use a "rescue" inhaler more than twice a week. On the other hand, wheezing may come on suddenly if your child is exposed to inhaled allergens such as peanut "dust" on board the airplane.

Keep your child's asthma medication, especially the "rescue" medication, with you at all times. Older children should carry their medication with them.

Younger children, who usually receive their medication by nebulizers requiring a source of electricity, may do very well on meter-dose inhalers (MDIs) administered with the aid of a spacer or holding chamber. However, if any changes are to be made, these changes should be made some time before your departure, and your physician should check on your child's technique when using MDIs and spacers.

CHILDREN WITH DIABETES

Travel, even to far-off and lesser-developed lands, is not contraindicated if your child has diabetes as long as the diabetes is stable. You should also have a good understanding of the illness, diabetic medication, and how to recognize and treat the complications of diabetes, including hypoglycemia and hyperglycemia. Even if you have a good understanding of your child's diabetes, it is preferable to select countries that have good medical care.

It is not wise to travel with a newly diagnosed diabetic, as the insulin requirements often vary greatly from week to week and you are unlikely to be familiar enough with the necessary adjustments in insulin dosage. There are many facets to the care of a diabetic, and it takes time to acquire a good understanding of the disease.

Your child's diabetes will probably be more difficult to control while traveling owing to a combination of factors:

- Irregular mealtimes.
- Different foods, not all of which may be to your child's liking and so may not be eaten.
- Motion sickness.
- Excitement.
- Variable exercise levels. It is impossible to get sufficient exercise on a long flight. On the other hand, once you

are sightseeing or hiking, your child may be exercising far more than usual.

- Change in time zones and sleep patterns.
- Intercurrent illnesses such as upper respiratory infections, travelers' diarrhea, and so on.

What to Do before You Go

- Visit your child's diabetes physician or diabetic educator and discuss your proposed travels with him or her.
  - Request a letter stating that your child has diabetes and will need to carry syringes, needles, and medications with her. This letter must be written on office letterhead.
  - Get prescriptions for all your child's medicines, syringes, and so on. In order to board with syringes and other insulin-delivery devices, you must produce an insulin vial with a professional, pharmaceutical, preprinted label that clearly identifies the medication. If the prescription is on the outside of the box that contains the vial of insulin, take this along with you as well.
  - Ask for an antibiotic prescription for treating travelers' diarrhea. Discuss with your child's physician the advisability of taking along an antibiotic to treat other infections as well. If you are planning a sea voyage and your child is 12 years or older, ask for a prescription to treat motion sickness.

- Get a contact phone number that you can use for advice after hours and on weekends (most diabetics already have this). Remember, you may be calling from a different time zone.
- Ask for guidelines on adjusting insulin doses if you plan on crossing many time zones (more than five time zones). No adjustments are necessary for north-south flights.
- If your child's usual insulin regimen does not include short-acting insulin such as Humalog (insulin lispro), ask for a prescription for this and guidance on how to use it. This insulin has a rapid onset and short duration of action. It is ideal when your child may need extra doses of insulin, such as when crossing time zones or when your schedule, mealtimes, and exercise are unpredictable and erratic.
- Insulin pen injectors have insulin-containing cartridges that make the administration of insulin far more convenient while traveling.

Note: Any changes in your child's insulin regimen should be made weeks before travel and not just before you depart.

- Contact the FAA and the American Diabetes Association (www.diabetes.org) to find out the latest guidelines and restrictions concerning the carriage of medical equipment on board the aircraft. (You may take lancets on board if they are capped and they are carried with a glucose meter with the manufacturer's name embossed on the meter.)

- Make sure you have an adequate supply of insulin, insulin syringes, glucagon, and glucose test strips and an extra battery for the blood glucose meter (glucometer) or a spare meter. Include ketone urine test strips to detect and monitor ketones in the urine. It is a good idea to take extra quantities of insulin and other supplies in case there are unscheduled delays or other mishaps. Most authorities recommend that you take at least double the supplies you think you will need. You may not be able to purchase the identical insulin in other countries.

- If your child uses an insulin pump and you are traveling outside the United States, either take along a supply of insulin and syringes or contact your pump company and request a backup loaner in case the pump fails. Also, take along your pump manual and log book with basal rates. Insulin pumps are not harmed by metal detectors and will not trigger the airport metal detectors.

- If you intend to travel to areas with extreme climates, purchase an appropriate container in which to carry your child's insulin (contact Medicool Insulin Protector at 800-433-2469). Insulin can be stored for 30 days at room temperature. **Do not** expose it to extremes of temperature. It should not be left in luggage that is stored in the aircraft luggage hold, as it may freeze. Insulin that is frozen is useless. Nor should it be left in the trunk of your car or on the dashboard, where it may become too hot. Do not expose it to direct sunlight. Consider purchasing an appropriate carrying case to carry all your child's diabetic medication and equipment. Keep this with you while traveling.

- Purchase a supply of snacks to treat low blood sugar or to take the place of meals that do not meet your child's fancy.

- If your child is prone to motion sickness, purchase medication to prevent this (see Chapter 10).

- It is especially important to visit a travel clinic or travel physician if you intend to travel to countries where contracting illnesses such as travelers' diarrhea or malaria is likely.
  - Get appropriate advice on the prevention and treatment of malaria, travelers' diarrhea, and so on.
  - Get appropriate immunizations, including a flu shot and the pneumococcal vaccine.
  - Get further advice about medical facilities and diseases relevant to the countries you intend to visit.

- Make sure you have travel medical insurance. Ideally, this should be medical insurance with assistance (see Chapter 3). If you are traveling to remote or lesser-developed countries, consider purchasing evacuation insurance as well.

- Make sure you know how to locate reliable health care while away (see Chapter 3). The American Diabetes Association and the International Diabetes Federation (www.idf.org) may also be able to provide you with additional information and medical contacts while away.

Contact these organizations prior to departure and keep their phone numbers and addresses in a safe place with your other documents. If you have a Medtronic Mini-Med insulin pump, contact Medtronic to get the direct phone numbers for Medtronic MiniMed because the 800 number will not work outside the United States. The general phone number is (818) 362-5958. The 24-hour helpline is (818) 576-5555. Medtronic MiniMed has offices worldwide and can assist you in locating an endocrinologist internationally.

- Contact the airline before your departure date if you want to order diabetic meals for the flight. The airline's regular meal may be a better alternative but will require you to make appropriate choices for your child.

What to Do while You Are Traveling

- Ensure that your child wears her diabetic identification bracelet (MedicAlert bracelet) at all times.
- **Keep all you child's diabetic medication and equipment with you in your carry-on luggage.**
- Make sure you always have a supply of snacks with you. This is especially important while traveling as you may not know when your child's next meal will be.
- Carry with you, on your person, a letter from your child's doctor stating that she has diabetes and will need to carry her medication, syringes, and needles with her at all times. Have this letter easily accessible at check-in

and available for airport security. Notify the screener at airport security that your child has diabetes and is carrying her diabetic supplies with her.

- Try to regulate your child's meals. If your child is taking her insulin in relation to meals, do not give insulin unless you are sure that her next meal is right in front of her.

- While flying, keep your watch set to the time of your departure point. This will help you keep track of the time in relation to your child's insulin schedule. While crossing time zones, treatment schedules should be based on the time at the point of departure.

- If your child is prone to motion sickness, try to prevent this (see Chapter 10). If she has trouble keeping her meals down, it is far better to avoid large doses of long-acting insulin. Rather, use small frequent doses of short-acting insulin such as Humalog.

  - You may need to adjust your child's insulin dosage if you will be crossing many (more than five) time zones. When traveling west, the day will be longer, and your child may need an extra dose of insulin. When traveling east, the opposite happens—the day will be shorter, and your child may therefore need less insulin, especially long-acting insulin. You should have discussed all this with your child's diabetes physician prior to travel.

  - The secret to diabetic control while traveling is to check your child's blood glucose level *frequently*, at least every four to six hours. This cannot be emphasized enough.

- – You should not aim to keep as tight control as you do at home, but aim to avoid the extremes: too high blood glucose or, even more important, too low blood glucose. You may decide to let your child's blood glucose run a little higher than usual to avoid hypoglycemia.
- Be on the lookout for scratches and insect bites, which in a diabetic child tend to become infected more easily. Clean scratches, abrasions, and bites well and apply an anti-itch ointment and possibly a topical antibiotic as well. Keep your child's nails short to prevent further skin damage from scratching.
- Good foot care is essential. If your child is doing a lot of walking or hiking, keep an eye on your child's feet to make sure that blisters are avoided. This is not the time to try out new boots. Treat any foot problems promptly.
- Be especially vigilant regarding safe food and water precautions. It is important to prevent travelers' diarrhea in diabetics, as diarrhea and vomiting will make your child's diabetes more difficult to control.
- Avoid sunburn, as it may lead to dehydration and to blistering, which carries a greater risk of secondary infection in diabetes.
- Make sure your child drinks plenty of fluids and keeps well hydrated. Keep an eye on her urine output (both color and amount). This is especially important in hot climates and while hiking or climbing.
- Glucose meters may not give reliable readings at high altitudes. They tend to underestimate blood glucose levels.

- In diabetics at high altitudes, it may be difficult to differentiate hypoglycemia from high-altitude sickness.

In summary, it is safe for most diabetic children to travel providing the diabetes is under good control and they are supervised well during their travels. Do not aim for extremely tight control, but do check your child's blood glucose levels more frequently. Anticipate events that are likely to put your child's diabetes out of control, such as erratic mealtimes, motion sickness, and travelers' diarrhea.

 For Your Reference

For an excellent discussion on diabetes and travel, see the *International Traveler Health Guide*, by Stuart R. Rose and Jay S. Keystone—a *must read* for the international traveler who has diabetes.

CHILDREN WITH HEADACHES

We all tend to have an idyllic picture of vacation and travel: relaxation, tropical beaches, palm trees, cruise ships, sightseeing in fascinating cities, and so on. The reality is often far different: rushing to the airport, lining up to board the plane, uncomfortable seating, fussy children, a lack of sleep, trying to make yourself understood in foreign languages, and so on. There is nothing quite like the stresses of travel to trigger headaches in the chronic headache sufferer.

At least 5 to 10 percent of children suffer from chronic or recurring headaches, either tension headaches or migraine. This number is a lot higher in adults, especially women. If you or your child belongs to this select club, it is important to have a physician who understands headaches and knows how to treat them. Children who suffer from frequent headaches, particularly if they are disabling, should probably be on daily prophylactic headache medication. They will also need to have another type of medication, a "rescue" medication, to treat headaches acutely. Ideally they should have a *written* headache action plan detailing how and when these medications should be used. This plan should include the doses of all medicines.

 ### *What to Do before You Go*

- Make sure you take enough medication with you. Take extra medication to allow for travel delays, spoilage, or loss.
- Ask your physician for an extra prescription, including the generic or chemical names of the drugs.
- Have a headache action plan so that you know how to increase or add medication if necessary.
- Know how to locate medical care away from home and how to contact your physician back home.

What to Do while You Are Traveling

- Keep medications in the original containers in case they are inspected by customs officials.
- Keep the medication in your carry-on luggage so that it is both easily accessible and also less likely to get lost.
- If your child is on daily prophylactic medication, make sure this is taken.
- Keep his "rescue" medication on hand at all times.
- If he senses a headache coming (or you do), take time out from your activities. Have him take the "rescue" medication, and find a quiet and preferably dark place to rest. Do not attempt to fight a migraine—you will not win. Give in. Relax. Be sensible. In migraine sufferers, less is usually more.

Pay attention to the common triggers of headaches:

- A lack of sleep.
- Unwise food choices, especially an excess of caffeine-containing beverages, foods containing MSG (monosodium glutamate), found in many Asian foods, and other foods loaded with preservatives, such as hot dogs. You may be aware of other foods that trigger headaches in your child. Avoid these, especially when eating out.
- Hunger. Regular meals are important. Have a supply of snacks readily available. Children often become whiny

and fussy when hungry. A headache is next down the pike.

- Too much stress. Give yourself plenty of time to get to the airport, check in, and board the plane. Do not take unnecessary luggage. Label your luggage so that it is easily identifiable. Catch a cab to your hotel. Have local currency available for snacks for hungry kids, for tips, and so on. In other words, try to plan your vacation to be as stress-free as possible.
- Too much excitement. Do not try to do and see too much. Leave plenty of time for relaxation, afternoon naps, and strolls in the park.
- If your child suffers from allergies, be alert for allergic triggers that may cause sinus headaches. Continue regular allergy medication.
- Although too much caffeine can cause headaches, so can caffeine withdrawal. A not uncommon cause of headaches in adults who "head back to nature" and go on wilderness or "extreme" travel excursions is a lack of their usual morning caffeine fix!

CHILDREN WITH CHRONIC LUNG DISEASE AND CARDIAC DISEASE

If your child has a serious cardiac disease or a chronic lung disease, discuss the suitability of air travel with your child's physician. Extra oxygen may be required during the flight. Commercial airlines will not allow private oxygen tanks aboard the aircraft but will supply oxygen if contacted in advance.

If you plan to travel to high-altitude locations, have your child checked beforehand by a pulmonologist (lung specialist) and a cardiologist (heart specialist) and discuss with them the advisability of traveling to such a location. A child with chronic lung disease (other than asthma) and some cardiac diseases is especially prone to high-altitude sickness.

CHILDREN WITH RECURRENT AND CHRONIC EAR PROBLEMS

See the section "Ears and Flying" in Chapter 8.

CHILDREN IN WHEELCHAIRS

Contact the airline to make appropriate wheelchair and transportation arrangements. Some countries are not suitable for handicapped people, and you should research this beforehand. Most barriers are not insurmountable, but the stresses and hassles of travel will be increased.

CHILDREN WITH ECZEMA (ATOPIC DERMATITIS)

See Chapter 37.

CHILDREN WITH EPILEPSY

Make sure your child's epilepsy is well controlled prior to travel. If indicated, have anticonvulsant blood levels checked.

Take an adequate supply of medication, including medication to treat seizures acutely (such as rectal diazepam). Be sure you know how to use this medication. Discuss this with your child's physician beforehand and write down the directions and dosages.

CHILDREN WITH COLOSTOMY BAGS AND INTESTINAL DISORDERS

- Take along an adequate supply of colostomy supplies, as they may not be obtainable in other countries or may not be the right size. Be sure to apply a larger-than-usual bag when flying because the air inside the bag will tend to expand with air travel. Using a larger bag may prevent leakage.
- If your child has diarrhea and needs to go to the bathroom frequently, as many people with ulcerative colitis do, reserve an aisle seat. This will definitely make the flight less stressful for everyone.
- Children with intestinal disorders such as Crohn's disease, ulcerative colitis, celiac disease, and short gut, among others, are more prone to get travelers' diarrhea. If they do, it is more likely to be severe and may lead to dehydration. It is especially important for these children to be vigilant regarding safe food and water precautions to avoid travelers' diarrhea. It may be wise for these children to be on prophylactic antibiotics for travelers' diarrhea or possibly to take Pepto-Bismol on a regular basis. If they are not already on an antibiotic, it is a good idea

for them to have access to an appropriate antibiotic in the event that they do develop travelers' diarrhea. Discuss this with your child's physician prior to departure and take along the necessary medication (see Chapter 12).

• If your child is taking medication to suppress gastric acid production or to treat gastro-esophageal reflux (regurgitation of stomach contents up the esophagus), such as Zantac, Prevacid, or Prilosec, he may be more prone to travelers' diarrhea. Prophylactic antibiotics or prophylactic Pepto-Bismol may be indicated. Discuss this with your child's physician.

6

Traveling Teenagers

Adolescents are especially high-risk travelers. They seem to regard themselves as immortal and feel that "the laws of nature" do not apply to them. In truth, not only are they more prone to many of the common travel-related problems such as travelers' diarrhea and sunburn, but they have a number of problems specific to their age.

All the anxieties you may have at home when your teenager goes out at night with a group of friends are multiplied manyfold when he sets off on spring break to Fort Lauderdale, Cancun, or Ibiza, either on his own or with some high school or college friends. He may need to make decisions beyond his level of maturity, and he may have more independence than he can handle. Adolescents do not always seem to be aware of the consequences of their actions. They may be particularly carefree and more likely to take part in risk-taking behavior when away from home. Summer vacations especially may be seen as an opportunity to escape from the regimented life and social mores back home, to a life of adventure and romance. You will, understandably, worry that you will not be there to guide and protect them. Before your adolescent sets out on her travels, discuss your family values, your family morals, and your expectations with her. Stress safety issues and common sense.

Our teenage son frequently travels overseas on his own to visit relatives in France, Switzerland, or South Africa. One of my wife's standard reminders goes as follows: "Remember, David, you represent not only yourself but your family, your school, and your country."

It is not easy being a parent to an adolescent. Your "baby," who is striving for his independence, seems very sensible and mature at one moment and totally irresponsible at another. Traveling with adolescents requires a lot of patience, tolerance, and understanding. You will vacillate, one minute wanting to "strangle" them and the next agonizing about their safety and future. When talking to your teenager, it is important to be nonjudgmental, but do not abrogate your parental rights or responsibilities. You will need to balance firmness with understanding. Discuss your expectations and set clear-cut guidelines beforehand.

Much of the advice in this chapter applies to the adolescent whether she is traveling or at home.

TRAVEL PLANS AND THE ADOLESCENT

Medical, Travel, and Evacuation Insurance

Find out whether your adolescent will be covered by your health or travel insurance while he is away. Many insurance policies have an age limit, and your 21-year-old may no longer be covered. If that is the case, you will want to get insurance for him. It is also a good idea to have evacuation insurance, especially if your child is visiting a lesser-developed country.

Identification

Your adolescent will need her own passport and should carry a copy of it separately in case the passport is lost. It is also a good idea for her to carry a notarized letter from one of her parents giving permission for her to travel on her own.

Medical Kit

It is a good idea for your adolescent to take along his own medical kit. Do not forget sunscreen, insect repellent, non-prescription painkillers, and his usual medications. If your adolescent is sexually active, condoms are essential. If your adolescent is a girl and is sexually active, some other reliable form of contraception such as the birth control pill or patch, as well as condoms, is essential.

SPECIAL CONCERNS ABOUT ADOLESCENTS

Alcohol

Many countries have a far more casual attitude toward alcohol than the United States does. The legal drinking age may be lower, or not enforced, or even nonexistent. Teenagers often join their parents in a glass of wine around mealtimes. Even in the United States, consumption of alcohol by adolescents is a lot greater than their parents would like to believe. (Approximately 50 percent of high school seniors drink regularly.) Alcohol is one of the primary causes of fatal motor vehicle accidents involving adolescents. Drinking alcohol while participating in water sports contributes significantly to fatal drownings. Adolescents love to partake in exciting and dangerous sports such as jet skiing, parasailing, and scuba diving. Alcohol should never be consumed when participating in these sports. Adolescents and alcohol may be a lethal combination, but they do not have to be. For some, drinking in moderation may be an option. Discuss alcohol and drinking with your adolescent.

Drugs

Adolescence is often a time of experimentation. Up to one-third of high school students have tried marijuana. In no country are people under the age of 18 legally allowed to use or possess marijuana. There are also no countries in which the use of hard drugs is legal. In many countries, dire consequences await the person who is caught with hard drugs. Discuss with your adolescent the importance of not agreeing to carry parcels or packages from strangers through customs or across borders. Severe penalties may result if she is caught dealing or transporting drugs across borders. These penalties include the death penalty and imprisonment without trial. Your teenager needs to understand these facts before he ventures into foreign lands.

I am sure you also feel that your teenager should understand the consequences of taking recreational drugs even if she never leaves the United States. Drugs such as crack and Ecstasy are often readily available at parties and raves in the United States and even more so at "hot party spots" away from home. Drinks may be spiked with drugs, leading to unwanted and unprotected sex. Talk with your adolescent about all these issues.

Sexually Transmitted Diseases

Many people first become sexually active during adolescence. Many adolescents (and adults for that matter) view a vacation, especially a vacation abroad, as a time for romance and casual sex. The media frequently reinforce this point of view with suggestive pictures of seminaked vacationers on a tropical beach. Promiscuous sexual behavior carries many risks, particularly sexually transmitted diseases such as gonorrhea, chlamydia, herpes, and syphilis. Although many of these diseases can be cured, others such as hepatitis B and C may lead to chronic ill health, and still others may lead to permanent infertility. Some, such as AIDS, may ultimately be fatal. AIDS is a worldwide problem—you are guaranteed that wherever you travel, AIDS is already there. AIDS shows no respect for class or age. In Africa, a large percentage of the population is HIV-positive. In some countries up to 70 percent of prostitutes are HIV-positive. Teach your teenagers to avoid all casual sexual encounters, and discuss safe sexual practices, such as using condoms.

Pregnancy

In addition to the risk of sexually transmitted diseases, sex carries the risk of unwanted pregnancy.

Body Piercing and Tattooing

Hepatitis B, hepatitis C, and HIV can be spread through these practices. In addition, it is not uncommon for a bacterial infection to occur after piercing or tattooing, and the wound may take six weeks or longer to heal, sometimes with disfiguring results.

Motor Vehicle Accidents

Motor vehicle accidents are the leading cause of death for adolescents both at home and while traveling. Wearing a seat belt may save your life. Fatal accidents are often associated with alcohol consumption, and alcohol-related motor vehicle accidents are more likely to occur if the driver is an adolescent. Educate your teenagers about the dangers of drinking and driving. Ask them not to ride in the car if the driver has been drinking. Also discuss the risks of riding on motorcycles, mopeds, and scooters and in the back of open trucks. If they are riding a two-wheeled vehicle, whether a bicycle or motorbike, wearing a helmet is essential, and wearing bright and reflective clothing is also sensible.

Drowning

Drowning is the second commonest cause of death in children and adolescents when traveling. See the section "Alcohol" earlier in this chapter and also Chapter 61.

Mental Health Issues

Adolescence is a time of finding oneself, experimentation, and testing boundaries. It is often a very stressful time mentally. Suicide is a common cause of death in adolescents at home, and the stress and insecurity that occur with travel may tax an already insecure and vulnerable human being. Provide your child with the resources (such as a prepaid phone card) to call home if he needs help or is in trouble. Maintain contact with your teenager via cell phone, instant messaging, or e-mail.

THE TRAVELING ADOLESCENT'S HEALTH

Travelers' Diarrhea

Adolescents may be keen to experiment with new foods and drinks and are probably less likely to wash their hands before eating. They are often in a hurry and do not give much thought to the safety of the food they are about to eat. Travelers' diarrhea is more common in adolescent travelers than in adult travelers.

Sunburn

Many adolescents are sun worshipers and would probably regard their vacation as a failure if they returned home without "a really good tan." Stress sun safety. Remind them that sunburns can occur even on cloudy days and that sunscreens need to be applied at least 20 minutes before sun exposure and reapplied often.

Rabies

Teenagers are more likely to pet strange animals. Consider rabies immunization as part of your adolescent's immunization schedule if she will be spending time in an area where rabies is prevalent.

Snake Bites

Adolescent males are the prime target here as they "show off" to others by handling venomous and nonvenomous snakes.

Altitude Sickness and Extreme Sports

Adolescent males often do not display much wisdom when they tackle sports and activities such as rock climbing, scuba diving, bungee jumping, and whitewater rafting. Fitness, good instruction, and being in the company of experts may prevent a disastrous outcome. Do not assume that the companies in other countries that offer these activities are as well regulated and safety conscious as companies in the United States (see Chapter 11).

DESPITE ALL THE CAUTIONS IN THIS CHAPTER, we note that travel, especially to foreign lands, has tremendous benefits and will help your adolescent to expand his or her horizons, experience other cultures, and, one hopes, become more tolerant and understanding of other peoples and ideas. Travel will help your adolescent become a citizen of the world and encourage him or her to be more sensitive and caring toward our fragile world and its peoples.

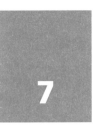

Camping and Other
Outdoor Adventures

If you love the outdoors and like to hike, climb, canoe, or

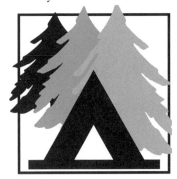

camp, you will want to teach your children to enjoy these activities. Start when they are young and you will be able to show them an exciting world that has no television and no computers. Without these distractions your children will be a captive audience, and you will interact on a different level.

WHERE TO GO

- Start close to home when your children are young. We started very close to home, and after a few nights in a tent in our own backyard our son was begging to try something more adventurous.

- Choose a location that is familiar to you.
- Be age appropriate. Remember that if you are carrying your child, the distance you travel will depend on your ability and stamina.
- Don't be too ambitious. Consider the skill level of the children.
- Have a backup plan and use it when appropriate.
- Choose a child-friendly destination.

WHEN TO GO

- Until your children are experienced, it is better to plan your activities for good weather. Check the weather forecast before you leave home.
- If you are going to high altitudes, read the chapter on altitude sickness (Chapter 11).

SAFETY

- Be well prepared.
- Use the best equipment you can afford.
- Take flashlights.
- Give your itinerary to a friend or family member so someone will know where you are.
- A cell phone is useful if you have a problem and need help.
- Supervise children and set clear guidelines for safe behavior.

- Arrive at campsites in daylight so you can identify potential hazards.
- Teach safe behavior around campfires and gas stoves.
- Remember that children are more prone to extremes of temperature.
- Use sunscreen when needed.
- Don't forget insect repellent and mosquito netting.
- Provide each child with a whistle so he or she can signal for help.
- Bells on the shoes worn by young children will keep parents aware of the children's location.
- Water safety is very important. Drowning is a common cause of death in childhood. Wear life jackets when boating. Teach your children how to swim.

CLOTHING

- Clothing should be appropriate for the activities and for the weather.
- Layering is a good principle.
- Hats are important. A brim will provide protection from the sun, and a warm head covering will prevent heat loss in cold weather.

SHOES

- Don't try out new shoes on a long hike.
- Take along an extra pair.

- High-top shoes will support ankles.
- River shoes protect feet in water.

FOOD AND DRINK

- Breast-feeding is the most convenient way to feed a baby.
- Powdered formula is convenient only if safe water is available.
- Children can carry their own snacks and drinks. Don't wait until they are thirsty or hungry. Encourage them to drink frequently.
- If you will be eating dehydrated food, let your children test these foods at home.
- S'mores are a tasty treat to enjoy around the campfire after a day outdoors.

FIRST AID KIT

- Check your kit before you set out. Have any of the medications expired?
- Make sure the contents are age appropriate.
- Don't forget sunscreens and insect repellent.

BACKPACKS AND CARRIERS

- Front carriers are suitable for babies up to 20 pounds.
- Back carriers are suitable for babies seven months and older, when their head and neck are more stable.

- Children can carry a light pack once they are three years of age.
- Children four feet and taller can carry a framed pack. Make sure it is comfortable and fits well.

GENERAL CONSIDERATIONS

- Have fun! Enjoy the journey.
- Be flexible.
- Respect the environment.
- Taking a friend along may ease your child's transition from the electronic world to the wilderness.
- Involve children in planning and preparation. Teach children necessary skills and practice them before leaving home. This may include pitching a tent, signaling when lost, and fire safety.

 For Your Reference

1. An entertaining and fun book for families to read is *Camping and Backpacking with Children*, by Steven Boga (1995).
2. And for the truly adventurous: *Field Guide to Wilderness Medicine*, by Paul S. Auerbach, Howard J. Donner, and Eric A. Weis (2003). This book is highly recommended for those going into the true wilderness far from medical care.

8

Traveling by Air

Flying, especially in today's aircraft with cramped seating, is seldom restful or relaxing, but good planning might make the experience more tolerable. It has been said that there are only two classes of air travel: with children and without!

Here are some general tips to make the flight slightly less nerve-wracking:

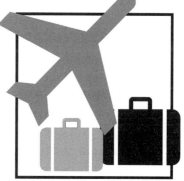

- If possible, try to select less crowded flights. This is becoming increasingly difficult, if not impossible, in this age of increased airline competition and cost cutting. Friday evening and Sunday afternoon and evening flights are often overbooked and crowded. It is especially stressful to travel over the very busy holidays of Thanksgiving, Christmas, and New Year's.

- Few airlines require booking a seat for a child under the age of two years, but having a seat for your child to stretch out in makes for a happier and more relaxed child and consequently a happier parent. Regardless of your child's age, it is preferable to book a seat for him if you can afford it. This way, you can also bring along an airline-approved infant seat, which can double as a car seat at your destination. When purchasing an infant car seat, look for one that has a label that reads as follows: "This restraint is certified for use in motor vehicles and aircraft." Choose one that is 16 inches or less in width, as many coach seats aboard aircraft are only 16 inches wide. The car seat must be placed in a window seat so that it will not block the escape route in the event of an emergency. Children weighing less than 20 pounds should be in a rear-facing car seat. From 20 to 40 pounds your child should be in a forward-facing car seat. Children over 40 pounds do not need to use a car seat but can be safely buckled up using the aircraft seat belt. It is not safe to share an adult's seat belt by squeezing your child in between you and the belt. Most airlines will provide you with an extension for your seat belt if you are sharing your seat with a young child. Contact the airline for its policy on child-restraint systems. For further information, you can also contact the Federal Aviation Administration (FAA) at (800) 322–7873.
- Remember that injuries often occur when the plane unexpectedly hits air turbulence and passengers are thrown

from their seats. This is particularly likely to happen to an infant or a child, so booking your infant or young child her own seat is not only a comfort issue but also a safety issue. Many infants and young children will cry and fuss more if confined to an infant car seat during a flight, so for these children using an infant seat during the flight may just not be practical. However, bringing an infant car seat along is probably worthwhile, even if your child occupies it only when napping.

- If you are traveling long distances with an infant, try to reserve the seats just behind the bulkhead. Many airlines will then supply you with an infant bassinet or cot. If your children are slightly older, this might not be a good location because in many airlines these seats have armrests that do not fold back, making it difficult for a child to stretch out and sleep across you. The flickering images of the movie screened on the bulkhead may also make sleep even more difficult for you and your child.

- If you have a toddler, reserving an aisle seat is often a good idea, as this will allow you and your toddler to take frequent walks around the cabin to ease the boredom and frustration of being confined to a seat for prolonged periods.

- Do not set out on your journey already sleep-deprived and exhausted. Do not leave too much to be done on the day of departure. Get a few good nights' sleep prior to departure and allow adequate time to get to the airport, check in, clear security, and board the plan. This will ensure that you "start off on the right foot."

- Limit carry-on bags to essentials, but do not forget your

child's teddy bear or favorite blanket, a supply of snacks, and boxes of juice.

- Carry essential medications with you.
- Prior to departure, prepare an activity pack with books, games, puzzles, and special treats to help entertain your child during the journey.
- Carry a change of clothing and sufficient disposable diapers for infants. Pack these items so that they are easily accessible during the flight.
- Children often get very thirsty during long flights. Offer them liquids frequently.
- For young children who have graduated from a bottle, take along a "sippy cup" (trainer cup or a cup with a spout) to limit spills and sticky fingers.
- When making airline reservations, it is a good idea to reserve a child's meal because many children do not appreciate the food served to adults. A hot dog or chicken nuggets may go down a lot better than a spinach quiche! (Adults may not appreciate airline food either.)
- Be careful when drinking hot beverages. Sudden movements can result in nasty burns.
- Do not let your children run in the aisles. This is not only inconsiderate toward other passengers and the flight attendants but also dangerous. With air turbulence (and even without) young children may fall and injure themselves.
- Make sure carry-on luggage is securely stored in the overhead luggage bins. Luggage falling from overhead bins is a common cause of injuries.

- Keep essential items under your seat to avoid having to repeatedly get up and search through the overhead bins.

HOW YOUNG IS TOO YOUNG TO FLY?

It used to be said that infants younger than two weeks of age should not fly because of immature lungs. It is probably quite safe for healthy, full-term infants of this age to fly in today's pressurized aircraft. However, check with your pediatrician first. As mentioned earlier, the first three months of life are not a good time to travel because of the risk of acquiring infection.

EARACHE

Earache is common in people of all ages when flying and is especially common in children. It is due to pressure changes within the middle ear and is most likely to happen when the aircraft is descending just prior to landing. To the young child who does not understand what is happening, this sensation may be alarming as well as painful.

 Prevention

The following strategies can minimize this discomfort:

- Allow an infant to nurse or suck on a bottle or pacifier during ascent and descent.

- Older children can be told to do the following—on ascent, hold the nose, close the mouth, and suck in; on descent, hold the nose, fill the mouth with air, close it, and try to force the air through the closed nostrils.
- Chewing gum may help older children and adults, as it helps contract the muscles around the eustachian tube (the tube draining the middle ear), allowing it to stay open and equalize the pressure within the middle ear.
- If you know that your child usually suffers from severe ear discomfort when flying, be prepared in advance. Give your child an adequate dose of ibuprofen or acetaminophen half an hour prior to flying. If the flight is long and sufficient time has elapsed, the dose can be repeated one hour prior to descent.
- If you or your child has nasal congestion from a cold, using an oral decongestant such as Sudafed prior to and during travel may help the nose and ears stay open. Topical nasal decongestants such as Afrin and Neo-Synephrine in the form of nasal sprays or drops can be particularly useful. Ideally, they should be used half an hour prior to take off and half an hour prior to descent. They can be used either on their own or together with oral decongestants. For infants older than six months, ⅛ percent or ¼ percent Neo-Synephrine may be used (one to two drops in each nostril every four hours as necessary).

CAUTION

Nasal decongestant sprays should never be used for longer than four days.

- If you or your child is prone to nasal allergies or hay fever, using a steroid nasal spray for a few days before and during the flight will also help to decrease the swelling in the nose, ears, and sinuses. The swelling can be further relieved by using oral antihistamines such a diphenhydramine (Benadryl) or nonsedating antihistamines such as Claritin, Clarinex, Zyrtec, or Allegra. Parents should not take sedating antihistamines during flights if they will be driving a car after landing.

- Although it is often said that children who have an ear infection should not fly, there is no good evidence for this. Fluid in the middle ear may partially protect the child from some of the pain and discomfort experienced on taking off and landing. Infants and children with aerating (tympanostomy) tubes can also fly. Pain will be minimized because the tubes will equalize the pressure on either side of the eardrum. However, there is no doubt that flying with an acute cold with nasal and sinus congestion will be uncomfortable and may lead to a middle ear infection. This is the ideal time to use topical and oral decongestants. It may be a good idea to postpone your trip if at all possible.

- Cabin atmosphere contains very little humidity, and mucous membranes dry out easily. Some of the crying and misery experienced by infants and children may be related to this discomfort. They can be nursed or offered other fluids frequently throughout the flight.

- Crying often helps unblock the ears. Distressing as this crying may be to you and to your fellow passengers, it often brings relief and a period of quiet.

- It is never a good idea to try out any medication for the first time during a flight. Many medications, especially cough and cold medications and antihistamines, may have unpleasant and unexpected side effects and may make your journey less pleasant. Always try a test dose of any medication a few days before you depart.

SEDATION

Generally speaking, it is not a good idea to sedate infants and children before a plane flight or other journey. A sedative for children such as chloral hydrate and antihistamines such a diphenhydramine (Benadryl) or promethazine (Phenergan) may have the opposite effect. Instead of ending up with a mellow and sleepy child, you may have an irritable, wide-awake, active child who cannot be pacified.

We made this mistake ourselves. We gave our three-year-old chloral hydrate to sedate him for a flight. He slept peacefully for two hours while the plane was held on the runway during a thunderstorm. He awoke as we took off. Our usually calm and pleasant little boy was transformed! For the next three hours we were the embarrassed owners of an uncontrollable, feisty, and badly behaved child. Nothing calmed him. It was an unforgettable flight.

If you feel you must try sedatives, discuss your plan with your child's physician prior to travel. Do a trial run several days before departure to assess the effect on your child. This will also enable you to establish the appropriate dose for your child. I want to repeat, however, that sedation is usually not a good idea and is not recommended during travel.

JET LAG

Jet lag occurs when traveling across time zones. The body's internal clock and biological rhythms get out of sync with the new time zone or "outside clock." Jet lag is worse when traveling from west to east. When traveling east, you may have difficulty falling asleep at the new bedtime and difficulty awakening in the morning; when traveling west, you may be sleepy in the early evening and awake before dawn.

The more time zones crossed, the more severe the effects. It is generally accepted that for each time zone crossed it will take at least one day for your body to adjust or recover. On a 10-day vacation to the Far East, much of the time may be spent adjusting to jet lag because of the 10 to 12 time zones crossed!

Symptoms of jet lag include excessive daytime sleepiness, nighttime insomnia, fatigue, irritability, poor concentration, and bowel upsets (especially constipation).

Jet lag is compounded by lack of sleep; the physical, emotional, and mental stresses of flying; erratic and often unhealthy meals; excess alcohol and caffeine consumption; and irregular toilet habits.

Unfortunately, there are no wonder medications or remedies that work for all children or adults, but the following strategies may help:

- Make sure you are well rested prior to travel. Try not to leave all your travel arrangements and preparations until the last minute. Get to bed early and get a few good nights' rest in the days preceding your trip.
- Two or three days before departure, try to schedule your routine daily activities earlier or later, depending on the time zone at your destination. For example, if you will be traveling from west to east, go to bed earlier and arise earlier.
- As you board the aircraft, set your watch to your new time zone. (If you are traveling with a diabetic child, however, you should keep your watch set to the time of your departure point in order to help you keep track of the time in relation to your child's insulin schedule, as discussed in Chapter 5.) Start adjusting your eating and sleeping habits to the new time zone.
- Keep well hydrated during the flight. Drink plenty of water and other nonalcoholic beverages. Avoid alcohol and caffeine-containing products.
- When you arrive at your destination, force yourself to adapt to the new time zone as quickly as possible. Stay awake during daylight hours and go to bed at night. Schedule your meals and activities appropriately for your new time zone.
- Exposure to bright sunlight at the correct time of the day may hasten your adaptation to the new time zone. If you've traveled from west to east, expose yourself to morning light. If you've traveled from east to west, expose yourself to afternoon light. For example, if you

catch the late-night flight from New York to London and arrive in London at 8 a.m. the following day, force yourself and your children to stay awake during the morning. Expose yourself to bright, outside light during the early part of the day. In the afternoon, avoid bright light, decrease activities, and cut back on caffeine-containing beverages and alcohol. Keep daytime naps short.

- Allow time to adapt to the new time zone at the other end of the flight. If at all possible, do not arrange too hectic a schedule for the first three to five days of your vacation, especially if you have crossed many time zones; this way, you and your family can adapt to the new time zone with less stress and fatigue. European travelers often seek somewhere peaceful to spend the first few days of their holiday so that they can relax and adjust to the new time zone. Nonretired American travelers, who typically get very little vacation time compared with Europeans, often do not enjoy this luxury, as they tend to schedule a trip over a brief holiday vacation, a child's spring break, or a one-week work reprieve. It is understandable that most Americans feel they need a vacation after the vacation. They do not recuperate from jet lag in either direction until several weeks after returning home.

- Occasionally, parents may have to resort to sleeping pills to help them sleep for a few nights in the new time zone. One adult should remain unsedated so that he or she can attend to the children if necessary. A very effective sleeping pill for adults is zolpidem (Ambien).

- As mentioned earlier in this chapter, it is usually not a good idea to sedate children. However, you may have to do this if your child is having a great deal of trouble falling asleep in the new time zone. A good sedative for children is a prescription medication called chloral hydrate; however, some children may get sufficient sedation from an antihistamine such as Benadryl to enable them to go to sleep. Discuss these possibilities with your child's physician before your departure. Remember, these medications should always be given a trial run at home first (see the section titled "Sedation" earlier in this chapter). This may avoid unpleasant surprises on your vacation.

- Numerous other remedies have been tried as sleeping aids. These include melatonin and a variety of herbal treatments. Melatonin, a hormone, has been shown in many studies to be an effective remedy for adults. Melatonin is available in the United States as an herbal supplement, but because of the lack of regulation by the Food and Drug Administration (FDA), no specific formulations can be recommended. In parts of Europe and many other countries where the herbal industry is more closely regulated, melatonin preparations are more likely to contain a specific amount of the active ingredient. The recommended dose of melatonin is 3 to 5 mg taken at the target bedtime, beginning three to four days before departure. No studies have been done with children, so melatonin cannot be recommended for them at present.

- Not everyone gets jet lag. You may be one of the lucky

people who are unaffected by it. Relax and enjoy your travels. Focus on the positives.

DEEP VEIN THROMBOSIS

You may well ask what a discussion on deep vein thrombosis (DVT; blood clot in the leg) is doing in a book on children's travel problems. Normal children rarely develop blood clots in their legs. However, children travel with parents and grandparents, and it is a tragedy if the adults become seriously ill or die from this largely preventable condition.

My mother-in-law developed a DVT and pulmonary embolus (blood clot that travels to the lungs) after a long flight from the United States to South Africa. She spent some days in intensive care recovering from this avoidable condition. A few minutes of counseling, a pair of compression stockings, and some leg exercises would have saved her weeks of illness and agony.

The term "economy class syndrome" was originally used to describe a condition of blood clots in the legs that some passengers developed during or after flying long distances in the coach section of the airplane. It is a misnomer because passengers in first class can also develop this condition, as well as people traveling long distances by car, bus, or train. Informally called "traveler's thrombosis," it may even occur after sitting for prolonged periods in a theater.

Small DVTs are not unusual after a long flight. Fortunately they seldom lead to major medical complications.

The tendency to develop blood clots in the legs on long journeys is due to a number of factors but especially the following:

- Immobility, which leads to sludging and pooling of the blood in the veins.
- Kinking of the blood vessels, related to the cramped position of the legs.
- Increased tendency of the blood to clot at high altitudes. Cabin pressure at cruising altitude is equivalent to an altitude of 6,000 to 8,000 feet.

Many other factors, such as those listed below, may also play a contributing role, but note that many people who develop DVTs after a flight do not have any of these risk factors.

Risk Factors

- A history of blood clots
- Age of 40 years and older
- Obesity
- Pregnancy
- Recent surgery, especially orthopedic surgery to the legs
- Dehydration
- Sedation
- Certain diseases, especially blood diseases, heart disease, diabetes, and malignancies
- Some drugs, important examples of which are the birth

control pill and tamoxifen (used in the treatment and prevention of breast cancer)

• Recent excessive exertion, such as marathon running

 ### *Prevention*

Traveler's thrombosis is a preventable disease. Here are some important ways to decrease the likelihood of developing it.

• Move your legs often.
  – Extend your legs as far as possible, flex your ankles, pulling up and spreading your toes, and then push down and curl your toes.
  – If there is not enough room to extend your legs, start with your feet flat on the floor and push down and curl your toes while lifting your heels from the floor. Then with your heels back on the floor, lift and spread your toes. Repeat this toe-heel cycle five times or more every 30 minutes.
  – Exercise your thigh muscles by sitting with your feet flat on the floor and sliding your feet forward a few inches, then back; repeat.
  – Change your leg position frequently.
  – Get up and walk around the cabin as often as possible.

Many airlines show a short film at the beginning of the flight describing the type of exercises you can do to minimize your risk of developing a DVT. Pay attention to this film. It may save your life!

- Do not cross your legs, even for short periods.
- Keep well hydrated. Drink plenty of water or electrolyte solutions such as Gatorade.
- Limit the intake of alcohol and caffeine-containing beverages, all of which tend to lead to dehydration.
- Avoid sedatives, which lead to more immobility.
- Wear graduated compression stockings during the flight. These are extremely effective in preventing thrombosis. They are available at many drugstores.
- Wear loose-fitting clothing.
- Anticoagulants ("blood thinners") are recommended for certain high-risk people. If you have had a prior leg thrombosis, discuss the use of these medications with your doctor before traveling. They are not without risk and should not be started just before travel. Aspirin is not particularly effective in preventing venous thrombosis of the legs.
- If traveling by car, stop frequently to stretch your legs.

Symptoms

The most common symptom of traveler's thrombosis is calf pain that develops during or soon after a long airplane flight. The pain is often mistaken for a muscle cramp. Other common symptoms are swelling of an ankle and later the development of a cough, shortness of breath, or chest pain. The chest pain may be so severe that it is mistaken for a heart attack. Rarely, a large clot breaks off, travels to the lung, and causes sudden death.

If you develop any of the these symptoms, seek medical care promptly. Be sure to inform your physician of your recent journey, as this information will aid him or her in making the correct diagnosis.

> *Note:* Swelling of the ankles and feet is not unusual after a long flight.

For Your Reference

For further information, see www.airhealth.org/prevention.

9

Cruise Ships

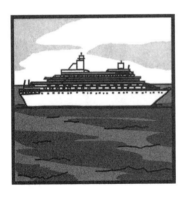

The growth of the cruise ship industry is a testament to the popularity of this type of vacation.

About 6 million people in the United States take a cruise vacation each year. About 5 percent of these people (about 300,000) seek medical attention while away on a cruise. Most of these medical problems are relatively minor. Even though health care aboard cruise ships has recently improved, do not assume that every modern cruise ship has sophisticated medical care and medical facilities on board.

If you or your child has significant medical problems, you should check before going on the cruise that the cruise ship has the medical capability to take care of these medical problems. Do not assume that you can be transported relatively easily to a sophisticated medical facility close by. Many of the locations that these cruise ships visit do not have sophisticated medical facilities.

Cruise ships are ideal locations for the spread of disease. They collect together people from many parts of the world in a confined environment. Some board with infectious diseases. Others are incubating them. The crew members also often come from widely diverse locations, frequently from developing countries where infectious diseases are common.

MEDICAL PROBLEMS WHILE ON BOARD

The following medical problems are the ones most frequently encountered aboard cruise ships:

- Gastrointestinal illnesses, notably travelers' diarrhea. Occasional outbreaks of hepatitis A have also been reported.
- Respiratory tract infections, mainly upper respiratory infections (coughs and colds), but also influenza. Flu may occur even in the summer months, as passengers from another hemisphere may bring their flu with them.
- Accidents, principally minor falls. These are more common on the first day or two after boarding and before you have had time to get your "sea legs."
- Motion sickness. See Chapter 10.

Suggestions for avoiding medical problems on a cruise are listed below. Even when precautions are taken, however, people sometimes get sick. Before you leave, check whether the medical insurance you have back home will cover medical expenses incurred while aboard ship. They are not usually covered. Purchase travel medical insurance with assistance.

 ## *Prevention*

- Make sure your immunizations are up to date, especially for hepatitis A. Consider getting a flu shot.
- Pay attention to safe food and water precautions (see Chapter 13). When you disembark at the various ports on your voyage, eat wisely. Even on board ship, avoid high-risk foods such as potato and egg salad, custards, and cream-filled pastries. Remember, much of the food served on the ship may have been taken on board at the last port of call. Wash hands before eating.

Despite all these warnings, most people do not get ill while on a cruise. They have a wonderful vacation with ample fresh air and sumptuous buffets. The cruise ship industry works hard to maintain good standards of hygiene. Medical care aboard cruise ships continues to improve.

Enjoy your trip!

10

Motion Sickness

Children are more prone to motion sickness than are adults. It is especially common between 4 and 12 years of age. It occurs less frequently in the first two years of life.

The typical symptoms of motion sickness are nausea, vomiting, sweating, and increased salivation. Your child may also look very pale. A common symptom in younger children is an unsteady gait.

General measures to prevent motion sickness include

- avoiding dairy products and heavy and fatty meals;
- giving your child a light meal two to four hours before your journey;
- distracting your child by telling stories or letting him listen to music with headphones;
- using medications to prevent and treat motion sickness; and
- avoiding others who are vomiting.

CAR SICKNESS

Many children get car sick. Car sickness may be minimized using the preventive guidelines below.

 Prevention

- If your child is older than 12 years, allow her to sit in the front seat.
- Try to get her to focus on the horizon.
- Booster seats allow younger children to see out the window.
- Keep the car well ventilated.
- Do not smoke in the car.
- Avoid video games and reading.
- Avoid tight clothing.
- Wearing dark glasses may help.
- If possible, avoid rough, winding, and hilly roads.
- Drive carefully and minimize rapid cornering, stopping, and acceleration.
- Try traveling at night.

If traveling by bus, sit toward the middle of the bus. Open the window slightly if possible.

Despite all these measures your child may still vomit. Have a plastic bag or container easily accessible. Wet wipes and a change of clothing are also a good idea.

AIR SICKNESS

Most children do not develop air sickness when traveling in large commercial aircraft. These fly above the altitude of maximum turbulence and usually are fairly stable.

Prevention

- If possible, avoid commuter flights; small commuter planes fly at low altitudes and are more prone to turbulence.
- Book seats over the wings. This section is the most stable part of the aircraft.
- If your child feels nauseated, encourage him to keep his head still and hold it firmly against the back of his seat.
- Have your child keep his eyes closed.

As mentioned earlier, have a container handy, as well as wet wipes and a change of clothing.

SEASICKNESS

Seasickness is more common than car or air sickness, especially when traveling in small boats and across rough stretches of water.

Prevention

- If traveling in a large ship, choose a cabin in the middle of the ship close to the waterline.
- If traveling by ferry, stay on the upper deck where there is ample fresh air. Tell your child to focus on the horizon. If this is not possible, choose one of the lower decks close to the waterline and near the middle of the boat. If possible, your child should lie down and close her eyes.

MEDICATIONS TO PREVENT AND TREAT MOTION SICKNESS

Sometimes the suggestions provided above are inadequate, and medication is needed to prevent or treat motion sickness. Three medications commonly used for children are diphenhydramine (Benadryl), dimenhydrinate (Dramamine), and promethazine (Phenergan). For the appropriate doses of Benadryl and Dramamine, see tables 8 and 10 in Part Five. Always consult the directions on the labels or manufacturers' packaging.

Promethazine (Phenergan) is a prescription medication in the United States. It is also available as a suppository.

Scopolamine patches are very effective for older children and adults. A prescription is required for these patches. Side effects include dry mouth, drowsiness, blurred vision, and difficulty with urination. Apply the patch four hours before departure. Each patch lasts up to three days. They are not approved for children younger than 12 years of age.

- Benadryl, Dramamine, and Phenergan should be taken at least half an hour before departure. It is easier to prevent motion sickness than to treat it. During long journeys you will need to repeat the dose.
- Dramamine is not approved for children younger than two years of age.
- If you need to use medications such as Benadryl, Dramamine, or Phenergan, try these medications prior to your trip, as they may have unpleasant and unexpected side effects. Discuss the use of these medications with your child's doctor.
- Ginger is a homeopathic remedy that may be effective for some people and is very safe.
- Simple measures are often all that is necessary. Plan ahead and be prepared!

Altitude Sickness

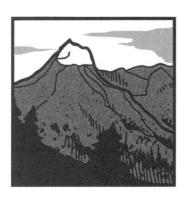

Few of us will climb Mount Everest or Mount Kilimanjaro, but if you decide to leave the sun and warmth of the beach and fly to Aspen to ski, your body will notice the difference. You will definitely be aware of the effects of altitude if you fly into Cuzco in Peru from sea level or ascend to the top of Pike's Peak in Colorado. Many a traveler has had the first day or two of a vacation at high altitude ruined by a severe high-altitude headache.

WHAT IS IT?

Altitude sickness is the term used to describe a spectrum of symptoms and syndromes that occur at high altitude. All the tissues of the body are affected by the lack of oxygen at high altitude, but the two organs most strikingly involved are the brain and the lungs. The milder manifestations of altitude sickness are known as acute mountain sickness. At the other end of the spectrum are two manifestations that may be fatal unless immediate measures are taken to treat them: one of these is high-altitude cerebral edema (HACE), a condition in which the brain swells and doesn't function properly, and the other is high-altitude pulmonary edema (HAPE), a condition in which the lungs may become very congested and "drown" in fluid.

The terminology relating to altitude sickness can be confusing: some authors use the term "acute mountain sickness" synonymously with the term "altitude sickness" to include the entire spectrum of symptoms and syndromes from the milder manifestations to HACE and HAPE. Other authors use the term "acute mountain sickness" to include only the milder manifestations of altitude sickness.

WHY DOES IT OCCUR?

Altitude sickness occurs when a person ascends to high altitudes, especially if this is done rapidly. At high altitudes, less oxygen is available to the body. The lungs and heart have to work a lot harder to supply the muscles and other tissues with enough oxygen to function.

WHO GETS IT?

Anyone can get altitude sickness; it is just as likely to occur in children as in adults. Being physically fit at sea level does *not* prevent altitude sickness. Even the most athletic teenagers and young adults who are in superb physical condition can develop fatal altitude sickness.

Both the likelihood of developing altitude sickness and the degree of its severity are related to several factors:

- The altitude. The higher you go, the greater the risk.
- The speed of ascent. The faster you ascend, the greater the risk. In other words, the less time you take to acclimatize, the greater the risk.
- Physical exertion. The more you exert yourself at high altitude, the greater the risk.
- Genetic factors. Some individuals are more susceptible to developing altitude illness than others.
- Predisposing factors. You are more likely to get altitude sickness if you
  - have had altitude sickness in the past;
  - are dehydrated;
  - are hypothermic (have a low body temperature);
  - have an infection such as an upper respiratory tract infection (URI);
  - usually reside at a low altitude; or

– have certain medical conditions such as chronic lung disease and some types of heart disease.

To reduce the chances of getting altitude sickness, make sure you ascend slowly and take time to acclimatize. Keep well hydrated, and eat a high-carbohydrate diet.

AT WHAT ALTITUDES DOES IT OCCUR?

The onset of altitude sickness is related to numerous factors, some of which have been mentioned above. Minor manifestations, those seen in acute mountain sickness, are common with rapid ascent to 8,000 feet. This is the altitude at which many ski resorts are situated. Rarely, acute mountain sickness occurs at lower altitudes. The altitude at which you sleep is most important.

Fortunately, the more serious forms of altitude sickness, HACE and HAPE (described above), are uncommon below 10,000 feet. However, individual susceptibility varies, and deaths have even occurred at this altitude.

In general, the higher you go, the greater the risk, especially if you rapidly ascend from sea level to high altitudes.

WHAT IS NORMAL AT HIGH ALTITUDE?

- All of us get breathless with exertion at high altitude. We may also feel light-headed.
- Virtually everyone develops a cough if they ascend high enough.

- You may not sleep as well at night.
- You may have periodic breathing. This consists of cycles of breathing at a normal rate, then holding one's breath for up to 10 to 15 seconds, and then breathing rapidly.
- Increased urination is also common. This may be another cause for waking frequently at night.
- Swelling of the hands, feet, and face may occur. This is more common in women.

WHAT ARE THE SYMPTOMS?

Symptoms of altitude sickness usually begin within 6 to 12 hours of ascending to high altitude and increase in severity over the next one to two days. They are usually worse at night. The symptoms of altitude sickness vary with the severity.

Acute Mountain Sickness

Acute mountain sickness is a common condition and affects up to 50 percent of people who ascend to altitudes of 8,000 to 10,000 feet.

You fulfill the criteria for acute mountain sickness if you have recently ascended to a high altitude (above 8,000 feet) and have a headache as well as one of the symptoms described below:

- Nausea, vomiting, and a decrease in appetite
- Fatigue
- Dizziness

- Insomnia
- Irritability

Adults who have experienced a hangover will tell you that acute mountain sickness is very similar. An altitude-related headache tends to be severe, throbbing, and located at either the front or the back of the head. It is often worse at night or early in the morning when you awake and is aggravated by bending over. This headache may initially respond to the administration of analgesics such as ibuprofen. As the severity of acute mountain sickness worsens, these drugs are less effective. The headache typically responds to the administration of oxygen or descent in altitude or specific medications for acute mountain sickness.

A good rule of thumb is if you feel unwell at a high altitude, it is altitude sickness until proven otherwise.

As altitude sickness increases in severity, other more alarming symptoms may emerge.

High-Altitude Cerebral Edema (HACE)

The following symptoms indicate the presence of HACE (brain swelling):

- Headache that does not respond to analgesics. This is serious!
- Confusion.
- Disturbances of gait (ataxia)—walking as though drunk.
- Poor coordination.

- A complete lack of motivation.
- Poor judgment. A person with HACE tends to have poor judgment, displays irrational behavior, and frequently denies that there is anything wrong with him. If treatment is not instituted, he may become stuporous and eventually lapse into coma.

HIGH-ALTITUDE PULMONARY EDEMA (HAPE)

Lung congestion (HAPE) is suggested by a cough that is accompanied by extreme fatigue and shortness of breath at rest. Much later the cough may produce phlegm that is pink and frothy. Although shortness of breath with exertion occurs in almost everybody at high altitude, breathlessness should disappear fairly rapidly with rest. If you are short of breath at rest, this is cause for concern.

HAPE often occurs suddenly at night and may or may not be associated with symptoms of acute mountain sickness or HACE.

ALTITUDE SICKNESS IN YOUNG CHILDREN

It is more difficult to diagnose any illness in very young children because they cannot vocalize their symptoms. Children younger than three years of age are often fussy anyway (especially if their routine is altered) and are more likely to get upper respiratory infections and to become dehydrated. For these reasons it is difficult to detect the early signs of acute mountain sickness in children, especially young children. Symptoms may include

- excessive irritability and crying;
- a loss of appetite;
- nausea and vomiting; and
- inability to sleep.

If your child has any one of these symptoms, he should be considered to have altitude sickness and be treated accordingly.

It is probably not a good idea to travel to high altitudes (certainly above 12,000 feet) with very young children.

OTHER ILLNESSES AND ALTITUDE SICKNESS

As mentioned above, upper respiratory tract infections, hypothermia, and dehydration all increase a person's chances of getting altitude sickness.

Children with asthma do not have any higher risk of developing altitude sickness. However, certain triggers can bring on an asthma attack at high altitudes; these include having a "cold" and being exposed to cold air and air pollution. Asthmatics traveling to Mexico City are more likely to be affected by the air pollution than the altitude! It is unwise for asthmatics to ascend to high altitude if their asthma is not well controlled. People whose asthma is poorly controlled should not stray far from medical care as a general rule—regardless of altitude.

Children with severe lung diseases such as cystic fibrosis should not travel to high altitudes before being assessed by a pulmonologist (lung specialist).

Children with Down's syndrome are more prone to altitude sickness, and people with sickle cell disease will almost certainly have problems at high altitudes.

If your child has a heart murmur, she should be evaluated by a cardiologist before traveling to high altitudes, as certain cardiac conditions predispose a person to altitude sickness.

 ## *Prevention*

Several steps can be taken to prevent or minimize altitude sickness, which in some situations can be life-threatening.

- If you intend to vacation at a high altitude, you should discuss your plans with your physician and your child's physician. A variety of prescription medications may help you prevent and treat altitude sickness.
- When planning a vacation at high altitudes, make sure that the resort you are staying at is equipped to deal with acute mountain sickness.
- If you are planning to trek or climb at altitudes higher than 11,500 feet, you need to learn a lot more about the prevention and treatment of altitude sickness than is discussed here. You should have a guide with you who is experienced in recognizing and treating altitude sickness.
- The most effective preventive measure is acclimatization. Plan a two- to three-day stay at lower altitudes and gradually ascend to higher elevations. For example, if you are planning to stay at a mountain resort at an altitude of 9,000 feet, it would be advisable to stay for two or three days at an intermediate altitude of 6,000 to 7,000 feet. However, this is not always possible—for in-

stance, if you reside at sea level and just plan the occasional skiing weekend in the mountains.

- An important dictum when climbing at high altitudes is to "climb high, sleep low." In other words, you may make daytime excursions to high altitudes but should return to a lower altitude to sleep. Altitude sickness tends to be worse at night when sleeping.
- Drink plenty of fluids to keep yourself well hydrated.
- Eat foods high in carbohydrates.
- Avoid alcohol.
- Use sleeping pills and other sedatives judiciously at high altitudes.
- Prescription medications to prevent and treat altitude sickness include acetazolamide (trade name Diamox) and steroids. Diamox accelerates acclimatization. Prophylactic Diamox is an especially good idea for those skiing weekends at high altitudes when you don't have time to acclimatize.

CAUTION
You should not take Diamox if you are allergic to sulpha medication.
Medications such as Diamox may decrease your risk of altitude sickness but not totally prevent it.

A further discussion of medications to prevent and treat altitude sickness is beyond the scope of this book. Discuss these with your physician, and ask for a prescription for one of these medications. Know the dose for each member of your party.

 ### *Treatment*

Treatment of altitude sickness depends on its severity, and early recognition is vital. Descent will treat all forms of altitude sickness.

If you or your child has developed any of the symptoms of altitude sickness, you should assume that altitude sickness is present and consider descending to a lower altitude. Certainly ascend no further.

Never leave someone with altitude sickness alone.

Acute Mountain Sickness with Mild Symptoms

- **Do not ascend any farther.**
- Rest, drink fluids, and take medications for headache and altitude sickness. You may have to rest at the same altitude for a day or two before ascending farther.
- If the symptoms persist, descend. It is often necessary to descend only 1,000 feet or so to alleviate the symptoms of acute mountain sickness. Sometimes you may have to descend to the altitude at which the symptoms first occurred to alleviate the symptoms.

HACE or HAPE

- This is extremely serious, and **treatment must be instituted immediately.**
- If at all possible, descend now. The best treatment for HACE and HAPE is descent.
- Other treatment includes the administration of oxygen, a pressurization bag (Gamow bag), and specialized medications. These may be necessary if descent is not possible.

IN SUMMARY

- Altitude sickness is common.
- Be cautious when traveling to high altitudes with children.
- The best medicine is prevention. Ascend slowly and take time to acclimatize.
- Take any symptoms at high altitude seriously. Assume they are due to altitude sickness until proven otherwise.
- Do not ascend any higher if you have any of the symptoms of altitude sickness. Descend if symptoms persist or are severe.

 For Your Reference

1. *Altitude Illness: Prevention and Treatment,* by Stephen Bezruchka, M.D. (2001).

2. "High-Altitude Illness," by P. H. Hackett and R. C. Roach, in the *New England Journal of Medicine* 345 (2001): 107–14.

3. www.high-altitude-medicine.com.

12

Travelers' Diarrhea

Refer also to Chapters 13 and 31.

What's in This Chapter

WHAT IS IT?

Travelers' diarrhea is diarrhea that occurs in the context of travel. It is by far the most common travel-related illness you are likely to acquire when visiting lesser-developed countries. Travelers' diarrhea is especially common in the first week of travel, but it may develop at any time during a trip or even after returning home. A person with travelers' diarrhea has frequent, loose bowel movements, abdominal cramps, nausea, and sometimes vomiting. Fever may also be present.

Having a bout of travelers' diarrhea does not immunize you or prevent you from getting it again, and repeated bouts of it may occur.

In adults, travelers' diarrhea usually lasts three to four days, but this may be enough to ruin a carefully planned vacation or business trip. In children, travelers' diarrhea frequently lasts longer than a week. Children younger than the age of three years are especially prone to a more severe form of travelers' diarrhea that carries an increased risk of dehydration. The elderly are also more prone to developing dehydration.

WHO GETS IT?

Anyone can get travelers' diarrhea, but it is more common in children than in adults. It is especially common in adolescents and in young children. At least half of the people who travel from an industrialized country, such as the United States, to a developing country will experience travelers' diarrhea. The chances that you or your child will develop it will depend on which countries you visit, the season, how long you stay, your type of travel (adventure/roughing it or luxury), and the precautions you take to prevent it. Individual factors such as deficiencies of the immune system (for example, people on chemotherapy, people with AIDS) and the presence of certain bowel diseases may predispose a person to the development of travelers' diarrhea. If you are prone to bowel disturbances, be sure to maximize your preventative measures.

Destination is the most important predictor of travelers'

diarrhea. The world can be divided into three zones according to the risk of getting travelers' diarrhea:

Low-risk areas: The United States, Canada, northern and central Europe, Australia, New Zealand, and Japan.
Intermediate-risk areas: The Mediterranean countries, the Caribbean, South Africa, and Korea.
High-risk areas: The rest of the world.

WHAT CAUSES IT?

A wide variety of bacteria, viruses, and parasites cause travelers' diarrhea. Most cases are due to bacteria. Very serious causes of diarrhea that may be acquired while traveling include cholera, typhoid, and amebiasis. Dysentery, diarrhea with blood and mucus in the stool, frequently accompanied by high fever and severe abdominal pain, may be caused by typhoid and amebiasis. Fortunately, these illnesses are rare. Cholera may cause life-threatening diarrhea. It is definitely advisable to limit travel to areas of the world experiencing cholera epidemics.

HOW DO YOU GET IT?

Travelers' diarrhea is acquired by eating contaminated food, drinking contaminated water or other beverages, or eating with dirty fingers or hands. Poor restaurant hygiene is a major contributor to travelers' diarrhea. Most travelers' diarrhea acquired while abroad is due to eating contaminated food.

However, if you get diarrhea while backpacking or camping in the wilderness in the United States, it is more likely that you got it from contaminated water.

 ## *Prevention*

It is extremely difficult to prevent travelers' diarrhea, but the chances of getting it can be decreased by paying attention to what you eat, drink, and touch, as well as taking preventive medication.

Before leaving on your travels and as part of the preparation for your trip, visit your physician or travel clinic to discuss measures to prevent travelers' diarrhea and how to treat it should it occur. Discuss the use of preventive medications. This type of preventive treatment is known as "prophylaxis" or taking a medication "prophylactically." If your physician or travel clinic recommends the use of antibiotics in either the prevention or the treatment of travelers' diarrhea, make sure you get a prescription for the appropriate antibiotic and fill this prescription *before* you set out on your travels.

General Preventive Measures

The adage "boil it, cook it, peel it, or forget it" is good advice but very hard to adhere to. Part of the fun of travel is trying different foods, but try to follow as many of the guidelines below as possible.

Hygiene

- Wash fingers and hands frequently, especially before eating.
- Have wet wipes or antibacterial towelettes available at all times. Hand sanitizer gels or lotions are effective in killing "germs" on your hands.
- Always wash hands thoroughly after using the toilet.
- Try to discourage children from putting their hands and other objects into their mouth.
- If your child uses a pacifier, fasten it to his clothing to keep it from dropping on the floor or ground. Wash the pacifier frequently.
- Do not brush your teeth with water from fountains, streams, and so on. In developing countries it may not be safe to brush your teeth with tap water. Have a container for toothbrushes so that you do not have to put them down on surfaces that may not be clean.

Liquids

- Drink only safe water and beverages. Boiled water is usually the safest, but properly chemically treated water and appropriately filtered water is usually safe.
- Commercially bottled carbonated water and beverages (without ice) are usually safe. The beverage should be opened in front of you, and the tops of bottles and edges of cans should be wiped clean and dry. Noncarbonated bottled water in developing countries is not necessarily

safe to drink, as the bottle may have been filled at the local stream or village faucet.

- Tap water in developing countries is usually not safe to drink. Do not drink water from fountains, streams, and so on.
- Do not add ice to a beverage unless the ice has been made from boiled water and stored in clean containers and handled in a clean fashion.
- Breast-feeding is obviously ideal for infants. If using formula, prepare it with bottled water or appropriately treated water (preferably boiled) or use "ready-to-feed" formula.
- For older children and adults, hot beverages such as tea and coffee are usually safe.
- Drink extra fluids if you are in a hot climate.
- Increase liquid intake at the first sign of diarrhea.

Foods

The following foods are usually safe to eat:

- Vegetables and meat that are well cooked and piping hot.
- Fruit that needs to be peeled, such as oranges and bananas. Peel the fruit yourself after washing your hands. Fruits and vegetables that do not need to be peeled should be properly washed prior to eating. Wash the surfaces of fruits such as apples, oranges, and melons before cutting into them.

- Bread and dry foods.
- Foods with very high sugar content such as syrups and jellies.

When you eat out, choose better-class restaurants and hotels, although this is no guarantee that the food will not be contaminated. Avoid restaurants with many flies and poor toilet facilities.

Remember that when you fly home, the food that has been prepared in a developing country for the airline may be contaminated, so continue to follow these guidelines until you are back in a developed country.

Foods and Liquids to Avoid

- Raw and undercooked meats and fish. Avoid raw shellfish—it may give you not only diarrhea but also hepatitis A. (Hepatitis A can be prevented by appropriate immunization before setting out on your travels.)
- Reheated foods.
- Unpasteurized dairy products, such as milk, cream, butter, and cheese. Ice cream is particularly risky.
- Raw and undercooked eggs.
- Custards, salads with mayonnaise, or foods that have been allowed to stand out for some time (such as salads and buffets). Quiches and hot sauces are ideal culture mediums for bacteria.
- Food from a street vendor, unless it is fresh and steaming hot, you have watched it being prepared, and it has

been handled minimally by the vendor after cooking. Particularly avoid "slushies," ice cream, fruit juices sold at fruit stands, and other similar foods that can be purchased on the street.

- Fruits and other vegetables such as strawberries and lettuce that are hard to wash properly. These are especially risky.
- Tap water and drinks containing ice. These are often contaminated.

Even if you adhere to these guidelines closely, you may still get travelers' diarrhea, as food may become contaminated during preparation, handling, and storage. Flies may also play a major part in the contamination of food.

Preventive Medications

As mentioned above, before you set out on your travels, discuss these medications with your physician or travel clinic and acquire them prior to your departure. Preventive medications are often recommended for people with underlying bowel diseases (inflammatory bowel disease such as Crohn's disease and ulcerative colitis), people with low stomach acid production (acchlorhydria) or those taking medication to decrease gastric acid production (such as Prilosec, Prevacid, and Nexium), people with defects in the immune system (for example, AIDS and congenital defects in immune function), and people with serious chronic diseases (such as unstable diabetes mellitus, kidney failure).

Pepto-Bismol

Pepto-Bismol is approximately 60 percent effective in preventing travelers' diarrhea.

Some experts believe that this over-the-counter medication should be taken prophylactically by adults and children older than three years of age when traveling to especially high-risk countries. Pepto-Bismol should probably not be given to children younger than three years of age. There are contraindications to taking Pepto-Bismol. See list below.

Do not take Pepto-Bismol if

- you are allergic to or cannot tolerate aspirin;
- you have bleeding disorders or take anticoagulant medications ("blood thinners");
- you have a history of peptic ulcer disease or gastrointestinal bleeding;
- you are taking aspirin; or
- you have chicken pox or a flu-like illness. See the comment on Reye's syndrome below.

Side Effects

Some of Pepto-Bismol's side effects, such as black stools or a black tongue, are medically insignificant.

Ringing in the ears, however, is a sign of overdosage, which can be very serious. Overdoses of Pepto-Bismol will have the same effects as salicylate (aspirin) poisoning; these range from gastrointestinal problems (especially hemorrhage from the gastrointestinal tract and into other organs), to rapid respiration (hyperventilation), to serious side effects on the central nervous system, including coma. Be sure to keep Pepto-Bismol in a safe place where young children cannot get to it.

Pepto-Bismol contains salicylates similar to the salicylates found in aspirin. There are 102 mg of salicylates in every 1 tablet of Pepto-Bismol and 129 mg of salicylates in every 1 tablespoon (15 ml) of Pepto-Bismol liquid. Approximately 3 Pepto-Bismol tablets or 2½ tablespoons (1¼ oz) of the liquid contain as much salicylate as 1 adult aspirin tablet.

The chronic use of Pepto-Bismol may cause constipation.

Reye's Syndrome

Reye's syndrome has never been reported as a complication of taking Pepto-Bismol. However, it is probably wise not to give Pepto-Bismol to your child if she has chicken pox or a flu-like illness.

Use with Antibiotics

Pepto-Bismol should not be taken at the same time as antibiotics, as Pepto-Bismol may interfere with the absorption of antibiotics. Wait at least two hours after taking Pepto-Bismol before taking an antibiotic.

Forms of Pepto-Bismol

Pepto-Bismol is available in three forms:

1. Pleasant-tasting chewable tablets—each tablet contains 262 mg of bismuth subsalicylate.
2. Caplets—each caplet contains 262 mg of bismuth subsalicylate.
3. Liquid—3 teaspoons (1 tablespoon, or ½ oz) of liquid contain 262 mg of bismuth subsalicylate.

The three forms are equally effective in the *prevention* of travelers' diarrhea. The liquid, however, is slightly more effective than the tablets or the caplets in the *treatment* of travelers' diarrhea. The tablets and caplets are obviously more convenient than the liquid when you are traveling.

Pepto-Bismol Dosage to *Prevent* Diarrhea

Pepto-Bismol is most effective when taken with meals. The fourth dose can be given at bedtime.

Children over 12 years and adults: 2 tablets or 2 tablespoons (1 oz) of liquid four times a day.

Children 3–12 years: 1 tablet or 1 tablespoon (½ oz) of liquid four times a day. (Many physicians believe that Pepto-Bismol should not be given to children younger than six years of age.)

Children younger than 3 years of age: Not recommended.

Antibiotics

Antibiotics are generally not recommended as prophylaxis for travelers' diarrhea for the following reasons:

- Antibiotics may have side effects. These include allergic reactions and the development of yeast infections.
- The bacteria that cause the diarrhea may develop resistance to antibiotics, which makes the treatment of travelers' diarrhea more difficult if it should occur.
- People taking preventive medications may be less likely to follow the other preventive guidelines such as choosing safe food and water and hand washing.

Prophylactic antibiotics may be indicated in certain high-risk individuals such as those listed at the beginning of this section on preventive medications. Discuss this issue with your physician.

Probiotics

Probiotics, dietary supplements or foods that contain beneficial bacteria or yeasts, such as lactobacillus have a modest effect in preventing travelers' diarrhea but cannot be relied upon when used by themselves; other preventive measures should also be taken.

IN SUMMARY

Here is a summary of the guidelines for preventing travelers' diarrhea:

- If you are traveling to a lesser-developed country, there is a good chance that someone in your party will get travelers' diarrhea—be prepared for it!
- Visit your physician or travel clinic before you depart to discuss the prevention and treatment of travelers' diarrhea. Get prescriptions for antibiotics. Purchase the antibiotics and Imodium and Pepto-Bismol (if recommended) and know the dosages for each member of your party.
- Pay attention to the general preventive measures especially with regard to hygiene and food and liquid precautions.
- If you have an infant, breast-feed if at all possible.
- Certain high-risk persons may need to take Pepto-Bismol or antibiotics prophylactically.

 Treatment

There is a wide range in the severity of travelers' diarrhea. Some people have a few loose stools a day. Other people become severely ill and pass large quantities of watery stool and have severe vomiting and may become dehydrated. Fortunately, travelers' diarrhea is not usually a dehydrating illness in adolescents and adults.

Infants and younger children (under three years of age) and the elderly are at greater risk of becoming dehydrated, but even adults may become seriously dehydrated if the diarrhea is severe enough. This is especially likely to happen if the person is also vomiting, is in a hot climate, or is not drinking enough fluid.

The younger the child and the more severe the diarrhea, the more vital it is to use ideal fluids such as commercially prepared electrolyte solutions. These should be used in the correct quantities. It is very important to observe your child carefully for signs of dehydration.

Treatment *consists* of the following:

- Fluids and nutrition
- Medications such as Pepto-Bismol, loperamide (Imodium), and antibiotics

Treatment *depends* on the following:

- Severity of the diarrhea
- Age of the individual
- Presence of complicating factors such as dehydration, fever, blood and mucus in the stools (dysentery), and abdominal pain

CAUTION

Under no circumstances should the administration of Pepto-Bismol, Imodium, or antibiotics take precedence over the administration of appropriate fluids to young children with diarrhea. The most common mistake in taking care of children with diarrhea is not giving them enough fluids. The next most common mistake is giving them inappropriate fluids and foods, making the diarrhea worse.

Fluids and Nutrition

As with all treatment for diarrhea, fluid and nutritional therapy for travelers' diarrhea varies according to the age of the person, the severity of the diarrhea, and the presence of vomiting or other complicating factors.

In all cases, you should

- increase fluid intake at the first sign of diarrhea;
- increase fluid intake on hot days; and
- continue giving extra fluids until the diarrhea has resolved.

A person's activity level or energy level and her urine color are usually good guides to the presence of dehydration. For further information on assessing dehydration, see table 3 in Chapter 31.

Infants and Children up to Three Years of Age

These guidelines apply particularly to children between the ages of six months and three years. Ideally, for infants younger than six months of age you should consult your child's physician.

- Continue with the usual diet (breast milk or formula) and your child's usual solids. Breast-fed children should be fed more often.
- Give extra fluids between usual feedings. These fluids should consist of water, diluted juices (one-third strength), diluted sports drinks such as Gatorade, or Jello (both half strength). As long as your child is not vomiting, give these fluids with the solids mentioned in the next item in this list.
- Offer foods such as cooked cereal, bananas, rice, and mashed potatoes, all of which aid in the absorption of water from the intestine. Bananas are also a good source of potassium.
- Children older than 18 months of age can be offered salty crackers or pretzels as a source of salt.
- If the diarrhea becomes more severe (profuse, watery, explosive), preferably use electrolyte solutions. Dehydration may occur very rapidly in such children (see also the section "Points to Note with Fluid and Nutritional Therapy," p. 153). The most important aspects of this therapy are the following:
  - Give appropriate electrolyte solutions, frequently and in sufficient amounts.

- Give extra fluids for each watery stool passed.
- Continue giving extra fluids until the diarrhea has resolved.
- Avoid fluids and foods that will make the diarrhea worse.
- Do not starve your child.
- Assess the degree of dehydration frequently.

Children Older Than Three Years of Age and Adults

- Unless the person is vomiting, continue with the usual diet, but avoid caffeine-containing beverages and alcohol.
- Consume extra fluids in the form of water, diluted juices and sodas (one-third strength), Gatorade (half strength), soup, or electrolyte solution. As long as vomiting is not present, give these fluids with the solids mentioned in the next item in this list.
- Saltine-type crackers (salted crackers), pretzels, lightly salted cooked cereal, and mashed potatoes are a good source of extra salt if the main source of fluid is water or diluted juices. Bananas are a good source of extra potassium.
- As the severity of the diarrhea increases, increase the amount of fluid consumed. Adolescents and adults may need as much as 4 or more liters (4 or more quarts, or 16 or more 8-ounce cups) of extra fluid in a 24-hour period. Electrolyte solutions are preferable as the diarrhea increases in severity, especially in younger children.
- With profuse, watery diarrhea, offer large volumes of

electrolyte solutions. Adolescents and adults may need to drink an extra 5 to 6 liters (5 to 6 quarts, or 20 to 30 or more 8-ounce cups) of fluid per 24 hours.

- Continue drinking extra fluids as long as the diarrhea continues and until the urine is a light color.
- Give additional extra fluids (up to 12 ounces) after each loose stool.
- Once vomiting has stopped, give appropriate solids. Do not starve your child.
- Observe for worsening symptoms and signs of dehydration.

Points to Note with Fluid and Nutritional Therapy

Concentrated Liquids

- Avoid giving young children concentrated juices and full-strength Jello, Gatorade, and sodas. These have a very high sugar content and little or no salt, and they will often make the diarrhea worse.
- Diluted versions of the above-mentioned fluids may be used for short periods for mild to moderate diarrhea, especially if supplemented with salty foods such as salted crackers or pretzels. Use one-third-strength fruit juices and sodas, half-strength sports drinks such as Gatorade, and half-strength Jello.
- Do not use chicken broth because it has too much salt and no sugar and is not suitable for rehydration in infants and young children.

- Avoid caffeine-containing drinks.
- The younger the child and the more severe the diarrhea, the more important it is to use appropriate electrolyte solutions. However, if commercially prepared electrolyte solutions are not available and you do not have the ingredients needed for a homemade electrolyte solution, it is still essential to give whatever fluids you have available. Water, half-strength sports drinks such as Gatorade, half-strength Jello, and one-third-strength juices can be given along with Saltine-type crackers.

Vomiting

- If your child is vomiting, stop all solids and liquids other than the clear liquids mentioned below for four to eight hours.
- Offer electrolyte solutions or other clear fluids such as water or diluted juices or sports drinks. Give as little as 1 teaspoon every minute. Even infants and young children who are vomiting will usually be able to tolerate small volumes of such fluids.
- You may need to use a teaspoon or medicine dropper for an infant.
- For older children, you may use a medicine cup. As the fluid is tolerated, increase the volumes offered. Children older than 18 months of age may suck on ice chips if vomiting is a problem. Electrolyte solutions may be frozen into Popsicle-type bars, which your child can suck, or into ice blocks, which can then be crushed and offered as ice chips.

- If your child continues to vomit, medical care should be sought.

Food

- If your child is vomiting, you should stop his normal diet for a period of four to eight hours and then try to reintroduce appropriate foods slowly.
- Do not starve your child. Cereal, mashed potatoes, rice, wheat, and bananas will actually aid in water absorption, shorten the period of diarrhea, and decrease its severity.
- It is usually not necessary or advisable to dilute milk or formulas unless your child is vomiting; even then, do it for only short periods.
- Avoid fatty foods for two to three days.

Medications

Medications used to treat travelers' diarrhea include Pepto-Bismol, Imodium, and antibiotics. These are probably not necessary if the diarrhea is only mild. If the diarrhea is more troublesome, then Imodium may be used in those at least two years of age, and Pepto-Bismol can be used at three years of age. If the diarrhea is more severe, and especially if there are other distressing symptoms such as nausea and severe cramping, then it is a good idea to give an antibiotic and, if the person is at least two years of age, Imodium. Give one dose of each and repeat in about 12 hours. If the symptoms persist, continue with a three-day course of both the antibiotic and Imodium.

CAUTION

Under no circumstances should the administration of Pepto-Bismol, Imodium, or antibiotics take precedence over the administration of appropriate fluids to young children with diarrhea.

Pepto-Bismol

Pepto-Bismol may be used in the treatment as well as the prevention of travelers' diarrhea (see the earlier section on the use of Pepto-Bismol as a preventive medication).

Pepto-Bismol Dosage to *Treat* Diarrhea

The **first dose** of Pepto-Bismol is as follows:

Children older than 12 years of age and adults: 2 tablets or 2 tablespoons (1 oz).

Children 9 to 12 years of age: 1 tablet or 1 tablespoon.

Children 6 to 9 years of age: 2 teaspoons.

Children 3 to 6 years of age: 1 teaspoon. (Many physicians do not recommend Pepto-Bismol for children younger than 6 years of age.)

Children younger than 3 years of age: Not recommended.

Subsequent doses: The doses listed above can be repeated every hour up to a maximum of eight doses in a 24-hour period.

Be alert for the development of *side effects* as discussed earlier.

Loperamide (Imodium)

Imodium reduces both the frequency of bowel movements and the duration of diarrheal illness.

Side effects of Imodium include drowsiness, constipation, abdominal distension, and vomiting. If these occur, **stop the Imodium immediately.** If the abdominal distension persists for longer than four to six hours, consult a physician.

CAUTION

Imodium should not be used if there is blood or mucus in the stools or if a high fever is present.

Imodium is available in three forms:

1. Liquid, which contains 1 mg of loperamide per 5 ml (1 teaspoon)
2. Chewable tablets, each of which contains 2 mg of loperamide
3. Caplets, each of which contains 2 mg of loperamide

Imodium Dosage to *Treat* Diarrhea

Adults and children over 12 years of age:
– 2 caplets or 2 tablets immediately.
– Then 1 caplet or tablet after each watery stool.
– Do not give more than 8 caplets or tablets in a 24-hour period.

Continued

Imodium Dosage to Treat Diarrhea *continued*

Children ages 9 to 11 years (or between 60 and 95 pounds):
– 1 caplet or 1 chewable tablet or 2 teaspoons after the first loose stool.
– Then ½ caplet or ½ tablet or 1 teaspoon after each subsequent loose stool.
– Do not give more than 6 teaspoons or 3 caplets or tablets in a 24-hour period.

Children ages 6 to 8 years (or between 48 and 59 pounds):
– 1 caplet or 1 chewable tablet or 2 teaspoons after the first loose stool.
– Then ½ caplet or ½ tablet or 1 teaspoon after each subsequent loose stool.
– Do not give more than 4 teaspoons or 2 caplets a day.

Children ages 2 to 5 years (or between 24 and 47 pounds):
– ½ chewable tablet or 1 teaspoon after the first loose stool.
– Then ½ chewable tablet or 1 teaspoon after each subsequent loose stool.
– Do not give more than 1½ chewable tablets or 3 teaspoons per day.
Use with caution in this age group.

Children younger than 2 years of age:
– Not recommended.

CAUTION
Never use diphenonxylate hydrochloride (Lomotil) to treat diarrhea in children.

Antibiotics

Antibiotics are often very effective in the treatment of travelers' diarrhea. This is because most cases of travelers' diarrhea are due to bacteria.

The traditional approach to the treatment of travelers' diarrhea in children has been *not* to use antibiotics or Imodium and to rely only on administering fluids. Although this approach may be correct in the management of childhood diarrhea that occurs at home, it may not be wise in the treatment of travelers' diarrhea. The combination of antibiotics and Imodium is usually very effective in stopping travelers' diarrhea. Antibiotics treat the *cause* of the diarrhea, whereas fluids prevent and treat dehydration.

Many different types of antibiotics are used in the treatment of travelers' diarrhea. Discuss your options with your physician prior to traveling. Which antibiotic is most suitable for you and your family will depend on a number of factors, the most important being your destination and the likely antibiotic susceptibility pattern of the causative bacteria. Recommendations change from year to year as the bacteria that cause travelers' diarrhea change and as the bacteria become resistant to different antibiotics. As of 2007, commonly used antibiotics include the quinolones (such as Cipro or Floxin), azithromycin (Zithromax), rifaximin (Xifaxan), and cefixime (Suprax). (Many of these medications may also be used to treat other infections such as ear infections, strep throat, and pneumonia.)

If the diarrhea and other symptoms settle rapidly, only one

or two doses may be necessary. A three-day course of antibiotics may be required for more severe and persistent diarrhea.

IN SUMMARY

Here is a summary of the guidelines for treating travelers' diarrhea:

- Give extra fluids at the first sign of diarrhea.
- If an infant who is breast-feeding develops diarrhea, breast-feed more often.
- If your child is *not* vomiting, continue to offer appropriate solids as well.
- Give electrolyte solutions if the diarrhea is very severe.
- Consider using Pepto-Bismol (in children three years of age and older) and/or Imodium (in children older than two years of age).
- If the diarrhea is more frequent or severe, or if there are distressing symptoms such as severe abdominal cramps, administer one dose of an appropriate antibiotic. In persons older than two years of age consider adding Imodium. If the symptoms persist, continue with a three-day course of antibiotics and possibly Imodium.
- Watch out for signs of dehydration. Seek medical help early, especially in the first six months of life.

When to Seek Medical Attention

Reasons to seek medical care are similar to those mentioned in Chapter 31. Finding medical care while traveling is not always easy, but the presence of any of the following criteria indicates that you need to seek medical care:

- If your sick child is an infant six months old or younger. Generally, the younger the child, the earlier you should seek expert medical advice.
- If your child is limp and lethargic or appears very ill.
- If your child has moderate or more severe dehydration.
- If dehydration worsens despite appropriate fluid therapy.
- If there is persistent vomiting.
- If your child will not take fluids by mouth.
- If your child has a stomachache lasting longer than two hours. Note, however, that many children have recurrent bouts of abdominal pain or cramps, especially when passing gas or stools. Persisting pain (longer than one or two hours) or worsening pain indicates the need to seek medical attention to rule out more serious causes of pain such as appendicitis, bowel perforation, or obstruction.
- If the stool contains a large amount of mucus or blood or is black (and your child is not taking Pepto-Bismol).
- If the diarrhea is not improving after 3 to 4 days. It may take as long as 7 to 10 days before your child's stools are totally normal, but each day there should be improve-

ment. Your child should be eating and drinking well and be active, alert, and interested in his surroundings.

- If your child has a high fever (over 102°F [38.9°C]).
- If the diarrhea continues or recurs after returning home.
- You should seek medical attention earlier in any country where diseases such as cholera, typhoid, or amebiasis are common, especially if these countries are having epidemics or outbreaks of these diseases.

Homemade Electrolyte Solutions

Here are four recipes for making your own electrolyte solutions:

Sugar and salt mixture
   5 to 10 level teaspoons of sugar
   1 level teaspoon of salt
   1 liter of water (approx. 1 quart)

Rice cereal mixture
   1 level teaspoon of salt
   1 cup (50 grams) of rice cereal
   1 liter (approx. 1 quart) of water
   Dissolve the salt and water, gradually adding cereal to the water until the mixture is thick but still drinkable. Mix well.

Orange juice mixture
   8 ounces of orange juice (1 cup)
   1 level teaspoon of salt
   24 ounces of water (3 cups)

Continued

Homemade Electrolyte Solutions *continued*

Mashed potato mixture
 8 ounces of mashed potatoes
 ½ level teaspoon of salt
 ¼ level teaspoon of baking soda
 ¼ level teaspoon of salt substitute (provides potassium)
 1 liter (approx. 1 quart) of water

13

Selecting and Preparing Safe Food and Water

Refer also to Chapter 12.

One of the most important aspects of safe travel is preventing illness caused by contaminated food and water. In the developed world, the availability of safe, drinkable water is usually taken for granted. In fact, when you stop to think about it, the ability to turn on a faucet and get abundant clear water that is safe to drink is almost a miracle and must be regarded as one of the major advances of the twentieth century! In contrast, in many developing countries, the water is not safe to drink, even though it might come out of a faucet. The load of infectious organisms may be high because of inadequate water treatment or outdated plumbing. In general, all water in developing countries should be considered contaminated and capable of causing disease, usually diarrhea. Surface water is often highly contaminated with human waste. Much of the disease, malnutrition, and shortened life span in developing countries is related to poor sanitation and contaminated water. Unsafe drinking water causes millions of deaths a year, especially among young children, when repeated bouts of diarrhea lead to malnutrition and poor health.

Even in North America, all untreated natural water should be regarded as being contaminated. This includes water from mountain streams, rivers, and crystal-clear lakes. Contrary to popular opinion, fast-running, pristine mountain streams may also harbor disease-causing organisms, especially *Giardia,* which causes the disease giardiasis. Bloating, chronic diarrhea, and weight loss are some of the symptoms of giardiasis.

Although diarrhea and other intestinal illnesses are commonly caused by intentionally drinking water, sometimes water is unintentionally ingested while partaking in recreational activities such as swimming and boating. Many children and even adults swallow large amounts of water while swimming. Out-

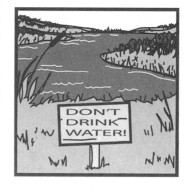

breaks of disease due to *Giardia, Shigella,* and hepatitis A and E and many other organisms have occurred in the United

States from exposure to recreational water. Infants and young children often swallow large amounts of water while taking a bath!

One does not have to drink water to acquire certain waterborne diseases. This applies particularly to a disease known as schistosomiasis, in which the organism enters directly through the skin. This disease is particularly common in Africa and certain parts of Asia. As in the case of giardiasis, this disease may not manifest for many weeks, months, or even years after acquiring it. Generally speaking, it may not even be safe to wade in most rivers in Africa.

People usually do not get infections from swimming in a sea, unless they swim in an area into which sewage flows.

Water may contain not only infectious organisms but also chemical pollutants that may be hazardous to people's health. These chemicals may come from industrial sources or runoff from farms where pesticides and fertilizers are used. Pollutants often seriously damage our environment, so it may be not only unsafe to drink the water but also unsafe to eat the fish swimming in the water. (Sadly, we are not doing a very good job of taking care of this planet for our children and our grandchildren.)

The risks of acquiring infectious diseases from water are related to a number of factors, including the number of infectious particles in the water (the infectious load), the virulence of the infectious organisms, and human (host) factors.

People at greater risk of acquiring diseases from contaminated water include

- young children (especially infants);
- people with certain gastrointestinal diseases such as inflammatory bowel disease (Crohn's disease or ulcerative colitis);
- people whose immune system isn't functioning properly (such as people who are on immunosuppressive drugs);
- the elderly; and
- pregnant women.

For these high-risk people, it is especially important to drink only safe water.

Infectious agents that may be present in water can be divided into viruses, bacteria, protozoa, and parasites. These vary greatly in size and in their ability to resist eradication.

PREPARATION OF SAFE (POTABLE) WATER

The preparation of "safe" water is known as *disinfection*. This is not the same as sterilization, as disinfected water may not be totally free of organisms. However, disinfected water does not contain sufficient numbers of organisms to cause disease.

Before embarking on disinfection of water, it is necessary to select the water and then to get it as clear as possible.

Selection

At times, water from a faucet may not be available, and you may have to rely on other sources of water. Spring water and collected rainwater are likely to be cleaner than surface water, such as water from rivers, streams, and ponds. Fast-moving water is preferable to stagnant water. Similarly, clear, colorless, odorless water is probably safer than discolored water that may contain debris. When collecting water from a lake or pond, try not to disturb the bottom. Select the clearer water just below the surface. When camping, choose water upstream of human habitation.

Clarification

If the water is very cloudy, it is a good idea to clear the water before proceeding with further disinfection. Clarifying the water not only makes it more aesthetically pleasing but also makes further filtration or chemical treatment a lot easier. Clarification can be achieved by one of these three methods:

1. Sedimentation. Allow the water to stand for several hours and pour off the clean upper portion for further treatment.
2. Filtration. Filter the water through a commercial paper filter, a coffee filter, or a clean cloth.
3. Flocculation. Get the organic impurities to clump together by adding a pinch of alum to the water and mixing.

Disinfection

Three methods are commonly used to disinfect water:

1. Heat treatment
2. Chemical treatment
3. Filtration

Each of these methods may be used alone or in combination with another method. The method you choose depends on a number of factors, including the type of organism you wish to eradicate, the amount of water you need to prepare, and the resources available. A full discussion of disinfecting water is beyond the scope of this book. For further information, consult the references listed at the end of this chapter. If you are planning a prolonged stay in a developing country or traveling in the wilderness, it would definitely be a good idea to do further reading on the subject.

Heat Treatment

Boiling Water
Boiling water is the most reliable way to purify it. However, it is not always feasible to do this because a source of electricity or other fuel is necessary. If you are staying in hotels, all you may need is a small electrical heating coil or a portable kettle. Remember that the electrical current and electrical outlets in many countries differ from those in the United States. It is a good idea to take a selection of electrical outlet adapters with you.

It is necessary only to bring the water to a boil to kill all offending organisms. For an extra margin of safety you can let the water boil for one minute or, alternatively, keep the water covered so that it retains its heat for a longer time.

Pasteurization

Microorganisms vary in their heat sensitivity. It is not necessary to bring water to a boil to kill most bacteria and viruses. Most bacteria and viruses are killed at much lower temperatures (60–70°C, or 140–160°F) as long as they are exposed to heat for longer periods (30 minutes or longer). This is the principle of pasteurization. In practice, when you are traveling and you don't have a means of checking the water temperature, it is usually easier just to bring the water to a boil. It is also much safer, as some organisms are more resistant to heat.

Hot Tap Water

If you have no other means of disinfecting water, hot tap water is probably safer than cold. There will be far fewer organisms in hot tap water than in cold tap water, but the safety of the water cannot be guaranteed.

Generally, in most countries it is safe to use water from a tap to clean your teeth. Although the water may contain organisms, you are unlikely to ingest enough of them to cause disease. However, **the high-risk groups mentioned above, especially young children, should use only totally safe water.**

Water that is boiled often has a rather flat taste. You can improve the taste of treated water by following these steps:

1. Add a vitamin C tablet or vitamin C powder to the water and shake.
2. Pour the water back and forth from one clean container into another to aerate it.
3. Allow the water to stand for a while in a clean, partially filled container.
4. Pass the water through a charcoal filter.

Chemical Treatment of Water

The chemical disinfection of water is usually accomplished by adding chlorine dioxide, chlorine, or iodine.

Many different preparations of these three chemical agents are available. Follow the directions on the bottle. Be aware of expiration dates.

The efficacy of the various methods of chemical disinfection is affected by many factors but especially by the concentration of the chemical agent, the turbidity of the water, and the temperature of the water.

Chlorine Dioxide

Chlorine dioxide is a fairly recently marketed method of water disinfection. It is marketed in the United States under the trade names Pristine and Aquamira. Disinfecting water with chlorine dioxide is a quick and easy two-step process that renders the water completely safe without the disadvantage of the unpleasant taste imparted to the water by chlorine or iodine (discussed below). This method of water disinfection is highly recommended.

Chlorine

The chlorine is added to the water and left to stand for 30 minutes. If the water is cold or cloudy, either double the recommended dose of chlorine or double the contact time. Two chlorine formulations are commonly used—chlorine bleach and chlorine tablets.

Chlorine bleach is ordinary household bleach (e.g., Clorox); a 4–6% solution may be used. Add two to three drops of chlorine bleach to each liter (quart) of water.

Chlorine tablets are commonly marketed as Halozone tablets. Add two tablets to 1 liter (quart) of water.

Chlorine may not kill all organisms, especially *Cryptosporidium* and *Cyclospora. Giardia* cysts are also relatively resistant to chlorine. Chlorine may also impart a rather unpleasant taste to the water. The taste can be improved by adding a vitamin C tablet or powder to the water or by passing the water through a charcoal filter.

Iodine

Add the iodine to the water and allow it to stand for 30 minutes. If the water is cold or cloudy, either double the recommended dose of iodine or double the contact time. Several forms of iodine are available to disinfect water. Iodine is light-sensitive and should be stored in a dark bottle.

Iodine solutions include tincture of iodine (2%) and Lugol's solution (5%). If using tincture of iodine, add five drops to 1 liter (quart) of water. If using Lugol's iodine, add two to three drops to 1 liter (quart) of water.

The best-known brand of iodine tablets (tetraglycine hydroperiodide) is Potable Aqua. Add half a tablet to 1 liter (quart) of water.

As with chlorine, iodine may not kill all organisms (notably *Cryptosporidium* and *Cyclospora*) and imparts an unpleasant taste to the water that can be improved by adding a vitamin C tablet or by passing the water through a granular activated charcoal filter.

> ### CAUTION
> **Do not use iodine preparations for longer than one month, and do not use them if you are pregnant.**
>
> **Do not use iodine preparations if you have thyroid disease.**
>
> **Do not use iodine preparations if you are allergic to iodine.**

If there is concern that *Cyclospora* or *Cryptosporidium* may be present in the water, the water should be filtered either before or after chemical treatment. *Cryptosporidium* and *Cyclospora* may both be present in water in the wilderness in the United States.

Filtration

Filtration is another commonly used method of water disinfection. Be skeptical of claims made by manufacturers that their filtering devices render the water "completely safe." The principal disadvantage of filtration is that it does not remove viruses, the smallest infectious particles. Filtration, especially if the pore size is no larger than 0.2 to 1.0 μm (micrometer), will remove bacteria, parasites, and cysts but not viruses. Another disadvantage of filtering systems is that they often are bulky and tend to clog.

Filters made of porcelain (ceramic candles) that are commonly purchased in developing countries are not reliable.

> *Note:* If you are in a location where it is likely that disease-causing viruses are in the water and filtration is used as the method of disinfection, you must use another method besides filtration to destroy viruses. This would be the case if you were using surface water in developing countries where there is a high likelihood of contamination of the water by human fecal organisms. You should either boil the water or use one of the chemical methods mentioned above.
>
> In some situations, viruses may not be a problem, and filtration alone may suffice. An example of such a situation is in the remote wilderness where there is minimal likelihood of contamination from human fecal material and the primary concern is ridding the water of *Giardia* and other large organisms.

More details on filters and filtration can be found in the references at the end of the chapter or on the Web at www .nsf.org.

The bottom line is that to obtain completely safe water, you must drink either water that has been boiled or water that has been filtered and then chemically treated. The filtration will remove the larger organisms, and the chemical treatment will kill viruses.

If water is stored for a time, it should be covered and an appropriate dose of a chemical disinfectant added to prevent contamination.

ADDITIONAL REMINDERS AND COMMENTS

In developing countries, even water that comes in sealed bottles may not be safe to drink. Carbonated water is generally safer. Preferably the bottle should be opened in front of you.

Unless ice is made from safe water and handled in a clean fashion, it should be regarded as contaminated.

Water safety cannot be assessed by look, smell, or taste. Even pristine surface waters may contain *Giardia* cysts and other organisms. Remote lakes and streams that contain crystal-clear water may be contaminated by disease-causing organisms.

Chemical hazards are becoming an increasing problem and will not be removed by boiling or other methods of disinfection.

Be sensitive to the local population, who may not have access to clean food and water as you do.

FOOD PREPARATION

- Remember that most cases of travelers' diarrhea are acquired by eating contaminated food and not by drinking contaminated water.
- Foods to avoid:
  - Unpasteurized dairy products

- Undercooked meats and fish
- Reheated foods
- Lettuce and other leafy vegetables that are difficult to wash thoroughly. These are often fertilized with human waste in developing countries. (See Chapter 12.)
- If you intend to eat fruit and vegetables that do not need to be peeled, clean them in one of the following ways:
  - Wash them thoroughly in clean, soapy water, and then rinse them in disinfected (treated) water. (Just rinsing the fruits and vegetables in treated water may not be sufficient because it does not allow enough contact time for the chemical to kill any disease-causing organisms.)
  - Soak fruits and vegetables in treated water that has two to three times the concentration of iodine or chlorine than is recommended for water disinfection.
  - Dip the food in boiling water.
- Plates, cups, glasses, and eating utensils should also be washed in a way that disinfects them. This can be achieved by washing them in boiling water or by washing them in a very strong chemical solution, again using a solution two to three times stronger than that recommended for water disinfection.
- Storage. Water, food, and eating utensils, once cleaned, should be stored properly so that they are not contaminated by flies, which may carry disease-causing organisms.

- Remember to wash your hands well before and after handling the food.

TOXINS

Although most illnesses acquired by drinking water or eating food are infectious in nature, some are due to toxins, which will not be affected by the disinfection methods described.

- Staphylococcal food poisoning usually presents with severe nausea and vomiting two to six hours after eating contaminated food. High-risk foods include creamy desserts, salads, and meats, especially if they are not eaten soon after preparation.
- Fish and shellfish poisoning. Shellfish may contain toxins when they feed on certain algae that proliferate during the warmer months ("red tide"). Many tropical fish contain toxins that can cause severe illness, paralysis, and even death. Even commonly eaten fish such as red snapper and grouper may be unsafe to eat if they are caught at certain times of the year. A discussion on this topic is beyond the scope of this book, but you should always be cautious when eating seafood. Most of the toxins found in fish and shellfish are *not* destroyed by ordinary cooking. Foods and seafood that are contaminated by toxins or toxin-producing bacteria are difficult to recognize by appearance, odor, or taste. Avoid eating the skin and organs of fish. If you want to eat seafood,

eat it only at top restaurants or restaurants that specialize in fresh seafood.

- Chemicals, toxins, and heavy metals such as mercury are *not* removed by the disinfection processes described above. Select your water carefully. Be aware of industrial pollutants, fertilizer runoff from farmlands, and other toxic wastes. Passing the water through a charcoal filter may not only improve the taste but also rid the water of some of these substances.

 For Your Reference

1. *Wilderness Medicine*, by Paul S. Auerbach, 4th ed. (2001).
2. "Water Disinfection for International and Wilderness Travels," by Howard Backer, in *Clinics in Infectious Diseases* 34 (2002): 355–64.
3. *The Backpacker's Field Manual*, by Rick Curtis (1998).

14

Skin Problems

Refer also to Chapters 18, 38, and 39.

Skin problems are common and are one of the more frequent reasons travelers seek medical care both while away and after returning home. They are even more common when traveling in hot and humid environments. Most of these problems are relatively minor but can be extremely irritating and detract from the pleasure of your trip. Skin problems range from common ones such as insect bites and sunburn and complications from insect bites to exotic parasitic diseases rarely seen in developed countries. Many of the skin diseases encountered while traveling can be prevented by sensible sun precautions, good hygiene, and prevention of insect bites. Preexisting skin conditions may be exacerbated by the stress of travel or by exposure to the sun.

Sunburn is the most important travel-related skin problem and is discussed separately (see Chapter 38). Insect bites and their complications, a close second in importance, are also discussed elsewhere (see Chapter 39).

HEAT RASH, OR PRICKLY HEAT

Heat rash is a fine, pimply rash that is caused by the blockage of sweat ducts. The surrounding skin becomes inflamed, and so the appearance is that of small pimples surrounded by red skin. As you would expect, prickly heat is more common in hot climates. This rash frequently occurs on the back and chest, but it also occurs in areas that do not get enough ventilation, such as the armpits and the groin, and on any part of the body where there is friction from clothing. The neck creases of infants are another common site.

Prevention

- Dress your child in cool, loose-fitting, cotton clothing.
- Avoid friction from clothing, for example, baseball caps rubbing against the forehead.
- Bathe daily.
- Some people are more prone to prickly heat. These individuals should, if possible, spend more time in a cool or air-conditioned environment.

Treatment

Continue with the preventive measures listed above. In addition, follow these measures to relieve the itch and calm the rash:

- Take cool showers and baths with a soothing bath product like Aveeno. Antibacterial soaps often help but tend to dry the skin.
- Apply calamine lotion.
- Keep the skin well aerated.
- Try to avoid scratching the skin. This may lead to impetigo (see below).

FOLLICULITIS

Folliculitis, or infection of the hair follicles, often appears as clusters of bumps or little pimples. These may occur on any part of the body but especially on the buttocks, inner thighs, scalp, and face. Folliculitis also is common where the scalp comes in contact with a headband or hat; where the buttocks come in contact with a sweaty, dirty seat; or where clothing rubs against the body. It is more likely to develop in hot and humid climates and with excessive sweating.

Prevention and Treatment

See prevention and treatment of heat rash, or prickly heat, above. Additional treatment measures include the following:

- Keep the skin clean and dry.
- Antibacterial soaps may be helpful, along with the application of antibacterial creams or ointments.
- For severe folliculitis, oral antibiotics may be needed.
- If folliculitis develops into small painful boils, they may respond to hot compresses. If the boils increase in size, lancing of the boils and oral antibiotics may be needed.
- "Hot tub folliculitis" may be acquired from bathing in hot tubs or whirlpools that are not adequately chlorinated. This condition usually resolves without treatment over 7 to 14 days. You may want to avoid hot tubs altogether, particularly if you're not sure the water has been adequately chlorinated, and people whose immune system is compromised should definitely avoid them.

IMPETIGO

Impetigo is the name given to a common bacterial infection of the skin. It is contagious and is caused by bacteria called streptococci (strep) or staphylococci (staph). It can be spread to other parts of the body by scratching and can also be spread to other people.

Impetigo often follows the scratching of bug bites and also occurs in areas where the skin has been broken—for example, around minor cuts and abrasions. It is especially common around the nose.

Impetigo usually starts as flat, reddened areas that develop into small vesicles (little blisters). These blisters rupture and discharge a yellowish fluid that dries into honey-colored crusts. The surrounding skin is red. Red satellite lesions may develop wherever the skin is scratched.

In third-world countries, many children have persistent impetigo because of poor hygiene, heat, humidity, and scratching. Even in developed countries, impetigo is common and may recur frequently.

 Prevention

- Avoid insect bites (see Chapter 39).
- Good hygiene is very important. Frequent baths or showers will keep the bacterial population of the skin in check, especially if an antibacterial soap is used. Prevent the skin from drying out by applying a moisturizer afterward.
- Keep as cool as possible—wear loose-fitting, cotton clothing.
- Wash and dry abrasions and cuts and keep them clean. Apply an antibacterial ointment to cuts and abrasions three times a day until the skin heals. Don't cover minor bites and scratches with bandages because this will encourage infection. (Bacteria love dark, moist places.) Al-

low these lesions to air and dry out. If a large or deep cut or abrasion needs to be covered with a bandage or dressing, change the dressing at least once a day and allow the wound to air.

- Don't scratch insect bites. Unless the skin is broken, apply topical 0.5% or 1% hydrocortisone cream to the insect bite to reduce inflammation and help relieve the itch. An oral medication such as Benadryl or one of the nonsedating antihistamines will also help relieve the itch.

 Treatment

- Use an antibacterial cream or ointment (e.g., Bacitracin, Neosporin, Triple Antibiotic Ointment, Bactroban) on the lesion.
- If your child has many lesions, an oral antibiotic is recommended.
- For recurring impetigo, the following suggestions may be helpful:
  - Apply Bactroban to the inside of the nose, three times a day for 7 to 10 days. Staph and strep bacteria are often harbored in the nose.
  - Bathe your child once or twice a week in a tub of water to which ¼ cup of bleach has been added. This will tend to dry out the skin, so apply a moisturizer afterward. (Keep the bleach in a safe place.)
  - An appropriate oral antibiotic is often necessary. If your child is prone to impetigo and you are planning

to travel to a hot and humid country, it may be a good idea to request an antibiotic so that you can treat this condition should it develop.

FUNGAL INFECTIONS

Fungal infections are particularly common in tropical and subtropical areas, but they do occur worldwide. Areas of a person's body that are moist and not exposed to light, such as under the diaper and between the toes, are typical sites for the growth of fungi. The more common fungal infections are vaginal yeast infections, yeast diaper rashes in babies, athlete's foot, and ringworm.

Vaginal Yeast Infections

These are particularly common in women who are taking antibiotics. When taking an antibiotic, your likelihood of developing vaginitis (and diarrhea) can be reduced by eating yogurt that has a live culture.

Yeast Diaper Rashes

Yeast diaper rashes often appear as a bright red rash in the diaper area with surrounding red satellite spots. This rash responds to airing the affected area, keeping it clean and dry, and applying an antifungal cream such as clotrimazole (Lotrimin). Prevention of diaper rashes includes changing your child as soon as he is wet or dirty, keeping his buttocks clean and dry, and avoiding plastic, "waterproof" pants. If your child has a diaper rash that is not responding to the usual barrier creams and hygiene measures, an antifungal cream may help (see section on diaper rash in Chapter 37).

Athlete's Foot

This is the most common fungal infection seen in adolescents and adults and usually presents as an itchy, red rash between the toes.

Prevention

- Keep feet clean and dry.
- Change socks frequently.
- Aerate shoes at night.
- Alternate between two pairs of shoes.
- Wear sandals instead of closed shoes and boots.
- Sprinkle an antifungal powder into shoes and socks.
- Wear slippers or shower shoes in public places such as gyms and swimming pool showers.

Treatment

- Continue with the preventative measures listed above.
- Apply an antifungal cream or powder. Athlete's foot usually responds well to clotrimazole (Lotrimin) cream,

terbinafine (Lamisil) cream, or an antifungal foot powder such as tolnaftate (Tinactin).

Note: Do not set out on a hiking trip or vacation to tropical or subtropical climates without first taking care of existing athlete's foot because the heat and sweating will dramatically worsen the condition.

Ringworm

This is a fungal infection of the skin and is commonly spread between children and from pets to children. The lesions usually have a round or oblong shape, a clear center, and a scaly advancing edge. Treatment consists of the application of antifungal creams or ointments for many weeks. Ringworm and eczema (atopic dermatitis) often look alike. They are both very common, but their treatment is very different.

CONTACT DERMATITIS

Contact dermatitis is an inflammation of the skin caused by contact with an irritating substance (such as a chemical) or a substance to which a person is sensitive or allergic (such as a metal or a plant). Poison ivy is one of the most common causes of contact dermatitis and is discussed at greater length in Chapter 42.

Many people who react to poison ivy also react to mangoes, especially mango peel, and may develop a rash after eating and handling mangoes.

Contact dermatitis may be caused by cosmetics, suntan lotion, bracelets, watch straps, and earrings, among other things. Vacationers often purchase new jewelry or apply unfamiliar creams, lotions, and cosmetics, which may lead to irritant rashes. Contact dermatitis usually responds to steroid creams and the removal of the irritant. If the dermatitis is extensive, oral steroids may be needed.

HIVES

See Chapter 37, pp. 388–89.

ECZEMA (ATOPIC DERMATITIS)

See also Chapter 37, p. 388.

Eczema often gets worse during periods of travel, especially when traveling in hot and humid areas or in very cold and dry climates. Just the stress of traveling may worsen it. Prior to travel discuss with your child's doctor what you should do if your child's eczema becomes more troublesome while away. Take along a supply of medications to treat worsening eczema, including

- more potent steroid creams and ointments;
- a course of oral steroids; and
- a course of antibiotics appropriate for treating staph and strep infections.

Ask your child's doctor for an eczema action plan that sets out steps you can take to treat worsening eczema.

A RASH THAT APPEARS SUDDENLY AND SPREADS RAPIDLY

If your child (or anyone in your party) develops a rash that appears suddenly, does not blanch (whiten) when pressure is applied to it, and spreads rapidly, and if your child is ill (e.g., has a fever and is lethargic), seek medical care immediately. These symptoms may indicate a disease called meningococcemia, **which may be fatal if not treated promptly.** This disease occurs throughout the world but particularly in sub-Saharan Africa and requires immediate antibacterial treatment. Some of the more serious viral infections, such as dengue fever, may also cause reddish rashes that are scattered over the entire body.

CAUTION

If anyone in your party is ill and has a high fever and a rash, medical care should be sought immediately.

RASHES THAT DEVELOP AFTER SWIMMING OR BEING IN CONTACT WITH WATER

Seabather's Eruption ("Sea Lice," "Ocean Itch")

This occurs after exposure to seawater that has larvae of a specific type of jellyfish in it. These larvae become entrapped under a bathing suit or in areas covered with hair, such as the armpit, or areas where friction occurs, such as the inner part of the thighs and the chest and abdomen of a surfer. The larvae contain venom-filled barbs that release their venom into the skin. A prickling or stinging sensation is often the first symptom. A raised, itchy rash develops some hours later and can last up to three weeks. The rash may blister. Some people, especially children, may also develop other symptoms such as fever, chills, and vomiting and may generally feel unwell for a few days.

 Prevention

- The best way to prevent seabather's eruption is not to swim in waters known to contain the larvae. This is hard to do, though, because the larvae can be present in the waters of the Caribbean, Central and South America, Asia, and even the United States along the Atlantic coast. Peak times for seabather's eruption are April to July off the Florida coast and August to November off Long Island. Seabather's eruption is not infrequently seen along the mid-Atlantic coast during the summer and fall months.
- Do not wear a T-shirt while swimming in infested waters, as the larvae may become trapped underneath it.
- Wear wetsuits with tightly occlusive cuffs.
- Remove your bathing suit and shower as soon as possible after swimming.
- Wash your bathing suit thoroughly in a detergent.

Treatment

- Remove your bathing suit and shower, if possible.
- Immediately apply papain (a naturally occurring plant enzyme that can neutralize venoms) or a meat tenderizer powder or solution to the rash.
- Later, apply steroid creams or calamine lotion with menthol.
- Oral antihistamines (Benadryl or one of the nonsedating antihistamines) will help relieve the itch, which can be very severe, especially at night.
- Very rarely, oral corticosteroids are needed to control symptoms.

For Your Reference

"Envenomations by Aquatic Invertebrates," by P. S. Auerbach, in *Wilderness Medicine,* edited by P. S. Auerbach, 4th ed. (2001).

Swimmer's Itch

This occurs after swimming in fresh water, either lakes or rivers, and the skin is penetrated by the microscopic larvae (cercariae) of a parasite known as a schistosome. This parasite is present in many countries, including the United States.

The larvae usually penetrate the skin after a person has gotten out of the water and as the skin dries. A prickling or itching sensation is usually the first symptom. Within a few minutes a reddish rash appears that often becomes raised and evolves into blisters or pustules. This rash is very itchy and may last up to two weeks. Unlike seabather's eruption (discussed above), the rash usually occurs on exposed parts of the body.

 ### *Prevention*

- Do not swim or wade in waters known to contain the parasite. This is particularly important in Africa, Asia, and other parts of the world where schistosomes may cause later, far more serious symptoms involving the internal organs.
- As soon as you emerge from infested waters, dry yourself vigorously with a towel.

 ### *Treatment*

- Apply a steroid cream or calamine lotion to the rash.
- Antihistamines, as described above for seabather's eruption, may be useful to control the itch.
- Very rarely, in highly sensitized individuals, oral corticosteroids may be needed to control the symptoms.
- If the affected person scratches a lot, secondary bacterial

infection may occur, and this may require an antibacterial cream or an oral antibiotic.

• If you have spent some time in countries where the more serious human form of schistosomiasis occurs, and particularly if you have swum or waded in infested waters, you should be screened for this parasite on return to the United States.

Rashes Caused by Sponges, Jellyfish, "Blue Bottles" (Portuguese Man-of-Wars), "Fire Fern," Sea Nettles, Sea Anemones, and Other Marine Animals

See Chapter 41.

Note: As mentioned at the beginning of this chapter, there are many other, less common rashes that can be acquired when traveling. Bathing in tropical waters can result in painful rashes due to contact with marine creatures. Spider and insect bites may cause a variety of rashes. Physicians who work in Western, more developed countries may have difficulty diagnosing some of the less common and more exotic rashes that may be acquired in tropical climates. It may be necessary to consult a dermatologist or tropical disease specialist to diagnose and treat these rashes.

STEROID CREAMS

• Steroid creams help to relieve the itch associated with insect bites, contact dermatitis, and eczema.

- If the skin becomes infected, these creams may encourage the spread of the infection. Yeast infections spread more rapidly when steroid creams are applied to them. Ringworm may initially appear to respond to a steroid cream, but later the rash increases in size.
- Application of steroid creams may also make subsequent diagnosis of the skin disorder far more difficult.
- **Never** apply steroid preparations to the eyelids. Do not use strong steroid preparations on the face or underneath the diaper unless directed to do so by a physician.

Malaria

See also Chapter 39.

Malaria is a parasitic disease that kills more than 2 million people annually (mainly children) and is transmitted by the bite of the anopheles mosquito.

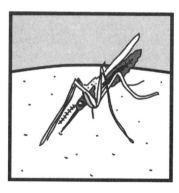

North Americans are particularly susceptible when traveling to malarial areas because they have never been exposed to malaria and therefore lack immunity to the malaria parasite.

If you intend to travel to an area where malaria is prevalent, it is essential to get advice on how to prevent it. If you intend to spend some months in a malarial area and especially if you do not have easy access to medical care, it is important to get guidelines on the self-diagnosis and self-treatment of malaria.

GETTING ADVICE ON MALARIA PREVENTION

The prevention of malaria is extremely complex. Recommendations vary according to

- the country you plan to visit;
- how long you intend to stay there;
- the location within the country (large cities versus rural areas, high-altitude areas versus low-altitude areas);
- the time of year you intend to visit the country, as many countries have a malarial season;
- the type of malaria that occurs in that country;
- the resistance pattern of the malaria parasite; and
- individual factors, especially the age and the health of the person traveling to the malarial area.

For these reasons, it is strongly recommended that you visit a travel clinic prior to your travels to discuss these issues. The physician at the clinic will assess your risk of malaria. Do this some weeks before you depart because some antimalarial medications need to be started at least one week before entering the malarial area. Visiting the clinic a few weeks before your departure will also give you and the physician an opportunity to assess any untoward side effects of the medication.

For Your Reference

Detailed recommendations for the prevention of malaria can be obtained from the following sources:

1. Centers for Disease Control and Prevention (CDC). Voice information service: (888) 232-3228. Fax: (888) 232-3299. Web site: www.cdc.gov.
2. World Health Organization (WHO). www.who.org.
3. Shoreland's Travel Health Online. Phone: (800) 433-5256. Web site: www.tripprep.com.

 Prevention

The prevention of malaria consists of two components: avoiding mosquito bites and taking antimalarial medication.

Avoiding Mosquito Bites

The single most important strategy in the prevention of malaria is to avoid mosquito bites. Guidelines are as follows:

- Choose your destination wisely, especially if you have young children. Within a country, certain areas have a higher malaria risk:

- High altitudes (above 1,000 meters) rarely have falciparum malaria (the worst type of malaria). This may
  change, however, with global warming.
- Malaria is less likely to be contracted in a large city
  than in a rural area.
- Traveling in the dry season is usually safer than traveling in or just after the rainy season.

If chloroquine-resistant malaria is present in an area you
intend to visit, you may want to reconsider your destination,
especially if you have young children.

- Choose the right clothing:
  - Wear clothes that cover as much of your body as pos-
    sible, such as long pants and long-sleeved shirts.
  - Light-colored clothing, such as khaki, is better than
    dark clothing.
  - Clothes can be impregnated with permethrin for
    added protection. This will not harm you or your
    child and will greatly help in deterring mosquitoes.
- Avoid using perfumes, scented soaps, scented deodor-
  ants, and other scented toiletries, which tend to attract
  mosquitoes.
- Use an appropriate insect repellent. Preparations con-
  taining DEET are the best. Reapply as necessary. (See
  Chapter 39, p. 415.)
- Choose accommodations that provide the best protection against mosquitoes and make your living and sleeping areas as mosquito-proof as possible:

- Select accommodations that have screened porches and screened windows.
- Sleep under mosquito nets. Infants and toddlers should definitely sleep in beds and cribs covered with permethrin-impregnated nets. Inspect mosquito nets for holes. If you detect any holes, repair them with thread or adhesive tape.
- Use a knock-down insecticide spray containing pyrethrin (such as Raid or Doom) in living and sleeping areas. Before retiring at night, inspect the walls and ceiling of your bedroom and kill any visible mosquitoes.
- Use an electric fan (if available) to keep the air moving. Moving air is an added deterrent to mosquitoes.

• Be outdoors as little as possible from dusk to dawn—the anopheles mosquito feeds almost exclusively during these times.

Antimalarial Medications

The second strategy in preventing malaria is to take appropriate antimalarial medication. This medication does not prevent mosquito bites; nor does it prevent you from acquiring the malaria parasite. Antimalarial medications work by preventing the later symptoms of malaria, but none are 100 percent effective.

Prescribing antimalarial medications appropriately is a real art and science. Consult an appropriate source such as a travel clinic, a travel physician, or an infectious disease specialist. It is especially important for your doctor to know whether chloroquine-resistant falciparum malaria is present in the area you intend to visit and then to prescribe prophylactic medication accordingly.

Some antimalarial medication needs to be started one week before departing from home and continued for some weeks after returning.

To assess the side effects and suitability of the medication for you, your physician may want you to try out the medication some weeks before your journey.

Do not skip any doses of your antimalarial medication.

Not all prophylactic medication may be administered to young children and infants. As mentioned before, it may be advisable to change your plans to avoid travel to a chloroquine-resistant malarial area if you are traveling with young children (most of the deaths from malaria occur in children younger than five years of age).

It is also important to be aware that some antimalarial medication may be extremely toxic if overdosed. Keep medication in a safe place away from infants and young children. Take syrup of ipecac along with you in case of accidental chloroquine ingestion—timely administration of this may literally be lifesaving.

Remember, taking antimalarial medication does not guarantee you will not get malaria.

A full discussion of antimalarial medication is beyond the scope of this book. Seek advice from an expert.

FEVERS AND ILLNESS WHILE IN OR AFTER LEAVING A MALARIAL AREA

The incubation period for malaria is at least seven days, so any illness in the first six days of travel to a malarial area is unlikely to be due to malaria.

Because most travelers do not spend many weeks in a malarial area, the symptoms usually present once they have returned home. Malaria may take many months or even years to manifest.

Any unexplained fever should be taken seriously. Until proved otherwise, it should be assumed to be due to malaria. Seek expert medical help.

If you or your children become ill while traveling in a malarial area, or on returning home from such a journey, seek medical care immediately. Inform your physician that you have been in a malarial area. Insist on blood tests for malaria. If these tests are negative and you remain ill, insist that these blood tests be repeated. Ask to be referred to an infectious disease specialist if your symptoms persist. Early treatment is essential.

SYMPTOMS OF MALARIA

Malaria often begins with a severe flu-like illness with fever, headache, and severe muscle aches. Other symptoms include nausea, vomiting, abdominal pain, and cough. Usually within a day or two the person develops paroxysms that have an abrupt onset and consist of chills followed by high fevers and profuse sweating. After the paroxysm, the person usually feels totally exhausted. If the illness is untreated, cerebral malaria may develop. People with cerebral malaria may have a depressed level of consciousness and convulsions. If they are not appropriately treated, death often follows.

People on antimalarial medication and those with partial immunity to the malarial parasite may have a less acute and less dramatic presentation.

THE ANOPHELES MOSQUITO is the most dangerous "animal" in Africa and is responsible for more deaths than lions, leopards, crocodiles, and other wild beasts! Do not underestimate the problem of malaria, especially in parts of Africa and Asia and especially in chloroquine-resistant malarial areas. **Malaria can be fatal.**

16

Other Mosquito-Borne Illnesses

DENGUE FEVER

Dengue fever is becoming an increasingly significant concern, not only for travelers but also for the populations in the countries where it occurs—in Central and South America, the Caribbean, Africa, and Asia. The number of cases of dengue fever is increasing at an alarming rate each year.

Dengue is caused by a virus that is transmitted to humans by the bite of the *Aedes aegypti* mosquito. Unlike the anopheles mosquito, which transmits malaria, the *Aedes* mosquito prefers urban areas and usually bites during the day or the early evening.

People who are infected by the dengue virus may have no symptoms at all or may be desperately ill. Common symptoms include

- fever;
- headache that is usually very severe and often just behind the eyes;
- severe muscle aches and backache (hence the name "breakbone fever");
- fatigue; and
- rashes.

A more severe form of dengue fever that occurs more commonly in children than in adults is known as dengue hemorrhagic fever (DHF). With DHF, bleeding occurs from the gums, nose and bowel, as well as into the tissues. **DHF may be fatal.**

 Prevention

Unlike malaria, which may be prevented with antimalarial medication, there are no specific medications that prevent dengue fever. There is also no vaccine to prevent this disease. Hence, it is essential to take protective measures to avoid mosquito bites:

- Wear protective clothing.
- Use appropriate insect repellents, especially during the daytime. Be especially careful if you like taking a nap outside after lunch and when relaxing outside in the late afternoon and early evening.

- Choose accommodations that provide the best protection against mosquitoes.

(See also Chapters 15 and 39.)

Treatment

There are no specific medications to kill the dengue virus. Good supportive care is essential, especially in DHF, where it may be lifesaving.

There are four separate dengue viruses, so a person can get dengue fever more than once. Subsequent attacks are often more severe and in children may lead to DHF.

YELLOW FEVER

Yellow fever is another viral illness transmitted to humans by the bite of the *Aedes aegypti* mosquito. It is a vaccine-preventable illness. Yellow fever occurs only in sub-Saharan Africa and tropical South America. It does not occur in Asia.

Symptoms of yellow fever may be minimal, but some people develop severe liver disease with jaundice and hemorrhage, **which may be fatal**. There is no specific treatment, but good supportive medical care may be lifesaving.

Yellow fever can be prevented by the yellow fever vaccine. This vaccine can be administered only by designated yellow fever vaccination centers, which will then issue an International Certificate of Vaccination for yellow fever known as "the yellow card." Proof of immunization against yellow fever is essential for entry into certain countries. This is an extremely important immunization—in fact, a "required" vaccination—for people traveling to areas where yellow fever is known to occur and to certain countries to prevent the importation of yellow fever by infected travelers leaving countries where the disease is known to occur. For further details, consult the CDC Web site at www.cdc.gov/travel.

Good personal protection measures against insects are vital for those who have not been vaccinated.

JAPANESE ENCEPHALITIS

Japanese encephalitis is a viral disease transmitted by the *Culex* mosquito, which feeds mostly during the evening and nighttime. It occurs in Asia, predominantly in rural areas where flood irrigation is practiced.

In some people, infection with the virus may not cause any symptoms. However, severe inflammation of the brain (encephalitis) may occur, leading to severe headache, confusion, coma, and even death. There is no specific treatment for Japanese encephalitis.

Japanese encephalitis can be prevented by vaccination. Vaccination is recommended for travelers who intend to spend some time in rural farming areas in Asia where Japanese encephalitis is known to occur.

Good personal protection measures against insects are also very important, especially for people who have not been vaccinated.

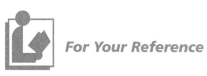

For Your Reference

For further information on the diseases discussed in this chapter, consult these Web sites:

1. Centers for Disease Control and Prevention (CDC). www.cdc.gov.
2. Shoreland's Travel Health Online. www. tripprep.com.

17

Emerging Infectious Diseases

Hardly a day goes by without a report in the news about a new and deadly infectious disease in some part of the world. In 2003/2004, it was SARS (severe acute respiratory syndrome). In 2005/2006, it was avian influenza. New contagious diseases seem to be emerging all the time.

These reports are especially troubling to travelers, particularly those about to set out for the country in question. The rest of the world cannot afford to be complacent—in the age of jet travel, diseases spread rapidly around the globe. We are all potentially at risk from these new emerging infections.

 For Your Reference

The easiest, and probably the best, place to find more information about these and other infectious diseases is the Centers for Disease Control and Prevention (CDC) Web site, www.cdc.gov. The CDC can also be contacted by telephone: (800) CDC-INFO/(800) 232-4636. It is definitely a good idea to consult this resource before undertaking travel to areas reporting outbreaks of infectious disease.

To avoid contracting infectious diseases while traveling, general measures should be taken before departure, during your trip, and once you return.

What to Do before You Go

- Consult the CDC Web site to see whether specific notices have been issued for the countries you plan to visit. The CDC issues different types of notices for international travel. Each type of notice describes the level of risk for the traveler and recommended preventive measures. These notices are as follows:
  - *In the news.* This type of notice provides information about sporadic cases of disease that may affect the traveler in the destination country. The risk for the traveler does not differ from the usual risk in that area.
  - *Outbreak notice.* This provides information about a disease outbreak in an area. The risk to travelers is "defined and limited," and the notice reminds travelers about standard or enhanced travel recommendations.
  - *Travel health precaution.* This notice provides travelers with specific information about a disease outbreak of greater scope and affecting a larger area. Specific preventive precautions are given with guidelines on

what to do should the traveler become ill while in the area.

- *Travel health warning.* This recommends against non-essential travel to an area.

If a travel health warning has been issued, postpone nonessential travel to these areas. Travel to areas experiencing epidemics may sometimes be essential for personal or other reasons, however. The CDC often gives more specific guidelines about locations or activities or food that should be avoided. Try to follow these. Also follow the guidelines below on how to avoid infectious illnesses while traveling.

- Make sure your routine immunizations are up to date. If you are due for a tetanus booster, ask for one of the newer combination tetanus boosters that will boost your immunity against whooping cough. Get recommended travel vaccinations. Ask your physician about other immunizations that may be advisable. These include the flu immunization and the pneumococcal immunization.
- Assemble a travel medical kit. This should definitely include an alcohol-based hand sanitizer spray or lotion. Include a thermometer, and consider purchasing face masks.
- Learn about health care resources in the countries you plan to visit. Know how to locate medical care while abroad.
- Review your heath insurance policy and consider purchasing supplemental health insurance and evacuation insurance.

What to Do while You Are Traveling

- Wash your hands frequently. This is one of the most important precautions you can take. Doorknobs, handrails, and elevator buttons may all be contaminated. You may not always have access to running water, so have easily accessible a bottle of bactericidal hand sanitizer lotion or alcohol-based wet wipes.
- Try to limit close contact with strangers. Avoid kissing, hugging, and even shaking hands.
- Avoid crowds and crowded spaces.
- Do not share eating and drinking utensils. Do not drink from water fountains.
- If you have close contact with an infected person, wearing a mask, eyeglasses, or goggles may be helpful because you will be less likely to rub your eyes or touch your nose. In addition, wearing a mask often suggests to other people that you have some contagious disease and may discourage other people from coming close to you. An N-95 mask is one of the more effective types of masks. The CDC does not recommend the routine use of masks or goggles.
- Wearing surgical gloves may help, too, but they often give a false sense of security. Even when you are wearing gloves, if you touch infected material and then rub your eyes or scratch your nose, you stand a good chance of transferring the infected material to yourself. The CDC

recommends the use of gloves only for health care workers who attend to patients suspected of having specific diseases.

- If you get sick, seek medical care.

 What to Do once You Return

Monitor your health. If you become ill, contact your health care provider. When you make your appointment, tell your health care provider that you have recently been in an area that has an outbreak of an infectious disease. Health care workers can then take the necessary precautions to avoid contracting the disease and spreading it to other patients.

SARS

Severe acute respiratory syndrome (SARS) is an illness that was first described in the winter of 2003. It began in Vietnam and China but spread fairly rapidly to other countries around the world, including the United States and Canada.

SARS is a viral disease that probably originated in animals, but the virus is able to thrive in humans as well. During the 2003 outbreak, more than 8,000 people worldwide developed SARS, and more than 800 of them died. Most of the people who were infected were adults, but a few children also became ill with the disease. Health care workers appeared to be particularly vulnerable. By August 2003, the disease appeared to be contained, with no new cases being diagnosed. Only time will tell whether SARS will reemerge.

How Do You Get It?

SARS is a droplet-spread infection acquired by close contact with someone who already has the disease or by touching objects contaminated with the virus. "Close contact" means living with or taking care of someone with SARS. It would include sharing eating and drinking utensils, touching the individual (shaking hands, kissing, or hugging), and talking to someone within three feet.

How Long Is the Incubation Period?

The incubation period may be as short as 5 days or as long as 15 days.

What Are the Symptoms?

The early symptoms of SARS are similar to those of many other infectious illnesses and include fever, headache, muscle aches, and often diarrhea. Later on (after two to seven days), the person may develop a cough and shortness of breath. If an X-ray is taken at this stage, it will show pneumonia. Some people may be only mildly ill, while others will be critically ill and require hospitalization, extra oxygen, intravenous fluids, and highly skilled medical and nursing care. Antibiotics will not kill the SARS virus (antibiotics do not kill viruses) but may be indicated for other reasons.

How Is It Diagnosed?

This is not an easy diagnosis to make because the pneumonia developed by people with SARS is very similar to many other types of pneumonia. SARS is suspected if the ill person has recently had contact with a known case or has recently traveled to an area where the disease is prevalent. Diagnostic tests for SARS are available only at more sophisticated and specialized laboratories.

 Prevention

Avoid unnecessary travel to areas that are experiencing SARS outbreaks. If travel to these areas is essential, follow the general guidelines for the prevention of infectious diseases outlined above.

What Did We Learn from the SARS Outbreak?

We learned how quickly infectious illnesses can spread around the world. With the advent of jet travel, a disease may be in China one day and the United States the next. We are all brothers and sisters on a very small planet and need to respect and take care of each other.

We learned that if we work together we can solve complex

medical problems much faster and stop the spread of disease. In the case of SARS, the World Health Organization (WHO) and laboratories around the world worked together to detect the SARS virus and contain the disease. Cooperation instead of competition between nations makes the world a better and safer place.

AVIAN INFLUENZA (BIRD FLU)

Bird flu is an infection caused by bird flu viruses. Bird flu viruses do not usually infect humans, but a number of cases of human infection with bird flu viruses have occurred since 1997. Most of these cases have resulted from contact with infected poultry or with contaminated surfaces. However, more recently, cases of bird flu caused by human-to-human transmission have been reported. Such cases have been rare, but there is concern that one of the bird flu viruses may mutate so that human-to-human transmission occurs more readily. This could lead to a flu epidemic.

As of 2007, most cases of avian flu in humans have occurred in Asia and the Middle East. However, cases affecting livestock and domestic poultry have occurred in many other countries.

Follow the guidelines below if you plan to travel to countries where bird flu has been known to occur.

What to Do before You Go

Follow the general guidelines for prevention outlined on pp. 209 through 210.

Check the CDC *and* WHO Web sites on avian flu:
www.cdc.gov/flu/avian/index.htm
www.who.int/csr/disease/avian_influenza/en

At present there is no immunization for avian influenza, but this is sure to change.

Discuss with your physician the advisability of getting an influenza antiviral drug and taking this along with you on your travels in case you develop an illness suggestive of flu while away. (Note that this is not a current CDC recommendation.)

What to Do while You Are Traveling

- Avoid all contact with poultry, both alive and dead. Avoid poultry farms and markets where poultry is raised or kept. Avoid surfaces that have been contaminated by poultry or their secretions or feces.
- Wash your hands well and repeatedly, especially if you have had contact with potentially infectious material. If you do not have access to water, use a waterless, alcohol-based hand gel to disinfect your hands.
- If you eat poultry or eggs, make sure they have been

thoroughly cooked. If you handle eggs, wash them well in warm, soapy water and then wash your hands.

- If a flu outbreak occurs among humans while you are away
  - stay away from crowds and crowded spaces;
  - limit close contact with strangers, including kissing, hugging, and shaking hands;
  - do not share eating and drinking utensils, and do not drink from water fountains;
  - wash your hands well before eating;
  - consider wearing a face mask and goggles (this is not a CDC recommendation);
  - try not to touch your eyes, nose, or mouth; and
  - wash your hands frequently.
- If you become sick, seek medical care. Symptoms suggestive of flu include fever; respiratory symptoms such as cough, sore throat, and shortness of breath; and headache and muscle aches. Try to limit the spread of your illness:
  - Cover your cough.
  - Limit contact with other people, especially young children and the elderly.
  - Avoid traveling by plane, bus, train, or cruise ship.

What to Do once You Return

- Monitor your health for 10 days.
- If you become ill with a flu-like illness as described

above, contact your health care provider. Inform your health care provider of your symptoms and your recent travel and possible exposure to avian flu. Also inform your health care provider of any direct contact with poultry.

SARS and Avian flu are in the news at present. These illnesses may eventually be controlled, but others will take their place. The principles of avoiding most infectious diseases spread by droplet are fairly similar. Contact the CDC Web site (www.cdc.gov) before all international travel, and keep washing your hands!

18

Bringing Your Internationally Adopted Child Home

What's in This Chapter

Coughs
Eye Problems
Gastrointestinal Problems
What to Do while You Are in Your Adopted Child's Country

Many U.S. citizens adopt children from outside the United States, commonly from China, Russia, Romania, and Guatemala but also from many other countries. Finally, after months or years of waiting, it is time for you to collect your child and bring him or her home! This is obviously a very exciting time for you and your family. Remember, you may be traveling to a lesser-developed country and you should plan appropriately. You do not want to spoil this special time by becoming ill. Your adoption agency will have provided you with helpful information about the country you will be visiting and will possibly have given you recommendations for preventing travel-related illness.

 What to Do before You Go

Visit *Your* Physician or a Travel Clinic

Especially if you are traveling to a lesser-developed country, it is essential that you get advice to guide you, particularly in regard to the prevention of travel-related illness. Make sure your routine immunizations are up to date, and get travel-related vaccines as well. It is important to get a tetanus booster every 10 years. Newer combination tetanus boosters are available that will also boost your immunity to whooping cough (pertussis). This is a good idea for most adults. Important travel-related vaccines include those against hepatitis A and B, but others may also be advisable. You should also get advice on how to prevent and treat travelers' diarrhea, which is by far the most common medical problem for travelers to lesser-developed countries. Your visit to your physician or travel clinic should take place at least six months prior to your departure date to allow sufficient time for your immunizations. However, if you have left it to the last moment, still make this appointment, as you may be able to prevent some very unpleasant illnesses.

If you are traveling to an area where malaria is prevalent, you will need to take precautions to prevent mosquito bites and you may also need to take prophylactic antimalarial medication.

Sometimes adopting parents take their own parents with them to share this exciting time or perhaps to help take care of siblings. If an elderly person accompanies you, it is especially important that he or she has travel insurance and has visited a travel clinic for advice and assessment. Elderly people should also get the pneumovax immunization, which gives protection against a very severe type of pneumonia. It is also a good idea for the elderly to get a flu shot. It is actually a good idea for everyone to get a flu shot.

Ask your physician for prescriptions for antibiotics to treat travelers' diarrhea. You may also want to ask for a prescription for a sleeping pill such as Ambien to help you get to sleep when you arrive in your destination country.

Do not bypass this visit!

Visit Your *Child's* Future Physician

You may have already met with your child's future physician to review the adoption records, your child's growth and development charts, and so on.

> *Note:* Most parents have medical and developmental questions about their future child. Some parents undertake an initial "first look" visit to assess their prospective child. If you are one of these parents, it is a good idea to meet with a pediatrician first. He or she can give you guidelines on what to look for, how to assess development, how to measure a child's head size (head circumference), and how to plot a child's measurements on a percentile chart. Take the following items with you on your "first look" visit: (1) percentile charts, (2) a Denver developmental chart, (3) a tape measure to measure head circumference, and (4) a camcorder to videotape your child. The information you obtain, along with birth and developmental history, will enable a pediatrician who specializes in adoption to help you assess a child. Keep in mind that there are few guarantees in life!

Even if you have already met with your child's future physician, another visit to discuss medications and supplies you may want to take with you is a good idea.

Medications that may prove particularly useful when collecting your child include the following:

- Analgesics and antipyretics such as acetaminophen (Tylenol) and ibuprofen (children's Motrin or children's Advil). (See Part Five, "A Medical Kit for Children," for dosages.)
- Diaper rash ointments and creams such as A&D, Desitin, or Triple Paste.
- Antifungal creams or ointments such as Nystatin (prescription) or clotrimazole (Lotrimin).
- Antibacterial ointment such as Triple Antibiotic Ointment, Neosporin, Bacitracin, or Bactroban (prescription).
- Hydrocortisone cream, either 0.5% or 1%, to treat itchy rashes, insect bites, or contact dermatitis.
- Nix cream rinse and a nit comb to treat head lice.
- Saline nose drops with a bulb syringe.
- Allergy medication such as Benadryl to treat itching, allergic reactions, and colds (for Benadryl dosage, see Part Five, "A Medical Kit for Children").
- Laxatives such as glycerine suppositories or Babylax.
- Rehydration salts such as Kaolectrolyte, Pedialyte, or Ceralyte. These need to be mixed with clean, drinkable water. Remember, if there is any doubt about the safety of the water, it should be boiled or treated chemically before use (see Chapter 13).
- A flexible digital thermometer.

- Vaseline to lubricate the thermometer (if used rectally) or to treat dry, chapped skin and lips.
- A course of antibiotics (prescription).
- Antibiotic eardrops (prescription).
- Antibiotic eyedrops (prescription).
- Elimite cream to treat scabies (prescription).

The last four medications are optional. Some physicians recommend them and others do not. Discuss these with your child's physician before you depart and get clear guidelines as to when the antibiotics should be used. Know the correct dose for your child.

If your child is ill when you collect her, the orphanage should be able to suggest a local physician to take care of the problem. If not, the U.S. embassy may be able to recommend a physician. Alternatively, your child's future physician may be prepared to accept a long-distance call from you to discuss the problem and advise you. Some agencies specializing in foreign adoption may be able to give you the phone numbers of local physicians in specific locations who are very qualified to help you take care of your child's problems. If you are working through such an agency, get the names and phone numbers *before* you leave home.

As part of the exit procedure, your child will require a physical examination to obtain a U.S. visa. This examination is usually fairly cursory and certainly does not take the place of a full medical evaluation when you get home.

For Your Reference

Information about international adoption and international travel can be found at:

1. www.travel.state.gov
2. www.cdc.gov
3. www.immunize.org
4. www.cdc.gov/travel
5. www.istm.org (to locate a travel clinic or travel physician)

It is often a good idea to contact people who have already adopted a child and discuss their experience. You could ask them for tips and what they would do differently if they were to do it again. There are a number of Web sites where you can chat with other families who have already adopted children internationally. One such site is www.rainbowkids.com. The agency handling your adoption will also often help you contact families that have already gone through international adoption. Many of these agencies have frequent "get-to-gether" functions where families that have adopted children and those planning adoption can meet.

Prepare Nonmedical Supplies You May Need for Your Newly Adopted Child

Depending upon the country you are visiting, it may be a good idea to take along three or four cans of infant formula. This could be a regular milk-based formula or a soy-based formula. Although many Asian individuals are lactose-intolerant, this generally develops only later in life, and so lactose intolerance is not usually a problem in the first one to two years of life. Do not make too many changes to your child's routine when you first receive her. Keep her on the formula or milk she is used to. This applies to the other elements of her diet as well. You will have ample time when you get back to transition her to a different type of formula, or if she is older than one year of age, to whole milk.

Other important items to take along are disposable diapers, wet wipes, toilet paper, and clothing. The orphanage will gratefully accept any items not used. The orphanage will also happily accept any medications that you do not need.

A car seat, child carrier, and stroller may be important, especially if you plan to do additional traveling with your child before you return home. (Regarding travel with your newly adopted child, many parents have told me what a difference it made having booked an extra seat on the return plane trip. This allowed for more space for all, and many parents have recounted how their child slept for a good part of the trip back home.)

Don't forget the fun stuff! Be sure to take along stickers, books, and toys.

Prepare Medical and Nonmedical Supplies for the Parents and Traveling Siblings

These types of supplies are detailed elsewhere in the book. They include basic analgesics, routine medications that you take, and medications to prevent and treat travelers' diarrhea. If you are traveling to a malarial area, antimalarial medications will be needed. If you are prone to constipation, include a suitable laxative in your medical kit.

When traveling to lesser-developed countries, it is always a good idea to have a good supply of antibacterial wipes or towelettes or a bottle of alcohol-based antiseptic hand spray for each member of the travel party. Remember, most infections are spread by poor hand hygiene. Wash your hands frequently; when you can't, use your alcohol hand spray or towelettes.

If traveling to an area where SARS, Avian flu, or some other similar contagious disease is known to occur, consider purchasing N-95 masks. Once a face mask is damp, it is no longer effective, so take along a good supply.

If you arrive jet-lagged and are unable to sleep, sleeping pills may help you get a few good nights' sleep before you collect your child. The prescription medication Ambien (zolpidem) is a suitable sleeping pill. Melatonin tablets may help jet lag, so consider getting these, especially if you are prone to jet lag (see Chapter 8, p. 105).

Refer to Part Five for suggestions on what to include in a medical kit.

COMMON MEDICAL PROBLEMS OF
FOREIGN ADOPTEES

Skin

Mongolian Spots

These are blue-green or slate gray marks in the skin, occurring particularly over the lower back. They are common in more deeply pigmented races, especially blacks and Asians. These marks may be mistaken for bruises. They often fade in later childhood.

Dry Skin and Eczema

Many adoptees have dry skin and sometimes patches of eczema (atopic dermatitis). These patches are usually worse on the cheeks but may occur anywhere. Sometimes the patches of eczema have a circular shape and may be mistaken for ringworm. Some children may have cracked and bleeding skin behind the ears (see Chapter 14, p. 188).

Impetigo

Impetigo, an infection of the skin due to bacteria (streptococci or staphylococci), is also relatively common. If a child scratches his skin too hard or repeatedly because of insect bites or eczema, the skin may break open, start bleeding, and possibly become infected with the bacteria that cause impetigo (see Chapter 14, p. 182).

Insect Bites

Insect bites are particularly common among children living in hot and humid countries (see Chapter 39).

Scabies

Scabies is a skin infestation caused by a tiny mite that burrows into the skin, leading to a red, bumpy, intensely itchy rash. The rash tends to concentrate on the hands and feet, between the fingers and toes, on the wrists and ankles, and in the genital area. Scabies in adults is often most severe where clothing comes into contact with the skin.

Scabies is common in children in developing countries. It often occurs in orphanages. It also appears in children and adults in the United States. If your child is scratching incessantly, "tearing" at the skin where a rash has occurred, she may have scabies.

If you suspect scabies, apply Elimite cream from head to toe. Leave it on for 8 to 12 hours. Then bathe your child and wash off the Elimite. Dress her in clean clothing. Your child is likely to continue scratching for some time, but this does not necessarily mean the mite has not been eradicated. Benadryl, steroid creams, and keeping your child cool may help reduce her discomfort. If your child continues to scratch, a second Elimite treatment or other medication may be needed. Scabies is very contagious. If you do not treat your child soon, you may develop scabies yourself. Also, laundering clothes and bedding in very hot water is crucial to eradicate these mites.

Lice (Nits)

Lice in the hair are not unusual in the United States. They are more common in lesser-developed countries and especially in children from orphanages or institutions.

The most common symptom of lice is itchiness of the scalp. You may see the adult lice moving in your child's hair, but you are more likely to see the eggs (the nits) attached to strands of hair. They are most commonly seen behind the ears and at the nape of the neck close to the scalp. They may be mistaken for dandruff, but dandruff is easily brushed off or combed out.

A good medication for treating lice is Nix cream rinse. This is applied as follows: Wash the hair with a regular shampoo. Towel off excess water so that the hair is damp but not wet and then apply enough Nix to soak the hair and scalp. Pay particular attention to the area behind the ears and the nape of the neck. Wash off the Nix after 10 minutes. Rinse the hair well with water.

Elimite cream can also be used to treat head lice. Rub the Elimite into the scalp and hair and leave on overnight. Wash out in the morning.

Ringworm

Circular skin lesions with a dry, scaly edge may be due to ringworm. Use an antifungal cream such as Lotrimin to treat this. The lesions may take weeks to disappear. As mentioned above, eczema is often misdiagnosed as ringworm.

Fever

Remember, most fevers are due to mild viral infections that are usually not serious (see Chapter 20).

Ear and
Upper Respiratory Tract Infections

Children everywhere have frequent colds and "runny noses," and international adoptees are no exception. Do not be alarmed if your child has yellow or green mucus streaming from her nose. This does not mean she has bacterial sinusitis (see Chapter 23).

Some children may have pus draining out of one or both ears. This indicates that they have an ear infection and the eardrum has ruptured. Children in lesser-developed countries commonly have this problem, which is known medically as "chronic suppurative otitis media." This condition does not usually cause pain or discomfort and does not have to be treated immediately. Treatment usually includes drying up the pus with many cotton swabs (such as Q-tips) and instilling antibiotic eardrops (such as Floxin or Ciprodex) two to three times a day for many days. Sometimes an oral antibiotic is also used. If the draining ear is a recent event, it suggests that the ear infection has just occurred, and an oral antibiotic is the appropriate treatment (see Chapter 25).

Coughs

Coughs commonly accompany a cold. There are many other causes of coughs, most of which are not serious (see Chapter 28).

Eye Problems

Your child may have "pink eye" or pus in the eye when you collect her. This is known as conjunctivitis (see Chapter 30, p. 313).

Gastrointestinal Problems

Vomiting

The occasional vomit or "spit-up" is normal in childhood. If vomiting is more severe, it may require treatment (see Chapter 32).

Constipation

Constipation is common in children and adults, especially when traveling (see Chapter 34).

Loose Stools and Diarrhea

These are also not unusual. Both constipation and diarrhea may be exacerbated by changes in diet and emotional stress (see Chapter 12 and "Management of Diarrhea" in Chapter 31).

Note: Most of the illnesses of foreign adoptees will be minor. Do not panic. There is usually no hurry to treat them. If you are concerned, call your pediatrician at home and ask for advice. Occasionally your child will have a serious problem that will need to be treated urgently.

As a physician who treats many international adoptees, I am constantly heartened by the resilience as well as the health and good nutrition of most of the children who enter the United States.

 ## What to Do while You Are in Your Adopted Child's Country

- This is a stressful time but also a very special time. Do not try to do too much. Don't feel you have to sightsee. Get as much sleep as possible, and try to keep a sense of humor and enjoy this happy time.
- Eat sensibly. Remember your travelers' diarrhea precautions. Watch out for constipation.
- You and your new child may be spending many hours in a hotel room. There may be safety concerns here—loose and unprotected electrical wires, windows that open easily to the road below, bathroom hazards such as very hot water. Don't forget about choking and poisoning. Your child's inquisitive fingers may reach medicines not intended for her.
- Pay attention to road and water safety. Although travel clinics often focus on giving advice relating to the pre-

vention of malaria and other exotic diseases, the most common serious travel-related events are motor vehicle accidents and drowning. (See Chapter 2.) Do not forget sun protection, and be wary of bites from unfamiliar animals.

- Keep important telephone numbers easily accessible, including the numbers of your own physician or travel clinic, your child's pediatrician, the adoption agency, the U.S. consulate, and other important contacts, family or otherwise.

Collecting an international adoptee is extremely exciting but also exhausting and stressful. Making the appropriate preparations, being well rested prior to travel, and not being rushed will help make the entire visit more enjoyable.

What to Do once You Return

Once you have returned home and you and your new child have had time to settle and adapt to the new time zone, you should make an appointment for your child to have a full physical examination. This initial examination should take place within the first two weeks of returning home. Later your child will need some screening blood tests, a skin test for tuberculosis, and some stool tests to look for intestinal parasites. She may also need a chest X-ray. Some of the blood tests may need to be repeated six months later. Immunizations will also need to be administered at some stage.

Congratulations!

For Your Reference

1. *The Handbook of International Adoption Medicine: A Guide for Physicians, Parents, and Providers,* by Laurie C. Miller (2005). This book is essential reading for all physicians involved in international adoption and an excellent guide for adopting parents.
2. "International Adoption: Medical and Developmental Issues," by Lisa H. Albers, Elizabeth D. Barnett, Jerri Ann Jenista, and Dana E. Johnson, in *Pediatric Clinics of North America.* 52 (October 2005). This provides an excellent review for all medical personnel involved in international adoption.
3. *How to Adopt Internationally,* by Jean Nelson Erichsen and Heino R. Erichsen (2003).
4. *The International Adoption Handbook: How to Make Foreign Adoption Work for You,* by Myra Alperson (1997).

PART TWO

Common Childhood Illnesses

19

Newborns and Infants to Age Three Months

One of the most exciting things that can happen to a person is bringing home a newborn baby. Babies do not come with instruction manuals, however, and a parent's excitement is often mixed with a certain amount of anxiety. Discussed below are some seemingly unusual but normal things about babies.

SKIN

Skin Color

Newborn infants and infants in the first few months of life often have very blue, even purple, hands and feet. Sometimes the upper lip has a bluish tinge. This is due to poor circulation but is normal. However, your infant's tongue should be nice and pink.

The skin in the first week or 10 days of life frequently is yellowish in color. The whites of the eyes may also be yellow. This condition is known as jaundice and occurs when a newborn's body has too much of a substance called bilirubin. Although this is not usually a problem, it is important to have an infant checked in the first three to five days of life to make sure that the level of bilirubin in the body is not too high—a very high level of bilirubin can cause brain damage.

Rashes

Although babies are usually born with a lovely soft skin, after a few days it often becomes dry and cracked and may even bleed in certain areas (particularly around the ankles). No treatment is usually necessary, but you can decrease the dryness by bathing your infant less frequently or by applying a hypoallergenic moisturizer to the skin. It is normal for the skin to peel.

Babies have very sensitive skin and develop a variety of rashes, which tend to come and go. They often have reddish bumps with a yellowish white center scattered over the body. (The medical term for this rash is *erythema toxicum*.) These spots last for a week or two and are usually of no consequence apart from the fact that they may be mistaken for infected pustules.

Small pimples on the face that resemble acne are known as neonatal or newborn acne. Neonatal acne usually develops around the third or fourth week of life, is common, seldom requires treatment, and may last for many months. White spots on the nose are called milia and are also normal.

Many infants are born with reddish or pinkish marks or blotches on the upper eyelids, base of the nose, and nape of the neck. These are known as salmon patches, or "stork bites," and usually fade with time (months to years).

Diaper rashes are common and are best prevented by keeping the genital area clean and dry. If your infant develops a rash in the diaper area, apply a barrier ointment, such as Desitin, A&D, or Triple Paste. If this does not clear the rash in two to three days, try an antifungal ointment such as Lotrimin or ask your pediatrician about a prescription for Nystatin.

Good hygiene is the most important way to prevent and treat diaper rash, so change your child's diaper as soon as he is wet or dirty. You may need to wash your baby with warm water and a mild soap. Do not use plastic pants because they tend to retain moisture and make diaper rashes worse. Most diaper rashes respond well to air (see Chapters 14 and 37).

 ## When to Seek Medical Attention

Occasionally, a rash in an infant may be a sign of a more serious medical problem.

- Large blisters may be a sign of a serious underlying illness.
- If your infant has a nonblanching rash (a rash that does not fade when you press on it) accompanied by symptoms of illness (e.g., lethargy, decreased drinking, fever), consult a physician immediately.

- Redness around the umbilicus that is spreading outward over the belly area indicates an urgent need to visit a physician.

BREATHING

Newborn babies often sneeze, and this does not mean they are getting a "cold" or have allergies. They will often sound very "snuffly" from breathing through narrow nasal passages that contain mucus. If this interferes with feeding, it may be helpful to instill saltwater (saline) nose drops and then suction the mucus out with a bulb syringe. Do one nostril at a time. Your infant will object to this procedure, but it is effective. If the mucus contains a small amount of blood, don't be concerned. These nose drops may be purchased over the counter (Nasal, Little Noses, Ocean) or made up at home (dissolve ½ level teaspoon of table salt in 8 ounces of water).

Babies often make a lot of noise when they breathe. You will find this out if your baby sleeps in the same room as you! Babies also do not breathe evenly. They often have periods of very rapid breathing and then hold their breath for 10 to 15 seconds. This can be very disconcerting if your infant is sleeping right next to you. You may find yourself jumping out of bed to check whether your child is still breathing!

How fast do babies breathe? In the first few months of life, babies take 40 or more breaths a minute. At times, particularly after crying or feeding, they may breathe 70 or 80 or more times a minute! However, once they have settled, the respiratory rate should be around 40 times a minute or less.

(If you are concerned that your baby is breathing abnormally, see Chapter 62.)

EYES

As mentioned above, the whites of the eyes of a newborn infant often are yellow as a result of jaundice. This may last for one to three weeks, or even longer, but is no cause for concern if your baby's bilirubin level is not too high. Your baby's doctor may want to do a blood test to check the bilirubin level.

Some babies have red streaks in the whites of one or both eyes. These are hemorrhages that occur during the birthing process and fade over the ensuing two to three weeks.

"Sticky" or pus-filled eyes may be due to an eye infection (conjunctivitis) or to blocked tear ducts. The latter condition often leads to excessive watering of the eyes. If your baby's eyelids are red and swollen or are stuck together, he should be seen by a doctor. If there is just a small amount of eye discharge or one or both eyes are just tearing excessively, discuss this with your child's doctor at his next checkup.

YOUR BABY'S "SOFT SPOT"

Your baby will have a large "soft spot" (the anterior fontanelle) at the top of the head toward the front. This spot will get smaller over time and is usually closed by 18 months of age. The soft spot is usually slightly depressed but sometimes may appear fuller and tenser (for example, when a baby is lying down and crying or straining).

When to Seek Medical Attention

- A soft spot that is very sunken may be a sign of dehydration. If your infant is dehydrated, there will be other signs of dehydration (see Chapter 31).
- A tense, bulging fontanelle may be a sign of meningitis. In this case, your baby will also have a fever and be very irritable or very lethargic. Seek medical help immediately!

MOUTH AND TONGUE

A baby's tongue will often have a white coating on it, which can be wiped off easily. Usually the coating is just milk curds and typically occurs after feeding.

When to Seek Medical Attention

If the white coating extends to the inside of the cheeks, the gums, and the inside of the lips and continues for some hours after a feed, your baby probably has thrush. Occasionally thrush can interfere with feeding and cause fussiness. Thrush is a yeast infection that often needs treatment with an oral antifungal medicine. Discuss this with your child's physician. Thrush is not a medical emergency and may get better on its own.

SPITTING UP OR VOMITING

It is quite common for infants in the first few weeks of life to "spit up." Sometimes when babies spit up, the milk comes out through the nostrils. Do not be alarmed if this happens.

Many babies continue to spit up throughout the first year of life. As long as a baby is otherwise well, gaining weight, and happy, this is no cause for concern. The medical terminology for this is gastroesophageal reflux. Reflux tends to increase in severity and peaks at four months of age. It usually resolves by one year of age. While you have a baby around, there is not much point in wearing expensive silk shirts or blouses!

Some infants will have the occasional projectile vomit—when the vomit shoots out a few feet or more.

 When to Seek Medical Attention

- If your infant has repeated projectile vomits that seem to get more severe and occur with increasing frequency.
- If your infant "spits up" or vomits and does not gain weight adequately, or is always unhappy and fussy.
- If your newborn infant vomits green-colored liquid (bile), in which case medical attention should be sought immediately.

UMBILICAL CORD (AND "BELLY BUTTON")

It is important to keep the cord (umbilicus) clean and dry. Many physicians recommend cleaning the cord three or four times a day with rubbing alcohol. This is probably not necessary; allowing the cord to dry naturally may be just as effective.

The cord falls off within the first two to three weeks of life, but occasionally it stays on for up to two months. When the cord falls off, you may see a drop or two of blood around the umbilicus, which is not cause for alarm. There may also be slight drainage from the umbilicus for two to three days.

As mentioned earlier, redness of the skin at the base of the cord is not normal and may indicate a serious infection. Sometimes the cord develops an unpleasant odor, but apart from the odor this is not usually a problem.

 When to Seek Medical Attention

- If you notice redness of the skin around the base of the cord.
- If there is continued bleeding from the cord.

GENITALIA

Boys

No special care is needed for the uncircumcised male penis. It is especially important not to try to retract the foreskin forcibly.

Circumcised males often develop redness, swelling, a yellowish crust, and oozing at the circumcision site in the first week to 10 days after circumcision. The tip of the penis may look like it is infected, but this is normal at this stage. By 14 days the penis should be completely healed. Contact a physician if the circumcision site continues to bleed or if redness spreads up the shaft of the penis on to the lower abdomen.

Girls

Girls may have a whitish vaginal discharge in the first week of life, and sometimes this is blood-tinged. This is no cause for alarm and will settle by 10 days of age. You should clean the genital area with a cotton ball and warm water. When cleaning the genital area, always wipe from front to back.

WEIGHT LOSS AND WEIGHT GAIN

Most babies lose weight in the first few days of life. This is especially true of breast-fed babies because it may take up to a week for the mother's milk to come in fully. By 7 to 10 days of age, a baby should be back to his or her birth weight. After that your baby should gain 5 to 7 ounces every week for the next two to three months. Most infants double their birth weight by four to five months and triple it by their first birthday.

BOWEL MOVEMENTS

Your infant's initial bowel movements may be almost black in color. These first stools are known as *meconium*.

The stool color may vary from bright yellow to bright green to brown or be various shades in between. Sometimes the stools have a seedy texture.

Breast-Fed Babies

Breast-fed babies may have 7 to 10 loose to watery stools a day. A stool is often passed each time the infant feeds. As long as the infant is gaining weight, this is normal. In the second or third month of life, breast-fed babies may pass only one to two stools a week. As long as the stools are soft, this is nothing to be concerned about.

Bottle-Fed Babies

Bottle-fed babies tend to have fewer stools than those who are breast-fed, and their stools tend to be firmer in consistency.

Straining, Grunting, and Groaning during a Bowel Movement

Many infants appear to have trouble passing a stool—they grunt and groan, strain and grimace, and go red in the face while attempting to have a bowel movement. They may seem to be uncomfortable and appear relieved after the stool is passed. Usually the stool is soft and of normal consistency. This is normal, and the difficulty passing the stool is probably related to poor muscle coordination. This is not constipation.

You may sometimes feel it is necessary to aid your infant by rectal stimulation. Do this by using a well-lubricated rectal thermometer or by using infant glycerin suppositories, but these techniques should not be overused. Some infants may have less difficulty passing a stool if given 1 ounce of water once or twice a day. If this does not help, try giving ½ ounce of prune juice mixed with ½ ounce of water once or twice a day. This apparent difficulty with passing stools tends to resolve by three months of age.

Consistency of the Stool

The consistency of the stool is more important than the frequency of the stools. Hard stools indicate a problem. Constipation is the passing of hard stools (which are often small and pebble-like). The number of stools or frequency of stools does not necessarily define constipation. An infant may be constipated even if he or she is passing several stools a day, and an infant who passes only one stool a week may not be constipated. Discuss this issue with your child's doctor.

Initial treatment for constipation in the first few weeks of life may be to offer the infant 1 to 2 ounces of water once or twice a day or to give diluted juice once or twice a day. Diluted prune or pear juice is often very effective in relieving constipation. If the juice or extra water does not help with the constipation, try rectal stimulation or infant glycerin suppositories (or both).

For additional information about constipation, see Chapter 34.

When to Seek Medical Attention

- If there is blood in the stools. (A common cause of blood in the stools is a little tear in the anus. This is known as a fissure.)
- If the stools remain hard despite trying the measures suggested above.

URINATION

A newborn infant's urine may be concentrated (dark) until feeding is well established. When the urine dries on the diaper, it quite frequently has a pinkish color to it. This is not due to blood in the urine but to the presence of urates. The number of wet diapers will give you some indication of how your infant's fluid intake (feeding) is going. Most infants pass urine four to six times a day. (Stools may be a better indicator of the adequacy of fluid intake.)

INFECTIONS AND FEVERS

Newborn infants are especially prone to infections because of an underdeveloped and immature immune system. You may decrease your infant's chances of developing an infection by limiting his or her exposure to the outside world, as infections are usually acquired from other people.

It is especially important to limit your infant's contact with people who have infections such as coughs, colds, and diarrhea.

Insist that people wash their hands before they touch or pick up your infant.

Do not expose your infant to large crowds of people in shopping malls, churches, and other gatherings in the first two to three months of life.

Breast-feeding will also help decrease your infant's chances of developing an infection.

Fever

If your infant develops a fever (defined as a rectal temperature higher than 100.3°F or 38°C), you should seek medical attention. Any fever in the first three months of life needs to be discussed with your child's physician as soon as possible, preferably within a few hours.

Note: An infant does not have to have a fever to be ill. The way your infant is acting and feeding is usually more important than how high his temperature is. If your infant seems unduly lethargic or sleepy or is reluctant to feed, contact his doctor.

For further details on fever, see Chapter 20.

CRYING

All babies cry—even healthy ones cry! Babies cry for many reasons—because they are hungry or tired, are wet or dirty, or just have some vague bodily discomfort. Often we don't know why babies cry; they may just be extra sensitive to their environment.

Many infants cry for up to two hours a day, which is normal. Some infants cry for three or four hours a day, and even this may be normal for them. These infants are often called "colicky."

Colic typically occurs in the evening, a time when many infants have fussy periods. Colicky infants seem to be in pain, cry, and are frequently inconsolable for three to four hours at a time, but the rest of the day they are usually content and well. No one knows what causes colic, and the treatment of it is beyond the scope of this book. After a week or two, you will recognize your infant's typical pattern of crying.

Change in the Type or Length of Crying

If there is a change in the character of your baby's cry, or if your normally content infant starts crying a lot more, you should try to find out the cause. Check your infant's temperature. Your child may be in pain (see Chapter 21) or may be developing an illness.

Your Reactions to a Crying Child

An infant's cry is designed to get attention. Repeated crying often exhausts the parents and leaves them feeling tired, angry, tearful, and inadequate.

- If you feel you cannot cope with or tolerate your baby's crying, it is urgent that you seek help. It is natural for a new parent to feel helpless and even resentful at times.
- Try to remember that the crying is not your fault and it is not your baby's fault. You *do* need a break from your infant.
- If you cannot cope and there is no help at hand, just leave your baby in her crib, close the door, and give yourself "time out." Phone a relative, a friend, or your child's doctor.
- If you are a parent of one of these difficult, colicky infants, I suggest you buy Dr. Harvey Karp's book *The Happiest Baby on the Block,* which goes into great detail on how to calm a crying infant. Better still, buy the DVD with the same title, so you can see exactly how to swaddle and soothe an unhappy baby.

> **CAUTION**
> Never shake an infant! If you should lose control and shake your infant, seek medical care immediately so that permanent brain damage does not occur, and explain to the doctor exactly what happened.

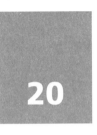

20

Fever

Fever is a common childhood symptom and usually occurs in response to infections, most of which are harmless viral infections. Young children get from 6 to 10 infections a year. Each infection may cause a fever for three to four days, so fevers are a common part of growing up. Fever is the body's normal response to infection and activates the body's immune system to help fight the infection. Many experts feel that fever helps your body fight infection. In other words, fever may be your friend, not your foe!

If your child has a fever, her behavior is a more important indication of how ill she is than the temperature reading on the thermometer.

NORMAL TEMPERATURE RANGES

A child's temperature will vary slightly with age, time of day, and activity. A child has a fever if the rectal temperature is equal to or higher than 100.4°F (38°C), the oral temperature is higher than 99.5°F (37.5°C), or the axillary (armpit) temperature is higher than 99°F (37.2°C).

HIGH FEVERS

Most fevers in childhood, including fevers as high as 104°F (40°C), are usually due to harmless viral infections. The likelihood that a fever is due to a bacterial illness increases with the height of the fever, but even then most high fevers are due to a viral illness. The height of the fever does not necessarily correlate with the severity of the illness. For example, roseola, a viral infection that is not usually serious, may cause a temperature of 104°F or higher, whereas a serious bacterial infection that may require urgent therapy may cause a fever of only 102°F (38.9°C) or lower.

Parents often worry that a high temperature will cause brain damage. It is extremely unlikely that temperatures below 106°F (41.1°C) would cause brain damage. However, a high fever may be an indication of a serious medical problem that needs attention.

> **CAUTION**
> Temperatures higher than 106°F (41.1°C) may be due to heat stress caused by overbundling a child who already has a fever, leaving a child in a hot car, or exercising on a hot day. Heat stroke and heat exhaustion are extremely dangerous and should be treated immediately (see Chapter 57).

Unless your child is overbundled, confined to a heated environment, or exercising excessively, the fever does not continue to rise. Before the temperature reaches 106°F (41.1°C), the body's thermostat will reset the temperature to a lower level and the fever will drop one or two degrees or more. If your child is overclothed or swaddled in blankets, however, the fever could continue to rise to dangerous levels. So keep your child lightly dressed!

YOUR CHILD'S BEHAVIOR

As mentioned earlier, how a child acts is far more important than the height of her fever in determining how ill she is. A child with a temperature of 104°F who is alert and active may be less ill than a child with a temperature of 102°F who is extremely lethargic and not showing any interest in her surroundings.

Many children with a fever are lethargic and irritable. Some children with a high fever may be confused and may even hallucinate. They often breathe faster than usual. However, once the fever is reduced, your child should perk up and be more alert. He may even have periods of playfulness. The breathing rate should return to normal. If your child is not acting normally once the fever is brought down, he should be seen by a doctor because the underlying illness may be serious and require treatment.

Four percent of children may develop a short seizure, or convulsion, with a fever. This is known as a febrile seizure and does not cause brain damage, although it may age the parent! Your doctor should be notified because the cause of the fever should be identified (see Chapter 36).

HOW TO TAKE YOUR CHILD'S TEMPERATURE

A child's temperature may be taken with a glass thermometer (oral or rectal), a digital thermometer, or an ear thermometer. Digital thermometers are much easier, quicker, and safer to use than glass thermometers and are much cheaper than ear thermometers. Temperature-sensitive strips are not very accurate.

Before using a glass thermometer, remember to shake it down well. It should be left in the rectum for at least two minutes, in the mouth for three minutes, or under the arm for four minutes.

A rectal temperature is the only reliable way to measure an infant's temperature in the first three months of life. Rectal temperatures are more reliable for older children as well.

Ear temperatures are acceptable, except in the first six months of life, when they may be less accurate.

CAUTION

Glass thermometers may contain mercury, which is extremely poisonous. This is a serious hazard if a thermometer is broken.

Rectal Temperature

- Place your child on your lap, lying on his stomach.
- Lubricate the thermometer tip using Vaseline or KY Jelly.
- Gently insert the tip into the rectum about one inch. Hold it in place for two minutes if using a glass thermometer. A digital thermometer will beep when it is time to read the temperature.
- Remove the thermometer, read it, and wash it.

Oral Temperature

- Make sure your child has not had hot or cold food or drinks within the past 30 minutes.
- Slide the clean thermometer alongside and under the tongue.
- Hold the thermometer in place and make sure the mouth remains closed.
- If using a glass thermometer, remove and read the temperature after three minutes.
- A digital thermometer will beep when the temperature has been recorded.

Underarm Temperature

- Place the thermometer tip in a dry armpit.
- Hold the arm against the chest for four minutes if using a glass thermometer.

- A digital thermometer will beep when ready to be read.

Treatment

Clothing and Environment

- When your child has a fever, keep her lightly dressed—ideally, stripped down to a diaper or underpants.
- If your child shivers, cover her with a light cotton blanket or cotton T-shirt.
- Keep your child's room comfortably cool.

Fluids

- Encourage your child to drink extra fluids. Give small amounts of liquids frequently.
- If your child is nauseated or vomiting, let her suck on ice chips.

Medicines

- **Never** use aspirin to treat fever in a child. It may cause a serious illness known as Reye's syndrome.
- Use fever-reducing medication (acetaminophen or ibuprofen) if your child is uncomfortable and his temperature is higher than 102°F (38.9°C). Both medications are extremely safe if used appropriately.

- Unless your child's temperature is only mildly elevated, neither acetaminophen nor ibuprofen will return your child's temperature to normal. They will only reduce the fever by two or three degrees—for example, from 104° to 102°.
- Neither medication will work if your child is overbundled or overclothed.
- You may need to give repeated doses of these medications because their effects will wear off after a specified number of hours, and the fever will continue to go up and down as the illness runs its course.
- Give the correct dose of the medication. If you underdose, the medication may not be effective; if you overdose, there is an increased risk of side effects. Refer to the manufacturer's recommendations and to Part Five for dosages.
- Do not continue either medication for longer than three or four days without consulting your child's doctor. Long-term use of acetaminophen may cause liver damage, and ibuprofen may cause stomach upset, stomach bleeding, and kidney damage.
- Some experts feel it is better not to treat a fever because it is helping the body fight the infection.

Acetaminophen

Acetaminophen is available as infant drops, children's suspension, chewable tablets, tablets, and suppositories. To administer the infant drops, use the infant dropper supplied with the medication.

Many over-the-counter medications contain acetaminophen, particularly cold medications. Check to be sure that the medications you choose do not contain acetaminophen, as it is very easy to overdose your child if you are using several different medications.

The temperature-lowering effects of acetaminophen usually last three to four hours.

Ibuprofen

Ibuprofen is available as infant drops, children's suspension, chewable tablets, and tablets. To administer the infant drops, use the infant dropper supplied with the medication.

Ibuprofen is longer-acting than acetaminophen; its effects usually last six to eight hours.

Ibuprofen is not approved for use in the first six months of life.

Sponging

Sponging can be used in addition to medication. Unless your child is allergic to or cannot tolerate acetaminophen and ibuprofen, give him a dose of one of these medications first. Use lukewarm water for the sponging, and never put alcohol in the water.

You may want to sponge your child if

- his temperature is higher than 104°F (40°C);
- he has had seizures during past fevers;
- he is confused and refuses to take medication by mouth (acetaminophen suppositories would be an alternative); or
- he is vomiting and can't keep oral medication down (acetaminophen suppositories would be an alternative).

When to Seek Medical Attention

It is extremely difficult to give hard-and-fast guidelines regarding fevers in children. A child who has a relatively low fever may have a serious cause for the fever that requires early and expert medical care. On the other hand, a child with a high fever may just have a minor viral illness and not require any special care.

Generally speaking, the younger the child, the more seriously you should take the fever. This definitely applies to the first three to six months of life and to a lesser extent to the first two years of life. Some experts feel that any child in the first two years of life who has a fever lasting longer than 24 hours without any obvious cause (such as a "cold," earache, sore throat, or diarrhea) should be seen by a physician.

Here are some guidelines to help you decide when to seek medical care:

- If your child is younger than three months of age and has a rectal temperature equal to or above 100.4°F (38°C).

- If your child has an underlying, preexisting condition such as an abnormality of the urinary tract (e.g., kidney reflux), an abnormality of the immune system, or other chronic disease.
- If your child is excessively lethargic or drowsy or has other worrisome symptoms such as abdominal pain, severe headache, neck stiffness, a rapidly spreading rash, or repeated vomiting and diarrhea.
- If your child still looks very ill after the temperature has been brought down to below 100.4°F (38°C).
- If your child has a fever that lasts longer than three to four days.
- If your child has a seizure. If your child has a short seizure and is acting normally after the seizure, it may not be necessary to see a physician, but it is wise to discuss the episode with one.
- If your child develops a fever during or after a stay in a malarial area, as she may have malaria. Malaria has an incubation period of at least seven days, so if your child gets a fever within the first week of visiting a malarial area, it is unlikely to be due to malaria (see Chapter 15).

Note: How your child acts is more important than how high his fever is. Treat your child, not the fever!

If, despite reading these guidelines, you're still concerned about your child's condition, seek medical care. There is no substitute for getting your child assessed by a competent medical professional.

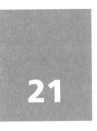

21

Pain

Pain is a common symptom of many childhood illnesses and is discussed in more detail in the chapters on the various causes of pain—for example, earache is discussed in Chapter 8 ("Traveling by Air") and Chapter 25 ("Earaches and Ear Infections"), bellyache in Chapter 33 ("Stomachache, Bellyache, and Abdominal Pain"), and head pain in Chapter 35 ("Headache").

It is especially difficult to determine the cause and severity of pain in children in the first three years of life because they have trouble vocalizing their symptoms and the location of the pain. A young child who pulls and tugs on his ears may be teething, or perhaps he has just "discovered" his ears! Tugging on the ears rarely indicates an ear infection.

In children of any age symptoms may be misleading, as pain is often referred from one part of the body to another. A child with pneumonia may complain of bellyache, and a child with a hip problem may complain of knee pain.

When assessing a young child who is fussy and seems to be in pain, it is important to undress the child completely and examine him or her closely for the cause.

RASH

Are you able to see any rashes? Nonblanching rashes that spread rapidly may be a sign of a serious infection. A nonblanching rash is one that doesn't whiten or fade when pressure is applied to it with a fingertip.

LUMPS OR SWELLING

Can you detect any lumps or swellings? A lump in the groin may indicate a hernia, and a swelling in the scrotum may indicate a strangulated testicle.

BELLY

Is the abdomen distended? Does your child cry or resist when you push on his abdomen? Sit your child on your lap and distract him by telling a story or reading a book while you feel his abdomen.

FINGERS AND TOES

Always check fingers and toes carefully. A thread of cotton or a piece of hair may have become entwined around a finger or toe and be cutting off circulation.

ARMS AND LEGS

If you move your child's limbs, does she cry out in pain? If your child has learned to walk, get her to walk. Watch how she moves her arms and legs. A child who refuses to stand or walk may have a painful hip (e.g., from a hip infection) or a fractured leg (which may be caused by a seemingly minor fall or injury). On the other hand, the child may have a serious abdominal condition such as appendicitis. Children with severe belly pain will usually refuse to hop and if asked to walk will often walk "bent over."

MEDICATIONS

Is your child on any medication? Many cough and cold medications may make children fussy and inconsolable. Some antibiotics (e.g., erythromycin) may cause severe abdominal pain.

 When to Seek Medical Attention

If your child is older than six months, it is acceptable to administer an appropriate dose of acetaminophen or ibuprofen and see if this settles your child. If the pain continues for more than three to six hours or is unresponsive or poorly responsive to the acetaminophen or ibuprofen, medical care should be sought. Seek medical attention immediately if your child is in severe pain or has other symptoms, such as breathing difficulties, repeated vomiting, scrotal swelling, or cold extremities.

22

Teething

The primary (milk) teeth usually begin to erupt between 4 and 12 months of age, but some infants do not get their first teeth until 18 months of age.

WHAT SYMPTOMS AND SIGNS DOES TEETHING CAUSE?

- Most infants who are teething drool more than usual and may get a mild rash on the chin.
- Many infants gnaw or chew on their hands or fists.
- The gums may be swollen or red.
- Some infants are a little fussier than normal and may have a mild elevation in temperature, say to 99° or 100°F.
- Many infants pull or tug on their ears. (If your child does not have a cold or a fever, an ear infection is less likely.)

WHAT SYMPTOMS ARE NOT CAUSED BY TEETHING?

- Fever. Remember, the definition of a fever is a rectal temperature equal to or higher than 100.4°F (38°C). Teething does not cause fevers!
- Diarrhea and colds. These may be present when your child is teething but are not caused by the teething. Teeth appear at the peak ages for early childhood infections. Children between 6 and 24 months of age may get 5 to 10 colds, the occasional bout of diarrhea, respiratory syncytial virus (RSV; see Chapter 26), coughs, and pink eye. All of these may cause a fever, which just happens to occur at the same time that your child is teething.

 Treatment

Most children do not need any treatment for teething symptoms. If your child seems unduly fussy and appears to be bothered by teething, try the following:

- Rub or massage the gums gently with a finger.
- Offer your child a teething ring to gnaw on.
- Offer teething biscuits to chew on. Avoid foods that are choking hazards.
- Some infants will be comforted by drinking a cool liquid. Cold water is a good idea. Avoid juices and other liquids that may cause tooth decay.

- Occasionally, it may be necessary to give your child a dose of acetaminophen (Tylenol) to settle him.
- If your child has a fever or other worrisome symptoms, consult his physician.

23

Colds, Upper Respiratory Infections, and Nasal Congestion

Refer also to Chapter 28.

In the first few years of life, most healthy children get between 5 and 10 colds a year. This is a normal part of growing up and does not mean that your child has something wrong with her immune system.

A typical cold in a young child lasts about 10 days. It usually begins with a low-grade fever (99° to 102°F [37.2° to 38.9°C]), nasal congestion, clear nasal discharge, and fussiness. Usually within two to three days, the fever will settle and the nasal discharge will turn yellowish or green and become thicker. This does *not* mean your child has bacterial sinusitis and needs an antibiotic. (Physicians frequently misdiagnose colds as bacterial infections and prescribe antibiotics inappropriately.) This colored nasal discharge will last for five to eight days before becoming clear again and then will disappear. Often your child will have a loose cough that is worse when lying down, when waking up, or when active. The cough may persist for a week or so after the cold has disappeared and is usually more prominent in the evening.

 Treatment

"Colds" are viral infections and will not respond to antibiotics. In other words, antibiotics should *not* be taken for a "cold." There are no wonder medications for colds, and nothing will turn a 10-day cold into a 5-day one.

There are a number of things you can do, however, to make your child more comfortable:

- Encourage your child to drink fluids. This includes your child's usual formula or milk.
- Use a cool-mist humidifier in the room at night. This will moisten your child's mucous membranes and help to get rid of the mucus. The humidifier should be discontinued once the cold is over.
- If your child has a fever or is very fussy, it may be worth trying a dose of acetaminophen (Tylenol). This may relieve some of the discomfort.
- Over-the-counter cough and cold medicines make very little difference and may make the nasal secretions

thicker. They may also make your child fussy and irritable. It is preferable *not* to use these during the first six months of life.

- If your child's cough is very troubling, try giving her Benadryl in the evening before she goes to bed. This will not get rid of the cough but may decrease it. There are many other over-the-counter cough medications you can try, but none of them are very effective and may have unpleasant side effects.

- If your baby has trouble feeding or breathing and the nasal secretions are very thick, administer nasal saline (saltwater) drops into one nostril at a time and aspirate the mucus with a bulb syringe. Your infant or child will not appreciate this, but it often opens up the nasal passages. It is especially helpful to do this just prior to feeding. Nasal saline drops are extremely safe and may be purchased over the counter or made up at home by dissolving ½ level teaspoon of salt in 8 ounces of water.

- Nasal decongestant drops, such as 0.25% ephedrine nose drops, are often very effective in relieving nasal congestion, but they should never be used for longer than four to five days continuously. Do not exceed the recommended dose. These drops can also have very unpleasant side effects.

When to Seek Medical Attention

You should seek medical care if any of the following occur:

- Your child is lethargic, extremely fussy, or refuses to take liquids.
- Your child appears sicker than you would expect from a simple viral "cold."
- Your child complains of earache or severe headache (a young child or infant is not able to vocalize symptoms; an indication of an earache or severe headache in children of this age may be extreme fussiness).
- Your infant in the first three months of life has a rectal temperature above 100.3°F, or 37.9°C.
- Your child has symptoms suggestive of a complicating bacterial sinusitis:
  - a fever that lasts longer than four continuous days
  - a fever that disappears and then recurs a few days later
  - a fever higher than 103°F (39.4°C)
  - a colored nasal discharge that persists beyond 14 days (Another cause for this is your child may already have another cold!)
  - a daytime cough that lasts longer than 14 days
  - a severe headache or facial or dental pain
  - extreme irritability or lethargy

- Your child seems to have trouble breathing that does not improve after suctioning of the nose (see the "Treatment" section earlier in this chapter).

Note: Just because your child has a yellowish green nasal discharge does *not* mean that he has bacterial sinusitis and needs an antibiotic.

If you are traveling and you are concerned your child may have an ear infection as well as a cold but you do not have access to medical care, do not despair—80 percent of ear infections will resolve without antibiotic treatment (see Chapter 25).

If your child has a persistent, foul-smelling discharge from just one nostril, you should suspect a foreign body in the nose and have your child seen by a doctor.

Allergies are usually the cause of a prolonged clear and watery discharge from both nostrils.

24

Sore Throats

A sore throat (pharyngitis or tonsillitis) is common in childhood and is usually due to a viral infection, although strep (a bacterium) is also a common cause. (See Table 1, pp. 278–79.)

A viral sore throat does not respond to antibiotic treatment, so antibiotics should not be used to treat one. The pain and fever will not go away any faster if an antibiotic is used. Viral sore throats are often accompanied by a cold or a runny nose, a cough, and hoarseness. They tend to come on gradually.

Strep throats are rare under the age of one year. Usually someone with a strep throat does not have a runny nose or cough. A child with strep throat will often appear ill and sometimes have a headache, abdominal pain, and swollen and tender glands in the neck. Another clue that the sore throat may be due to strep is a faint reddish rash that is usually more noticeable in the groin, armpits, and elbow creases. Strep throats often come on suddenly, and sometimes there is a history of contact with someone with strep.

A child with a strep or viral sore throat may have a fever, and white spots may be seen on the tonsils. The presence of white spots on the tonsils, however, does not necessarily mean strep. The only reliable way to tell the difference between a viral sore throat and a strep throat is with a rapid strep test or a throat culture.

A fairly common cause of a viral sore throat in a young child (six months to four years of age) is herpangina, also called hand, foot, and mouth disease (see Chapter 26, p. 289).

 ## *Treatment*

Neither viral nor strep throat is a medical emergency. Strep throat does not have to be treated right away.

Home treatment consists of giving analgesics (acetaminophen or ibuprofen) and fluids. Sucking on ice pops or ice chips is often soothing. An older child (six years of age and over) may be helped by sucking on lozenges or gargling with salt water. (Mix ½ level teaspoon of salt in 8 ounces of water.)

Antibiotics are indicated for strep throats but not for viral sore throats. One of the hallmarks of a strep throat is that the patient improves rapidly (usually within 24 hours) after antibiotics are started.

When to Seek Medical Attention

If you suspect strep throat, have your child seen by a medical professional within two to three days. However, if you are traveling and have no access to medical care or antibiotics, don't panic: most strep throats will get better even without an antibiotic; the symptoms just take longer to go away. If your child is not improving in three to four days or is becoming sicker, seek medical care.

The main reason antibiotics are used to treat strep throat is to prevent the later development of rheumatic fever. This is fortunately very rare in the United States. Studies indicate that as long as antibiotics are started within nine days of the onset of the illness, rheumatic fever should be prevented. The other reasons antibiotics are used to treat strep throat are to limit the spread of the infection and to make the patient feel better sooner. If you are traveling and do not have access to medical care, symptomatic care may be sufficient.

Extremely rarely, strep may cause an abscess to develop in one or both of the tonsils and cause obstruction of the airway. If this happens, the person will be seriously ill, be drooling, and have trouble swallowing and probably difficulty breathing. Urgent medical care is needed.

Remember, four out of five sore throats are due to viruses and do not require antibiotic treatment.

Please help your child's doctor to practice good medicine by not insisting that an antibiotic be prescribed for probable viral illnesses—colds, most sore throats, and bronchitis.

Table 1. Differences between Viral and Strep Sore Throats

Viral	Strep
Frequency	
Very common, accounts for 80 percent of sore throats	Common, but less common than viral sore throats
Age	
Any	Rare in the first year of life Not common in the second year of life
History of strep contact	
Not usually present	Often present
Onset	
Usually gradual	Frequently sudden
Fever	
May or may not be present	Almost always present
Other features	
Nasal congestion, cough, and hoarseness often present	May have headache and abdominal pain, typical strep rash, and/or enlarged and tender neck glands
Throat findings	
May have white spots on tonsils	May have white spots on tonsils Throat often a beefy red color May have minute red spots on hard and soft palate

Continued

Table 1. Differences between Viral and Strep Sore Throats

continued

Viral	Strep
Treatment	
Analgesics and fluids TLC	Antibiotics, analgesics, and fluids
Response to antibiotic	
None	Rapidly gets better on antibiotics

25

Earaches and Ear Infections

There are two common types of ear infection: middle-ear infection (otitis media), and outer-ear infection (otitis externa, also known as "swimmer's ear"). It is common to have ear pain with both types of infections.

Many young children complain of earaches even in the absence of ear disease. The apparent earache is commonly due to other causes such as teething or a sore throat. Pulling or tugging on the ear by infants and young children is a very unreliable sign of ear disease and rarely indicates that an ear infection is present. Children older than three to four years of age can usually report accurately when they have an earache.

MIDDLE-EAR INFECTION (OTITIS MEDIA)

Infection of the middle ear is the most common type of ear infection and the most common cause of ear pain. It is particularly common in infants and young children and is usually associated with a cold or upper respiratory infection (URI). The pain is often worse when the child is lying down.

Common symptoms are fever and fussiness, the latter often being worse at night. The symptoms of the associated viral URI, such as nasal stuffiness, often are more impressive. Some children have no apparent symptoms at all, and the ear infection is discovered incidentally at a routine medical examination.

 Treatment

- Analgesics (usually acetaminophen or ibuprofen) in appropriate doses.
- Antibiotics. Even though antibiotics are usually prescribed for middle-ear infections, most of these infections will get better without antibiotics. In many countries antibiotics are not routinely prescribed for ear infections. However, the infection and symptoms will usually resolve faster with antibiotics. They should probably be used if
  - your child is younger than two years of age;
  - your child has a fever above 102°F (38.9°C);
  - your child has a severe earache; or
  - your child's symptoms last longer than two to three days.

Sometimes the eardrum perforates as a result of pressure behind the drum, and yellowish pus may discharge from the ear canal. Although this discharge of pus is often alarming to parents, a perforated eardrum is not an emergency, and the pain should immediately lessen. The eardrum will usually heal on its own within a few days, but you should follow up with your child's doctor to check that it has healed completely.

At times a child will wake in the middle of the night with a severe earache. This may be helped with an appropriate dose of acetaminophen or ibuprofen, by propping up the head of the bed (e.g., with extra pillows) so that the child's head is elevated, and by instilling drops of warm oil (such as olive oil) in the affected ear. Do *not* put oil drops in the affected ear if the eardrum is already perforated or if your child has had tubes inserted.

Middle-ear infections are not contagious, but the cold that leads to the ear infection is contagious.

OUTER-EAR INFECTION (OTITIS EXTERNA), OR "SWIMMER'S EAR"

Swimmer's ear is an infection of the ear canal that leads from the outer ear to the eardrum. It is more common in older children and more common during the summer months, as this usually is the time they are swimming.

Symptoms include earache, a sense of fullness in the ear, and often itching. The pain is increased if the ear lobe is pulled downward or pressure is applied to the tab covering the opening of the ear canal. This is a good way to distinguish swimmer's ear from a middle-ear infection. At times the pain may be very severe.

Prevention

Swimmer's ear tends to be recurrent, and prevention is extremely important. Keep the ears as dry as possible:

- After swimming, have your child shake his head and jump up and down to get rid of excess water in the ears.
- Dry the outer part of the ear canals carefully and gently, using a Q-tip.
- Administer eardrops. These may be purchased over the counter or made by mixing equal quantities of rubbing alcohol and white vinegar. Instill five to seven drops in each ear at the end of each day that your child has been swimming.

Note: Do not use this homemade preparation if the ear canal is already inflamed (it will sting), if your child's eardrum is perforated, or if tympanostomy tubes are in place.

Treatment

- Analgesics, as listed for middle-ear infection (otitis media).
- Eardrops, either over the counter or prescription. Sometimes oral antibiotics are needed as well. If the pain per-

sists beyond 24 to 48 hours despite treatment or is very severe, your child should be seen by a physician.

While your child has swimmer's ear, he should not submerge his head when swimming. Try to keep his ears as dry as possible. It is probably wise to avoid swimming for two to four days.

26

Common Infections Your Child Is Sure to Get

COLDS AND VIRAL UPPER RESPIRATORY INFECTIONS

Most children get between 5 and 10 colds a year in the preschool years, making these the most common infections of childhood (see Chapter 23).

RESPIRATORY SYNCYTIAL VIRUS

Almost all children have had an infection caused by a respiratory syncytial virus (RSV) by two years of age. These infections can affect the lungs, causing bronchiolitis (a type of bronchitis) and pneumonia, or the upper respiratory tract, causing rhinitis (nose infection), croup, laryngitis, and otitis media (middle-ear infection). In the first two to three months of life, the initial manifestation of RSV may be apnea (a stop in breathing). RSV infections tend to cluster in the winter and early spring.

The younger the child, the more likely it is that RSV will affect the lungs and cause more severe illness. Infants with RSV bronchiolitis or pneumonia often wheeze and have difficulty breathing (fast respiratory rate, flaring and retractions). These infants also usually have a very congested nose that contributes to the breathing difficulty. Older children are more likely to be less ill and have involvement mainly of their upper respiratory tract. They may also wheeze but do not tend to have such severe respiratory distress as the infants.

The diagnosis of an RSV infection is suggested by the presence of one of the illnesses mentioned above, particularly bronchiolitis, with wheezing and nasal congestion, occurring at the typical time of the year. Children can get RSV infections more than once, but subsequent infections tend to be milder.

 Treatment

Infants with severe disease may require hospitalization and need oxygen therapy, close attention to their fluid intake, and skilled nursing. Antibiotics do not help RSV because it is a viral illness. Most children do not require hospitalization, but they may need smaller and more frequent feeds, nasal suctioning, and close observation for worsening respiratory distress (see Chapter 62, p. 556). Some children with bronchiolitis respond to nebulized bronchodilators.

CROUP

The term *croup* usually refers to a viral infection of the larynx (voice box) and trachea (windpipe), which leads to a barky cough (resembles the barking of a seal) and stridor (a high-pitched, raspy noise on inspiration). The airways narrow with croup, and this may lead to severe breathing difficulties (see Chapter 62, p. 556).

Croup tends to come on suddenly at night and may be extremely frightening for everybody. The barky cough is very typical, and stridor may be present as well. Signs of respiratory distress such as nasal flaring and retractions may be present. Your child may have a fever.

 Treatment

If your child has just a mild case of croup (hoarseness and a croupy cough), he may require only adequate fluids, a cool-mist vaporizer in his bedroom, and possibly a dose or two of Tylenol or ibuprofen for fever. Don't overdress your child. You may want to sleep in the same room as your child because croup can worsen rapidly. If your child has a more severe case of croup, try the following:

- Cold air. Croup often responds to breathing cold air. Wrap your child up warmly and go outside into the cold night air and walk around for 5 to 10 minutes. If it is not cold outside, hold your child in front of an open refrigerator or freezer door, and let him inhale the cold air.

- Warm, moist air. Croup may also respond to breathing warm, moist air, but this is not usually as effective as breathing in cold air. Take your child into the bathroom and turn on the hot faucets and steam up the bathroom. Sit with your child in the bathroom until her symptoms have eased.
- Medications. If your child has a nebulizer, it may be worth trying a nebulization of albuterol or saline, as this may lead to some improvement. High-dose inhaled corticosteroids, either by nebulization or metered dose inhaler (MDI), may also help. If you have oral steroids at home, administer an appropriate dose, but do not expect to see any benefit for two to three hours. Discuss all these medication options with your child's physician.

In most cases, croup will settle down by daybreak; in the morning your child may appear just fine but will still have a barky cough and hoarseness. Croup often tends to recur every night for three to four nights, however, so it is worth contacting your child's physician to discuss treatment to lessen the symptoms. Even if you got through the night without using steroids, your pediatrician may suggest using them to abort or lessen the symptoms, which are sure to recur the next night. It is also a good idea to use a cool-mist vaporizer in your child's bedroom for the next few days. Encourage fluids.

When to Seek Medical Attention

If none of the treatment suggestions help and your child is having significant breathing problems, you should head for the nearest ER, as your child may need extra oxygen and an epinephrine nebulization. If your child turns blue, passes out, or stops breathing, call 911 immediately. Start CPR if necessary.

HERPANGINA, OR HAND, FOOT, AND MOUTH DISEASE

Herpangina is an infection caused by the Coxsackie virus. It is particularly common in young children in the summer and fall. Symptoms include fever, a sore throat due to ulcers in the back of the mouth, drooling, and a reluctance to drink or eat. Other symptoms that are often present are loose stools and a rash on the hands and feet and sometimes also on the trunk. Children with this infection are often very whiny and miserable.

Treatment

Treatment consists of analgesics (Tylenol, Advil, or Motrin) for fever and pain; a bland, soothing diet; and the avoidance of fluids and foods that may cause pain (salty or acidic foods). Some physicians prescribe a mixture of Benadryl and Maalox to coat the mouth to relieve the pain.

The entire illness may last five to seven days, but the first three to four days are the worst with regard to the fever, drooling, and misery. Infants and young children may become dehydrated because of diarrhea and a reluctance to drink.

STREP THROAT

See Chapter 24.

ROSEOLA

This viral illness usually occurs between 6 and 18 months of age. It begins with a fever that is often very high (104° to 105°F) and that lasts three to five days. In some children the first sign of roseola may be a febrile seizure, a short seizure that is triggered by a fever. The diagnosis of roseola is not usually made until the fourth or fifth day, when a rash *appears* and the fever *disappears*. The rash consists of flat, faint pink or red spots that cover the body. The rash lasts from a few hours to days, but at this stage your child will probably be feeling much better. No treatment is necessary, apart from management of the fever in the early stages.

GASTROENTERITIS, AND DIARRHEA AND VOMITING

See Chapter 31.

ORAL THRUSH

This is a yeast infection of the mouth caused by the fungus *Candida albicans*. It is particularly common in the first year of life but may also be seen in children on antibiotics or on inhaled steroids. Infants often have a white tongue, especially after feeding. If this persists for some time after feeding, and if the white plaques extend to the inside of the cheeks and lips and on to the gums, a yeast infection is present. Milk curds tend to wipe off easily, but thrush tends to cling to the mucous membranes. Sometimes there may be an associated yeast diaper rash.

 Treatment

Treatment consists of antifungal medication, commonly mycostatin (Nystatin). It is important to sterilize pacifiers and the nipples of feeding bottles. Breast-feeding mothers should also treat their nipples with an antifungal agent. Oral thrush tends to recur, and occasionally a more potent systemic antifungal agent may be necessary.

FIFTH DISEASE, OR
"SLAPPED CHEEK DISEASE"

This illness, also called erythema infectiosum, is caused by the human parvovirus B19 and is most common in school-aged children. In the early stages of the infection very few symptoms are present—perhaps just a low-grade fever and a few body aches. A few days later, however, the child will develop a bright red rash on her face, making her cheeks look like they have been slapped. Often a lacy rash may be present on the upper arms and thighs, also. Once the "slapped face" rash appears, the child is not usually ill and is not contagious. Later symptoms include joint pain.

The diagnosis is seldom made in the early stages of the disease when the person is contagious. The greatest risk is to an unborn fetus. If a pregnant woman is exposed to a person with fifth disease, she should consult her obstetrician.

No treatment is usually necessary for the child with fifth disease.

> *Note:* Another illness that may cause very red cheeks is strep infection. However, children with strep infection usually have a fever and are ill when their cheeks are red.

MIDDLE-EAR INFECTIONS (OTITIS MEDIA)

See Chapter 25.

OUTER-EAR INFECTIONS (OTITIS EXTERNA), OR SWIMMER'S EAR

See Chapter 25.

SINUSITIS

Most children and adults who are diagnosed with sinusitis probably have a cold or a viral upper respiratory infection. Bacterial sinusitis usually follows a cold and is caused by the same bacteria that cause a middle-ear infection. Antibiotics may be needed.

See Chapters 23 and 28.

IMPETIGO

See Chapters 14 and 18.

HOW MANY INFECTIONS ARE TOO MANY INFECTIONS: Does My Child Have Something Wrong with His Immune System?

Many preschool children get 8 to 10 infections a year. These include simple upper respiratory infections, ear infections, pink eye, and bouts of vomiting and diarrhea caused by gastroenteritis. This number may be even higher among children in day care. Toward the end of winter, when your child is on his fifth or sixth cold of the winter, and has had perhaps a similar number of ear infections, you may well be wondering whether he has a defect in his immune system. The following illnesses and findings may suggest problems with the immune system:

- A child who is not thriving (i.e., not gaining weight and growing).

- A child who is not active and not interested in his environment.
- Infections due to unusual organisms.
- Infections that do not respond to appropriate antibiotics, or a need for intravenous antibiotics to clear infections that usually respond to oral antibiotics.
- Recurrent skin abscesses.
- Recurrent pneumonias. (The most common cause of recurrent "pneumonias" or recurrent "bronchitis," however, is asthma.)
- Persistent thrush in the mouth of a child not on antibiotics.
- A family history of immune deficiency.

If any of these situations apply to your child, a visit to your child's physician may be indicated.

27

Antibiotics

Antibiotics are one of the most significant advances in modern medicine. Along with immunizations, they have greatly reduced infectious diseases. Antibiotics do have their limitations, however, and they are not without side effects. Abuse of antibiotics has contributed to the development of resistance to antibiotics by bacteria. Some bacteria are now resistant to almost all antibiotics.

Because of the possibility of side effects and the problem of antibiotic resistance, antibiotics should be taken only for bacterial infections. *They are not effective for treating viral diseases.* And most infectious diseases (and fevers) in childhood are due to viruses, not to bacteria. Common viral illnesses in childhood include the following:

- Colds, most upper respiratory infections.
- Most sore throats. (Strep throat, which is due to the bacterium called streptococcus, is responsible for only about 20 percent of sore throats.)

- Gastroenteritis (which causes vomiting and diarrhea). In the United States gastroenteritis is most commonly caused by viruses.
- Bronchitis, which is usually caused by viruses. (Bronchitis in older adults, especially if they are smokers, may be caused by bacteria.)

In other words, most of the infections listed above should not be treated with antibiotics. Antibiotics will not make the disease go away any faster and may just cause unpleasant side effects.

COMMON SIDE EFFECTS

- Diarrhea. Usually the more powerful the antibiotic, the worse the diarrhea.
- Nausea, vomiting, and abdominal pain.
- Diaper rashes, often due to a combination of irritation from diarrhea and overgrowth of yeast (fungal infection).
- Vaginal yeast infections (at any age).
- Rashes.
- Bacterial resistance. This may be one of the worst side effects, because if it occurs, the next time your child is prescribed an antibiotic, it may not work. Overuse of antibiotics creates resistant bacteria. Each time you take antibiotics, the sensitive bacteria, including beneficial bacteria, are killed, and the resistant ones are left to grow and multiply. These bacteria may cause your next infection and may spread to those around you, causing illness that is difficult to treat.

Antibiotics may have many other, far more severe, side effects. Fortunately these are rare. They include severe allergic reactions including anaphylaxis (generalized rashes and swelling of the face and body, difficulty breathing and swallowing, a drop in blood pressure, collapse, and even death), joint pain and swelling, liver disease (hepatitis), and kidney failure.

 Prevention of Side Effects

- Take antibiotics only for legitimate reasons—in other words, for bacterial infections that require antibiotic treatment.
- Give your child yogurt that contains live culture, or probiotics, when she is on an antibiotic. This may decrease the risk of secondary yeast infections.
- If your child gets diarrhea, limit fruit juices. Encourage her to eat bananas and rice and offer more liquids (see Chapter 31).
- Take the antibiotic as prescribed. Complete the course. Do not keep some of the antibiotic to self-medicate future infections. Not taking all of the antibiotic as prescribed can mean failure to cure the infection and can lead to the growth of bacteria that are antibiotic resistant.

Unfortunately, some physicians prescribe antibiotics for viral infections. They do so for a variety of reasons, including the following:

- Time constraints. It takes only a few seconds to write a prescription for an antibiotic but 5 to 10 minutes to explain why you are not prescribing an antibiotic.
- Misdiagnosis. A physician might misdiagnose a cold as a bacterial sinusitis because of the common misconception that a yellow or green nasal discharge indicates a bacterial infection.
- To prevent a viral infection from developing into a bacterial one. Using antibiotics, however, seldom prevents this from happening.
- To avoid being sued. We live in a litigious society where, if the patient has a bad outcome, someone will be held responsible. Physicians are not infallible. Sometimes, what had been diagnosed as viral infection may have been a bacterial infection and would have resolved faster or with fewer complications on an antibiotic.

Please help your physician to practice good medicine by not insisting on an antibiotic for viral infections.

28

Coughs

A cough is a common symptom in childhood. Its most common cause is a cold. A cough is a protective reflex—it ejects foreign material and secretions from the airway. Coughs often disturb the parent more than the child!

A cough is called "chronic" if it lasts longer than three weeks. The following are common causes for chronic coughs in childhood and adolescence:

- Repeated colds
- Asthma
- Sinusitis
- Pertussis (whooping cough), which is often not diagnosed because of the common misconception by physicians that it is only a disease of infancy. (In fact, it is not unusual in adolescents and adults.)
- Exposure to tobacco smoke
- Allergies

There are many different types of coughs and even more causes of coughs. The following are some of the more common causes of coughing in children.

COUGHS FROM COLDS

The cough associated with the common cold is typically a loose, "junky" cough. It lasts for the duration of the cold (7 to 10 days) and often for one week afterward. The cough will occur on and off throughout the day but is usually more severe in the early evening and in the first hour or two after going to bed.

The cough tends to subside in the middle of the night, but as soon as your child awakens and stands up in the morning, the cough will return and be more severe for an hour or two. Frequently, the mucus is swallowed and then vomited up later.

When you hold your child, his chest may feel "rattly," and you may think that the cold is in the chest or that he has pneumonia. The rattle that you are feeling is the vibration and gurgling of the mucus in the back of the throat that is being transmitted to the chest. If your child is not in respiratory distress (breathing very fast or retracting) when the coughing bouts are over, it is less likely that he has pneumonia. For a discussion on retracting and assessment of respiratory distress, see Chapter 62.

During coughing bouts, your child may become red in the face and may even seem to be choking on the mucus. This is common and will settle when the mucus is swallowed or coughed up or vomited.

It is common for a child to have 5 to 10 colds a year, so it is quite possible that he may cough for 10 to 14 weeks a year! Many colds occur back to back, resulting in coughs that appear to last for three to five weeks. This makes recurrent colds the most common cause of a chronic cough. This is particularly likely if your child is in day care.

 ### *Treatment*

A cough associated with a cold usually does not require specific treatment.

- It is important to keep your child well hydrated.
- Using a cool-mist humidifier in the room at night for a week or two may help. The humidifier should be discontinued once the cold has resolved.
- If the cough is extremely troublesome, an appropriate dose of Benadryl may help to suppress the cough. There are many other cough medicines on the market, and ones containing dextromethorphan are usually safe. Most cough medicines are not particularly effective in stopping coughs: they are usually of more help to the company that manufactures them, or the pharmacy that sells them, than to the person who takes them!
- In young infants, using nasal saline drops and a bulb aspirator is often very useful in keeping the nose clear and so enabling your child to breathe more easily.

COUGHS FROM SINUSITIS

Sinusitis is also a very common cause of coughing. The features of a sinusitis cough are often very similar to those of the cough associated with a cold: the cough occurs when lying down and often has a loose, "junky" quality (see also Chapter 23). However, with sinusitis, the cough tends to be more troublesome during the daytime and often persists for longer.

Often there is not much drainage from the nose, and you may think that the mucus that your child coughs up is coming from the lungs. However, with sinusitis, the mucus usually drains from the sinuses and down the back of the throat. The cough reflex is then triggered, and the mucus comes back out through the mouth.

Symptoms that suggest your child's cold has turned into bacterial sinusitis are the duration of the cough (longer than 10 to 14 days) and a persistent daytime cough. The color of the mucus is not helpful in diagnosing sinusitis because it tends to be yellow or green with both a viral cold and sinusitis. Facial pain or painful teeth are sometimes present in older children and adults with bacterial sinusitis. Halitosis (bad breath), high fever or persistent fever, or a fever that disappears and then recurs also suggest the possibility of bacterial sinusitis. Children with bacterial sinusitis also tend to be sicker than those with "just a cold," but this is not always so. Some children with sinusitis are just "below par" and have very few other symptoms.

Treatment

A sinus cough will respond to an appropriate antibiotic, but it may take a week or two for the antibiotic to relieve the symptoms. Antibiotics may need to be continued for three to four weeks to totally clear the sinusitis. Additional medications that may be necessary include oral antihistamines and decongestants and decongestant nose drops. Occasionally a nasal steroid spray may be necessary, not only to help cure the sinusitis but to prevent a recurrence.

Like ear infections, most cases of sinusitis will resolve without antibiotics, but the symptoms may persist longer. A child with a persistent severe headache, a persistent fever, or tenderness over the forehead or cheekbones should definitely been seen by her doctor.

COUGHS FROM CROUP

A croup cough has a distinctive barking quality, suggestive of the barking of a seal. Your child may be in significant respiratory distress. See Chapter 26, p. 287, for a more detailed description and treatment measures.

COUGHS FROM ALLERGIES

Allergies may cause a cough that is due to a postnasal drip or irritation of the upper airway, or they may cause a cough by triggering asthma. If the cause of the cough is an allergy to house dust mites, the symptoms may be worse at night and the early morning. Hoarseness is sometimes present in the morning. Often nasal stuffiness is present as well. A cough due to allergies to pollens tends to be seasonal.

 ### *Treatment*

An allergic cough will respond to removal of the trigger and to the administration of an antihistamine such as Benadryl or one of the newer, nonsedating antihistamines. Nasal steroid sprays and occasionally oral steroids may be needed. Montelukast (Singulair) may also be helpful in treating the cough associated with allergies, as well as other allergy symptoms. Paying attention to the environment and avoidance of allergens is very important. Immunotherapy ("shots") may be needed and is often very successful if done correctly.

COUGHS FROM ASTHMA

Asthma is probably the second most common cause of a chronic cough in childhood. It tends to be worse in the middle of the night (12 midnight to 3 a.m.) and after exercise.

Note: Your child does not have to be wheezing to have asthma.

A child who has recently had a cold and continues to cough in the middle of the night for several weeks after the cold has run its course likely has asthma. In contrast, the cough associated with a cold usually lasts only two to three weeks.

A child with asthma often has had eczema in the past, and frequently other family members have allergic diseases such as asthma, allergic rhinitis, and hay fever. Children with asthma are frequently misdiagnosed as having pneumonia or bronchitis.

The many triggers for asthma include upper respiratory infections, cold air, exercise, allergens, and irritants such as cigarette smoke. Exercise in cold air is a particularly potent trigger for an asthmatic cough.

 Treatment

An asthma cough will respond to appropriate asthma medications. These should include a preventative/controller drug, as well as a rescue drug. It is also essential to identify and avoid asthma triggers. (See section on asthma in Chapter 5.)

COUGHS FROM IRRITATION

An "irritation" cough is often started by a viral infection, but then the cough continues to be triggered once the underlying viral infection has resolved. Triggers include cigarette smoke, perfumes, paint fumes, smoke from fires and stoves, and cold air.

This type of cough tends to be dry and does not produce mucus.

Treatment

Remove the trigger. Humidifying the air, sucking on cough lozenges, and cough suppressants often help. Keep your child away from cigarette smoke.

COUGHS FROM FOREIGN BODIES

If your child starts coughing after choking on food, he may have inhaled some food. This is particularly likely when eating foods such as peanuts, raisins, and hot dogs. Your child may also inhale foreign bodies such as small toys and beads.

 Treatment

If you suspect your child has inhaled a foreign body, seek medical attention immediately (see Chapter 63).

COUGHS WHILE TRAVELING

It is not unusual to develop a cough while traveling. Causes may include

- the dry air of the aircraft cabin;
- exposure to cigarette smoke, noxious fumes, and so on;
- the development of an upper respiratory infection (a cold);
- activation of preexisting asthma;

- altitude sickness if you are at a high altitude (see Chapter 11); or
- a chest infection, such as bronchitis or pneumonia.

When to Seek Medical Attention

If you have spent some time in a lesser-developed country and you or your child develops a chronic cough that persists for some weeks after you return home, seek medical care. Tuberculosis may be the cause.

PSYCHOGENIC COUGH

Some children may have a cough that has a psychological basis. The cardinal feature of a psychological cough is that it disappears once the child is asleep. Many coughs, especially coughs due to asthma and reflux, get worse at night. A psychological cough magically disappears once the child falls asleep. This type of cough often has a honking quality and is more prominent if there is an audience. Determining why a child has a psychogenic cough requires teamwork between the parents and the child's doctor.

SEVERAL TYPES OF COUGH AT THE SAME TIME

Many children have more than one cause of a cough and more than one type of cough at any one time. For example, an asthmatic child with a cold may have a loose, "junky" cough in the evening when he first lies down, followed by a tight cough between midnight and 3 a.m. As he awakens in the morning, the loose, "junky" cough returns. Later on that day, the asthmatic child will often cough with exercise. Children with asthma frequently have nasal allergies and sinusitis as well. They are also more likely to have gastroesophageal reflux (regurgitation of stomach contents up the esophagus, or "swallowing tube").

A child with a cold or postnasal drip will often cough more with exercise.

Children exposed to cigarette smoke cough more than other children. Exposure to cigarette smoke makes all coughs worse and makes them last longer.

When to Seek Medical Attention

- If your child has signs of respiratory distress, such as breathing very fast, retractions, and so on (see Chapter 62).
- If you suspect an inhaled foreign body.
- If a cough lasts longer than three weeks.
- For a cough during the first few months of life.
- If your child is sicker than you would expect just from the cough.

IN SUMMARY

By far the most common cause of a cough is a cold. Several colds in a row often lead to a cough that seems to last for months. Remember, coughs are often protective. They stop the mucus from going down into the chest.

29

Nosebleeds

Nosebleeds occur frequently in children and have many causes. The most common cause is nose picking. Other causes include colds, allergies, sinusitis, and exposure to very dry air, especially in heated homes in winter. Nosebleeds are very common at high altitudes because of the dry, cold air.

When you suction your infant's nose with a bulb aspirator (to help clear the nasal passages), a small amount of bleeding may occur.

 Prevention

- If the air in your home is too dry, use a humidifier and try to keep the humidity around 40 percent. Remember, if your house or bedroom has high humidity for prolonged periods, you will encourage the growth of molds and replication of house dust mites, which in turn may lead to allergies.

- Use saltwater (saline) nose drops frequently while traveling. The dry air of the aircraft cabin and dusty air while traveling on country roads will lead to a dry and stuffy nose. Each person should have their own bottle of saline drops.
- If your child has repeated nosebleeds, coat the lower part of the nasal septum (the part of the nose dividing each nostril) twice a day with a petroleum jelly (e.g., Vaseline).
- Discourage nose picking.

 ## *Treatment*

Have your child sit up, lean forward, and breathe through the mouth. Pinch the soft fleshy part of the nose tightly closed for about 10 minutes. (Hold a basin under the chin to catch any blood or mucus that drips through the mouth.) After the nosebleed has stopped, instruct your child not to pick his nose or to blow it too vigorously, otherwise the bleeding may restart.

 ## *When to Seek Medical Attention*

- If your child's nose continues to bleed after applying pressure to the nose for 20 minutes. (If you do not have access to medical care and you have nasal decongestant nose drops such as Neosynephrine or oxymetazoline [Afrin], use these, as they constrict blood vessels and will often help to stop the nosebleed. You may need to use two or three times the recommended dose to stop the bleeding. Never use nasal decongestant drops or sprays for longer than five days.)

- If your child has a foul-smelling or bloody discharge from one nostril for some days. This may be due to a foreign body up the nose.
- If your child has a tendency to bleed in other areas as well—for example, from the gums or into the skin.
- If your child gets recurrent nosebleeds despite using preventive measures.

30

Eye Problems

Eye problems in children are a common cause for concern among parents and a common reason for visits to the doctor. Discussed below are some of the more common eye problems seen during childhood.

When parents, teachers, and day care providers talk of "pink eye," they are usually referring to an infection involving the conjunctiva, the transparent outermost covering of the front of the eye and the inner eyelid. The correct medical term for this type of "pink eye" is infectious conjunctivitis. It is important to realize that there are many causes of pink or red eyes besides infectious conjunctivitis, some of which are far more serious than infectious conjunctivitis.

What Causes Pink or Red Eyes?

- Inflammation of the conjunctiva (conjunctivitis)
  - Infectious conjunctivitis is the most common cause of "pink eye" and is discussed in detail below.
  - Allergic conjunctivitis is more common in people who have allergies. It usually involves both eyes and is very itchy. If an eye discharge is present, it is usually clear. Common triggers are pollens, which tend to cause seasonal allergies, and cats, which usually cause problems all year. The child with allergic conjunctivitis usually has other allergy symptoms, such as nasal congestion and itching and frequent sneezing.
  - Chemicals and irritants may also cause red eyes. Common causes are shampoos, soap, and chlorine. Most people can remember getting red and sore eyes after swimming in an overchlorinated swimming pool! A person may also get red and irritated eyes when exposed to a smoky environment.
- Inflammation of the cornea (keratitis). The cornea is the clear part of the eye in front of the pupil (the dark spot in the center of the eye) and the iris (the colored part of the eye).
- Inflammation of the iris (iritis).
- Raised pressure within the eye (glaucoma).
- Eye injuries.
- Foreign bodies.
- Tumors.

INFECTIOUS CONJUNCTIVITIS

This is the most common cause of "pink eye" and is very contagious. It may be caused by viruses, bacteria, or a combination of the two. Children with infectious conjunctivitis usually have red eyes and often an eye discharge. On awakening in the morning, the eyelids are often matted together. Sometimes the child may be sicker and have a fever as well as other symptoms, such as sore throat or earache.

Good hygiene is important to prevent the spread of infectious conjunctivitis to other family members.

- Wash your hands well after touching your child's eyes and after instilling eyedrops or ointment into the eyes.
- Wash your child's hands frequently.
- Use disposable cotton balls to clean your child's eyes instead of a washcloth.
- Use a separate washcloth and towel for your child.
- Avoid kissing your child on the face while he has conjunctivitis.
- Do not share utensils or food while your child is infected.

The highly contagious nature of infectious conjunctivitis is a concern for teachers and day care personnel, and a child who has it may be sent home from school or day care to avoid spreading it to other children.

It is often very difficult to differentiate between infectious conjunctivitis caused by bacteria, which responds quickly and dramatically to antibacterial eyedrops or ointment, and infectious conjunctivitis caused by viruses, which usually gets better more slowly and often without any specific treatment.

In practice there is so much overlap between bacterial and viral conjunctivitis that it may be impossible to tell the difference between the two. This is one of the reasons why both are usually treated with antibacterial eyedrops or ointment. Sometimes oral antibiotics are needed as well. Most day care centers and schools will allow your child back once he has been on treatment for 24 hours.

 Treatment

Topical Medications

These include eyedrops and eye ointments. A prescription is needed for these. Eyedrops are generally easier to instill. Ointments are often prescribed for infants. These medications are usually used three times a day. Twice a day may be sufficient if one of the newer preparations is used, as these are very fast acting and effective.

The duration of treatment will depend on the cause of the conjunctivitis, the severity, and the response to treatment and will usually be from three to seven days. It is generally a good idea to continue the treatment for a day or two after the eye discharge has cleared.

It is easier to instill the medication if you first clean away the eye discharge with a wet cotton ball.

Putting eyedrops or eye ointment in the eyes of young

Table 2. Differences between Bacterial and Viral Infectious Conjunctivitis

	Bacterial	Viral
Age:	Usually younger (average 3½ years).	Usually older (average 8½ years).
Eye discharge:	Usually thick and "goopy." Often yellow or green. Eyes often glued together in the morning.	Usually thinner and more watery.
Associated illnesses:	May also have an ear infection.	May also have a sore throat.

children can be quite a challenge. Fortunately, most of the newer preparations do not sting, but despite this you may need two well-coordinated adults to instill the medication. If your child refuses to open her eyes, put one or two drops of the medication in the corner of her eye while she is lying down. When she opens her eyes, the drops will go in.

Oral Antibiotics

These are often prescribed for associated ear infections. They are also used alone for children who resist topical medication. They seldom work as fast as topical treatment. Sometimes both oral and topical antibiotics are prescribed.

IF YOU HAVE NO ACCESS TO MEDICAL CARE or medication, it may be reassuring to know that most cases of infectious conjunctivitis will get better on their own but just take longer to do so. Even the ear infection that is often associated with infectious conjunctivitis frequently resolves on its own. Bathing the eyes with cotton balls soaked in clean water or in a weak salt solution (½ level teaspoon of table salt to 1 cup of water) will soothe the eyes and help clear away the discharge.

Note: Do not use contact lenses when the eyes are infected.

Never put steroid eyedrops or steroid ointment in the eyes without consulting an eye doctor.

When to Seek Medical Attention

Seek medical care if any of the following are present:

- Pain. Most cases of infectious conjunctivitis are associated with mild discomfort. Many people with viral conjunctivitis feel like they have a foreign body in their eye. Severe eye pain, however, warrants immediate medical attention (see also "Herpes Conjunctivitis," below). In young children who are unable to vocalize their pain, crying or extreme irritability may be an indication that they are in pain.
- Blurred vision or loss of vision. Any difficulty seeing should be taken very seriously (see also "Herpes Conjunctivitis," below). Sometimes a large amount of pus in the eye will cause blurry vision, but once this is wiped away, the vision should be normal. Eye ointments may also cause blurry vision. This is one of the reasons why

it is preferable to use eyedrops rather than ointment when treating anyone older than one year of age.

- Severe light sensitivity (photophobia). This often indicates corneal involvement.
- Trauma. Any history of eye injury is of concern.
- Foreign body. Seek treatment if you think there is a possibility that your child may have something in his eye.
- Irregular pupils (the "black spot" in the center of each eye).
- The pupils are not of equal size.
- The cornea is cloudy.
- Increasing redness with treatment. This suggests that your child may be allergic to the eyedrops or ointment or that the diagnosis is incorrect.
- Persistence of "pink eye." In most cases, bacterial conjunctivitis begins improving within 24 hours of starting treatment and is much improved after 48 to 72 hours of treatment. In contrast, viral conjunctivitis usually takes longer to resolve—in some cases, it may be several days before any improvement is seen. If your child does not get better after a few days, she should be examined by her physician to rule out more serious causes.
- Marked swelling around the eye. This may indicate an infection of the skin and underlying tissues (cellulitis) or sinusitis. Allergies may also cause marked swelling around the eye. In this case the eyes will usually be itchy, and there may be other symptoms of allergy such as nasal itching and sneezing. Such a child may be uncomfortable but not ill.

- "Pink eye" that involves only one eye. Although bacterial and viral infectious conjunctivitis may start in only one eye, usually within a day or two it has spread to the other eye. Symptoms affecting one eye exclusively may suggest a more serious problem (see also "Herpes Conjunctivitis," below).
- Blisters involving the surrounding skin. This often suggests the presence of herpes (see also "Herpes Conjunctivitis," below).
- One or both of your newborn's eyes are very swollen and pus is pouring out from between the eyelids (see "Newborn Conjunctivitis," below).

More Serious Types of Infectious Conjunctivitis

Some types of infectious conjunctivitis can result in vision loss or permanent eye damage if not treated. Two of these more serious types of infectious conjunctivitis are discussed below.

Herpes Conjunctivitis

This type of infectious conjunctivitis is caused by the same virus that causes "cold sores" (the herpes simplex virus). The following symptoms may indicate herpes conjunctivitis, particularly if they occur in someone who has had contact with cold sores:

- Only one eye is involved.
- Severe pain.
- Blisters surrounding the eye.
- Impaired vision.

However, a person who has none of these symptoms may still have herpes conjunctivitis. In other words, herpes conjunctivitis may look identical to other, less serious eye ailments that cause "pink eye." Specialized treatment is required to preserve the vision of a person with herpes conjunctivitis. Anyone who has persistent or recurring "pink eye" should see a physician.

Conjunctivitis in the Newborn

"Sticky eyes" are commonly seen in newborns (see below) and are not serious. Occasionally, however, newborns may develop a very serious type of infectious conjunctivitis. These babies usually present with very pussy and swollen eyes. Immediate and expert treatment is necessary (see "Newborn Conjunctivitis," below).

AS MENTIONED AT THE BEGINNING OF THIS SECTION, there are other causes of "pink eye" besides inflammation of the conjunctiva. Some of these are serious. The eyes are delicate structures. Don't delay in seeking medical advice or treatment.

EYE CONCERNS IN THE NEWBORN

Red Marks in the Newborn's Eye

Many newborns have red, flame-shaped marks in the white part of their eyes. These are hemorrhages that occurred during delivery. They are of no concern and fade over the ensuing two to three weeks. No treatment is necessary.

Yellow Eyes

The whites of many newborns' eyes turn yellow in the first few days of life. This is known as jaundice and is extremely common in the first week or two of life. Your baby should be checked by a medical professional in the first three to five days after birth to make sure the jaundice is not severe. Your child's bilirubin level may be checked. Occasionally your baby will need treatment (phototherapy lights) to lower the bilirubin level.

"Sticky" Eyes

Many babies develop slightly "sticky" eyes. You may notice a discharge from one or both eyes. This is often more marked in the morning and after naps. Usually the whites of the eyes are nice and clear, with no redness. Despite treatment, this "stickiness" or discharge tends to recur. In many cases, this recurring condition is due to blocked tear ducts involving one or both eyes. The tear ducts usually open spontaneously sometime during the first year of life, but occasionally surgery is required to open a blocked tear duct. This is usually done in the second year of life.

Newborn Conjunctivitis

Newborns may occasionally develop infectious conjunctivitis, most often caused by bacteria. One or both eyes will be pussy and red. Your child's doctor may want to prescribe antibiotic treatment.

> **CAUTION**
> **If your newborn's eyes are very swollen and pus is pouring out from between the eyelids, immediate treatment needs to be instituted. If the infection is not treated aggressively, permanent eye damage may result.**

STYES

A stye is a small abscess on the margin of the eyelid. It may be very irritating but is usually not serious. Treatment consists of warm compresses several times a day. Often antibiotic eyedrops or ointment is prescribed as well, and occasionally oral antibiotics. Styes frequently take days to weeks to resolve.

EYE INJURIES

Trauma is one of the most important causes of vision loss in childhood. Boys are more commonly involved than girls. Boys between 11 and 15 years of age are particularly at risk.

Corneal Abrasions

These are the most common type of eye injury. Your child will complain of severe eye pain and will also be light-sensitive and have tearing. Your child needs to be examined by a doctor, who will probably prescribe antibiotic eye ointment or drops as well as pain medication. Patching of the eye used to be standard treatment but is now infrequently done.

Foreign Bodies

Foreign bodies in the eye most frequently affect the conjunctiva or cornea. Common offending objects include specks of dirt, pieces of grass, hairs, and similar objects. Try the following to get rid of the foreign body:

- Blinking.
- Specks of dirt may sometimes be removed by lifting the upper eyelid up and outward and drawing it down over the lower lid.
- Try to gently wipe out the foreign body using a clean tissue or Q-tip.
- Flush it out of the eye using an eye wash.

If none of the these methods work, seek medical attention. Do not rub the eye.

Occasionally specks of metal may penetrate deep into the eye. This should be suspected if the person has been working around metal. Never attempt to remove objects deeply embedded in the eye. Seek medical attention.

Sports Injuries and Blows

These types of injuries can result in bleeding within the eye, and you may see blood layering within the eye. If you observe this or there is reduced vision or severe pain, seek medical attention immediately.

Apply cold compresses without excess pressure to help reduce pain and swelling. Do not use ibuprofen (Advil or Motrin) as an analgesic. It may increase the tendency to bleed.

Lacerations and Punctures

Do *not* try to wash out the eye with water and do *not* instill any eyedrops or ointment. Do *not* try to remove any object protruding from the eye. Cover the eye with paper or a polystyrene cup trimmed to fit and seek medical attention immediately.

Burns

Burns may be caused by hot objects or chemicals.

Hot Objects

Cigarette burns of the cornea may occur in children when a child accidentally runs into a cigarette dangling from someone's hand. The affected part of the eye often has a white appearance. Medical attention should be sought. Fortunately, the eye often heals without scarring.

Burns from fireworks are usually far more serious and often result in the loss of vision (see Chapter 59).

Chemicals

Both acids and alkalis can cause very severe eye injuries. These are true medical emergencies. Alkali burns are far more dangerous than acid burns and tend to penetrate deeply. Alkalis that are commonly found around the home include ammonia, bleach, drain openers, cleaning solutions, fertilizers, lime, and cement. **Immediate** treatment should be instituted: Irrigate the eye with copious amounts of water; you can use running water from a faucet, or you can pour water into the eye from a clean container. This irrigation should continue for 30 minutes. It should also help remove any particulate matter. **Seek medical attention**.

Prevention

Most eye injuries are preventable. The following precautions should always be taken:

- Store chemicals safely, out of reach of children.
- If you regularly handle chemicals, have an eye wash station readily available.
- Wear goggles when using jumper cables or handling

acids, alkalis, strong cleaning fluids, and chemical sprays Also wear goggles when handling batteries, and beware of sulfuric acid splashes onto your face and body.

- Don't allow young children to handle scissors, sharp pencils, and similarly dangerous objects.
- Teach your child not to run while carrying sharp objects.
- Do not let your child play with pellet guns, darts, and similar dangerous "missiles."
- When you mow the lawn, make sure your child is a safe distance away. Stones can be thrown for many yards by power mowers.
- When working with power tools, wear eye goggles.
- When teaching your child how to hammer nails, make him or her wear goggles.
- Never allow your child to play with fireworks. Keep a safe distance away when other people are lighting fireworks. Bystanders are frequently injured by bottle rockets.
- Wear protective eye guards or glasses when playing contact sports or sports involving ball "missiles," such as baseball, racquetball, and lacrosse.
- When fishing, make sure your child is a safe distance from you. Fishing hooks can be very dangerous.
- Be careful when opening champagne bottles. Their corks may become very dangerous missiles.
- Respect the sun. Wear sunglasses. Never look directly at the sun or at an eclipse of the sun.

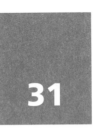

31

Vomiting, Diarrhea, and Dehydration Caused by Acute Gastroenteritis

What's in This Chapter

VOMITING AND DIARRHEA IN CHILDHOOD

Vomiting and diarrhea are two common symptoms in childhood. The most common cause of these symptoms is acute gastroenteritis, an infection of the intestines usually caused by a virus. The virus most often responsible for gastroenteritis is rotavirus, which causes winter gastroenteritis in many children. An oral vaccine is now available to prevent this illness. It is recommended that children in the first year of life receive this vaccine. Most young children get one or two bouts of gastroenteritis each year. Children in day care may have such illnesses more frequently. Bacteria can also cause gastroenteritis, more often in the summer months.

Children with gastroenteritis generally have a fever and are irritable. Their stools may be green in color and be foul smelling. They frequently have tummy cramps and intestinal bloating. The greatest concern for parents and physicians alike, however, is the risk of dehydration. It is the dehydration that leads to numerous physician and emergency room visits and to hospitalization. Gastroenteritis with dehydration is a common cause of death in childhood in lesser-developed countries when the illness complicates chronic malnutrition. In the United States, about 200 children die each year from gastroenteritis.

Most children with viral gastroenteritis first present with vomiting; diarrhea starts 12 to 24 hours later. Retching may precede the vomiting. Vomiting, unless it is prolonged, seldom leads to dehydration, but it is an extremely uncomfortable symptom. The vomiting usually settles by the second day of the illness. Diarrhea, especially when large amounts of watery stools are passed, is more likely to lead to dehydration. The diarrhea also tends to last much longer than the vomiting, often 7 to 10 days. The combination of persistent vomiting and explosive stools is particularly likely to lead to dehydration, especially if appropriate fluid therapy is not instituted.

The management of vomiting and the management of diarrhea are very similar in some respects but very different in others. With vomiting, fluid therapy should consist of stopping your child's usual diet and giving *very small* amounts (as little as 1 teaspoon) of fluids frequently. After the last vomit, a period of bowel rest—that is, a period when no food or fluids are offered—is often a good idea. This period may be as short as 15 minutes (for an infant) or as long as 4 to 8 hours for an older child. If your child has diarrhea or any of the signs of dehydration (see table 3), you need to begin administering appropriate fluids quickly. Most children with vomiting will tolerate clear fluids by mouth if the amount given is *very small*. (For details, see pp. 334–37.)

With diarrhea, *large* amounts of fluids are often necessary, and it is generally a good idea to continue with your child's usual feedings and solids. It is important not to give fluids and foods that will make the diarrhea worse. Certain solids aid in the absorption of fluids. (For details, see p. 350.)

When the child is both vomiting *and* having diarrhea, you will need to give small amounts of fluids frequently (often every minute or two) and repeatedly check your child for signs of dehydration (see table 3). Managing these symptoms is a real challenge—parents need to monitor their sick child constantly to prevent dehydration. Once the vomiting stops (and it usually does, unless the underlying cause is much more

Table 3. Assessment of the Degree of Dehydration

Factors Used to Assess Dehydration	Signs and Symptoms		
	Mild Dehydration	Moderate Dehydration	Severe Dehydration
Mental status and activity level	Normal: alert and interactive	May be normal but usually listless, less active, and irritable	Lethargic (apathetic, sluggish, very little interest in surroundings, drowsy) May be weak and limp May be comatose
Thirst	Slightly increased	Moderately increased	Very thirsty or too ill and lethargic to indicate thirst
Breathing	Normal	Normal to fast	Deep and sighing
Mucous membranes of mouth	Slightly dry	Dry Tongue will have a sand-papery feel	Very dry
Tears	Present	Absent	Absent
Eyes	Normal	Sunken	Very sunken
			Continued

serious than gastroenteritis), you can give larger amounts of fluid less frequently and later on add appropriate solids.

HOW TO RECOGNIZE DEHYDRATION

A child's behavior is a good indicator of the degree of illness. A child who is lethargic, lying around, and showing no inter-

Table 3. Assessment of the Degree of Dehydration *continued*

Factors Used to Assess Dehydration	Signs and Symptoms		
	Mild Dehydration	Moderate Dehydration	Severe Dehydration
Fontanel (soft spot)	Normal (a slight depression of the soft spot is normal	Sunken	Very sunken
Urine output	Slightly decreased and a little darker (more concentrated)	Decreased, very dark (very concentrated)	Very little to no urine, very dark

Note: Additional signs of severe dehydration include:
- Cool and mottled extremities
- Very weak pulses
- Tenting of the skin: if you pinch up the skin on the abdomen or chest, it stays up for a short while

est in the environment is probably severely dehydrated and significantly ill. An alert child who is interacting with his environment and crawling or running around is probably not significantly ill or dehydrated.

Refer to table 3 in this chapter for detailed information on the signs and symptoms of mild, moderate, and severe dehydration.

MANAGEMENT OF VOMITING

Acute viral gastroenteritis usually begins with vomiting, which in most cases lasts 12 to 24 hours. The following guidelines apply not just to vomiting caused by acute viral gastroenteritis but also to vomiting due to other causes (see Chapter 32).

- Assess your child's state of hydration (using table 3). If your child has signs of dehydration, follow the protocol on pp. 332–33.
- Stop all fluids and foods. If your child has just vomited, it is generally a good idea to stop all fluids and foods for a period of time in order to "rest" your child's bowel. The duration of this "rest" may be as short as 15 minutes or as long as 8 hours depending on the circumstances:
  - In certain cases, particularly in older children, and if your child has none of the symptoms of dehydration, and especially if there is minimal or no diarrhea, it may be prudent to "rest the stomach" for several hours. Encourage your child to keep quiet and try to go to sleep. This period of rest may be as long as eight hours in an older child, as such children do not usually become dehydrated even after a number of vomits. (If diarrhea develops, the situation may change.)
  - Infants who do not have diarrhea can usually tolerate going without feedings for four to five hours.
  - If your child has vomited only a few times, and/or if your child has any signs of dehydration, the period of bowel "rest" may be as short as 15 to 30 minutes.

Note: Do not delay giving fluids if your child has any of the signs of dehydration; has vomiting *and* diarrhea; vomits frequently (many times an hour); or has very large vomits.

- The further management of the vomiting child is influenced by the age of the child and whether she is breast- or formula-fed.

Children Younger Than One Year of Age

Breast-fed Babies

- Feed your baby for shorter periods and more often. (You may decide to let your baby nurse only on one side or to nurse for 4 to 5 minutes every 30 to 60 minutes.)
- If your baby is on solids, stop all solids.
- If your baby continues to vomit, stop breast-feeding and offer 5 ml (1 teaspoon or one 5-ml dropper) of electrolyte solution every one to two minutes.
- Once the vomiting has ceased, restart breast-feeding, again initially for shorter periods and more often.
- Once your child has not vomited for four hours, return to regular breast-feeding.
- You may offer your baby solids once she has not vomited for at least eight hours. Increase these very gradually.

Bottle-fed Babies

- Stop your baby's usual feedings and solids.
- Give *small* amounts (5 ml, or 1 teaspoon) of electrolyte solutions every one to two minutes.
- If your child vomits, wait 15 to 30 minutes and try giving the electrolyte solution again. Most infants and children, even if vomiting, will tolerate small amounts of clear liquids.
- If the electrolyte solution is tolerated, say after two to four hours, *gradually* increase the amount offered and the time between sips. (For example, offer 3 teaspoons, or ½ ounce, every three to five minutes.)
- Once your child has not vomited for four to eight hours, try her usual formula, but again start with small amounts. Increase the amount offered *gradually*.
- For infants who have already been introduced to solids (usually infants older than four months of age), gradually introduce solids such as cereal, strained bananas, and mashed potato. Increase the amounts *slowly*.

Children Older Than One Year of Age

- Stop your child's usual milk feedings and solids.
- Offer *small* amounts (1 to 2 teaspoons, or 5 to 10 ml) of clear fluids every one to two minutes. These fluids can be water, half-strength Gatorade or Kool-Aid, or flat soda. (Electrolyte solutions contain the ideal concentration of salts but are often not accepted by well-hydrated children of this age. They may be flavored or chilled to

improve their taste. See p. 347.) Children older than 18 months may prefer to suck on ice chips.
- As these liquids are tolerated, *slowly* increase the amounts offered, and lengthen the interval between feedings.
- After four to eight hours of no vomiting, add bland and starchy food such as crackers, pretzels, oatmeal cereal, mashed potato, or rice. Increase the amounts offered *very slowly.*
- Avoid fatty and greasy foods and orange juice.

Note: I cannot stress enough that the secret to success is giving *small* amounts (as little as 1 teaspoon, or one 5-ml dropper) frequently (every one to two minutes). Your child may be thirsty and will probably want to gulp down a full bottle of liquid, but doing so will almost certainly lead to further vomiting.

Even when you think you have the vomiting phase of the illness behind you, expect the occasional vomit. Do not get despondent; continue giving small amounts of fluids as described above. If your child vomits repeatedly, give her a rest for 15 to 30 minutes and then try again.

The younger the child and the more persistent the illness, the more important it is to use appropriate electrolyte solutions. This is particularly true if your child develops diarrhea.

Medications to Stop Vomiting

Older medications used to stop vomiting, such as promethazine (Phenergan), often have very unpleasant side effects. However, newer antiemetic (antivomiting) medications such as ondansetron (Zofran) may have a place in the treatment of the vomiting caused by acute gastroenteritis. They should *not* take the place of the other measures described above. Fluid therapy is the mainstay of the management of vomiting and diarrhea and is vital in the prevention of dehydration.

MANAGEMENT OF DIARRHEA

In acute viral gastroenteritis, diarrhea is usually the next phase of the illness. It tends to last longer than the vomiting, often for many days. The following guidelines apply not only to diarrhea and dehydration caused by acute viral gastroenteritis but also to diarrhea and dehydration due to other causes (see Chapter 32).

> *Note:* Diarrhea, especially if severe, is more likely than vomiting to lead to dehydration. The combination of severe diarrhea *and* vomiting is obviously more serious and requires more intensive treatment to avoid dehydration.
>
> You will need to give extra fluids as soon as the diarrhea starts. Continue giving extra fluids until the diarrhea has resolved.
>
> Check your child frequently for the symptoms and signs of dehydration (see table 3).

The management of diarrhea will vary depending on

- whether your child is dehydrated;
- the severity of the diarrhea;

- the age of your child; and
- whether your child is vomiting.

Assess your child's level of hydration—table 3 will help you determine which stage of hydration your child is in:

- No dehydration
- Mild to moderate dehydration
- Severe dehydration

Once you have assessed the stage of hydration, follow the guidelines below. Most children with diarrhea will fall into the first category—no dehydration (this isn't always the case, however, for children living in lesser-developed areas of the world, who may be chronically ill because of repeated bouts of gastroenteritis).

Mild Illness with No Dehydration

Your goal is to *prevent* dehydration. Make sure your child drinks extra fluids to replace the fluids she is losing. In most cases, well-hydrated children simply need to drink more of the fluids they usually drink. Continue with your child's usual solids unless she is vomiting.

Children Younger Than One Year of Age
- Continue your infant's usual feedings, either breast milk or formula. Offer these feedings more frequently. Other fluids that can be given in addition include water, di-

luted juices (one-third strength), or sports drinks such as Gatorade (half-strength). Ideally, for a child older than four to six months of age, these additional fluids should be given with the solids mentioned below. (Special electrolyte solutions such as those mentioned below are not essential in managing mild diarrhea in a child who is not dehydrated.)

- Unless your infant is vomiting, continue with her usual solids. Appropriate solids are cereals such as rice cereal and oatmeal, mashed potatoes, and strained bananas.
- Do *not* give full-strength juice or full-strength sports drinks, or full-strength sodas or full-strength Jell-O.
- If the diarrhea increases in severity, and especially if your child starts developing some of the symptoms or signs of dehydration, offer electrolyte solutions such as Kaolectrolyte, Pedialyte, Infalyte, Liquilyte, and Ceralyte. Children of this age will usually drink electrolyte solutions despite their salty taste. Liquilyte is one of the better tasting of these solutions.
- If your infant is vomiting, refer to the section on vomiting, p. 334.

Children Older Than One Year of Age

- Unless your child is vomiting, continue with her usual foods and fluids but give more of these foods and fluids. Give solids such as complex carbohydrates (rice, wheat, pasta, bananas, and potatoes), as well as meats, especially chicken. Fluids such as water, diluted juices (one-third strength), or half-strength sports drinks such as

Gatorade are acceptable if given with the foods listed above. Saltine-type crackers and pretzels are usually especially well tolerated.

- Avoid full-strength juices and full-strength sports drinks, and do not give sodas or Jell-O.
- Continue to offer extra fluids until the diarrhea has resolved.
- If the diarrhea increases in severity, and especially if large amounts of watery stool are passed, or if your child is starting to develop any of the symptoms or signs of dehydration, give electrolyte solutions.
- If your child is vomiting, refer to the section on vomiting, p. 334.

Note: Seek medical attention if your child (of any age) continues to vomit or shows signs of dehydration.

Mild to Moderate Dehydration

If your child is dehydrated, she is likely to be more ill. She will probably be thirstier than usual and, if the dehydration is moderate, have a dry tongue and sunken eyes. She will also pass less urine. (See table 3 for a more comprehensive list of signs and symptoms.) If your child is showing signs of dehydration, contact her physician. However, if you are on the road and don't have access to a physician, don't panic. Most children with mild or moderate dehydration can be successfully rehydrated orally if you follow the guidelines for fluid therapy outlined below. Remember: The more dehydrated your child gets, the more serious the situation becomes, so put aside all other activities and devote yourself to getting fluids into your child.

Fluid Therapy: What Fluids to Give and How Much
Once a child is dehydrated, it is preferable to give commercially prepared electrolyte solutions such as Kaolectrolyte, Infalyte, Pedialyte, Liquilyte, or Ceralyte. Liquilyte is one of the better tasting of these solutions.

Fluid therapy consists of two phases: (1) giving rehydration fluids (to replace fluid your child has already lost) and (2) giving maintenance fluids (to maintain hydration).

Rehydration Fluids
Children who are mildly to moderately dehydrated will need to get about 1 to 2 ounces of fluid for every pound they weigh (about 50–100 ml per kg). For practical purposes, you should aim to give your child about 1½ ounces of fluid per pound of body weight over the next four hours. More can be offered if your child will take it. However, if your child drinks too much, she may vomit. Adjust the amount of fluid you give according to your child's response and according to whether there is ongoing diarrhea and vomiting (see below for ongoing losses).

If your child is vomiting, it is essential to give very small amounts often. Follow these guidelines:

- For children less than 20 to 25 pounds (usually about one year of age), start by giving 1 teaspoon (5 ml) every one to two minutes. You may have to use a medicine dropper or syringe to do this.

- For children over 20 to 25 pounds (usually over one year of age), start by giving 2 teaspoons (10 ml) every one to two minutes. A medicine cup is a good way to give this fluid.
- If your child vomits these very small amounts of fluid, wait 10 to 15 minutes and then try again. If you offered 2 teaspoons (10 ml) before, try 1 teaspoon (5 ml) this time.
- After about an hour of giving fluids every minute or two, and once you are sure your child is tolerating these fluids, you may give slightly larger amounts less often.

Extra fluid will be required to replace fluid lost by continuing diarrhea and vomiting:

- For each watery stool in a child less than 20 to 25 pounds in weight (usually about one year of age), give an additional 2 to 4 ounces of fluid.
- For each watery stool in a child heavier than 20 to 25 pounds (older than about one year of age), offer an additional 4 to 8 ounces of fluid.
- Most vomits do not contain a large amount of fluid. However, if you feel your child had a large vomit, offer an additional 2 to 4 ounces of fluid for a child less than 20 to 25 pounds and an additional 4 to 8 ounces for a child heavier than 20 to 25 pounds.

For example, if your child is one year old and weighs about 20 pounds and is mild to moderately dehydrated, she will need to drink about 30 ounces over the next four hours (1½ ounces per pound of body weight) to replace the fluid she has lost. If she passes two loose stools and vomits once during the four-hour rehydration period, she will need an additional 6 to 12 ounces of fluid to make up for these losses. Over four hours she should receive about 36 to 42 ounces of fluid. You can achieve this by offering 1 teaspoon (5 ml) of fluid every minute (60 minutes × 4 hours × 5 ml = 1,200 ml = 40 ounces).

Maintenance Fluids

Once your child has been rehydrated, begin the second phase of fluid therapy: the administration of maintenance fluids. These are the fluids (both the types and the amounts) she usually consumes when she is well. Keep giving extra fluids, however, as long as the diarrhea continues. Urine output and color should help you to assess your child's state of hydration.

During this maintenance phase your child should also begin eating the food she usually consumes. Do not starve your child! Once she has stopped vomiting and the initial rehydration has been completed, offer her usual diet (see also the foods recommended earlier—for children both younger and older than one year of age—in "Mild Illness with No Dehydration").

Note: You will need to assess your child's level of hydration repeatedly (every one to two hours) and adjust the volume of fluid to be given accordingly.

Severe Dehydration

A child who is severely dehydrated will appear very ill. He will be lethargic and uninterested in his surroundings. He may be weak, limp, or unresponsive. His eyes will be very sunken, and he will have a very dry mouth. The tongue will have a leathery feel. He may not be able to drink. Often his hands and feet will be cold and mottled. There will be little or no urine output. His pulses will be weak.

CAUTION
Severe dehydration is a medical emergency, and immediate medical attention is required.

Medications to Treat Diarrhea

Antibiotics

Antibiotics make most cases of diarrhea worse and are usually not indicated. However, occasionally they may be needed—for example, in some cases of bacterial diarrhea and travelers' diarrhea.

Antimotility Agents

These agents slow the progression of food through your child's intestinal tract. They include loperamide (Imodium AD) and diphenoxylate hydrochloride (Lomotil).

- Lomotil should *never* be given to treat childhood diarrhea.
- Imodium AD may be used for older children and adults who do not have a high fever, abdominal distention, or blood in their stools. Imodium AD is often helpful for older children and adults with travelers' diarrhea. However, the use of this medication should not take the place of giving fluids by mouth. For the dosages and side effects of Imodium, see Chapter 12, p. 157.

Agents to Firm the Stools

Agents such as Kaopectate may firm the stools, but they do not shorten the illness and may detract from the primary objective, which is giving fluids by mouth. It is preferable *not* to use such agents.

Pepto-Bismol

Pepto-Bismol (bismuth subsalicylate) has been shown to be effective in preventing and treating travelers' diarrhea. It is seldom indicated, however, in the management of other types of diarrhea in children, even though it has been shown to decrease the frequency of unformed stools. There are side effects and contraindications to using Pepto-Bismol. (See Chapter 12, p. 144.)

MANAGEMENT OF DIARRHEA AND VOMITING

By far, the most common cause of diarrhea *and* vomiting is acute viral gastroenteritis.

As mentioned earlier, if your child is vomiting and also has diarrhea, there is a greater risk of becoming dehydrated.

Initially, follow the guidelines in the section "Management of Vomiting" and give *small amounts of fluids often.* As the vomiting settles (usually by the second day), give larger amounts of the appropriate fluids (as described in the section "Management of Diarrhea") and add in the appropriate solids once your child has not vomited for about eight hours.

Repeatedly assess your child's level of hydration, using table 3.

If your child is dehydrated, calculate the necessary rehydration fluids (see the guidelines in "Rehydration Fluids," above) and give these over four hours.

Do not forget to add in extra fluids to replace ongoing losses from diarrhea and vomiting.

MORE ON FLUID THERAPY

Fluids to Give

Electrolyte Solutions

These are sometimes known as oral rehydration solutions (ORS). Examples are Pedialyte, Kaolectrolyte, WHO-ORS, Liquilyte, and Ceralyte (of these, Liquilyte is slightly better tasting). These solutions are ideal for rehydrating children and adults.

Some of these electrolyte solutions taste very salty, but you can improve the taste by adding one or two drops of Nutra-Sweet or a little sugar-free Kool-Aid powder. You can also improve the taste by adding 2 to 3 teaspoons of apple or grape juice to every 8 ounces of electrolyte solution. Better tasting, fruit-flavored electrolyte solutions are commercially available.

Electrolyte solutions can be frozen and offered as Popsicle-type bars. Frozen bars made from electrolyte solutions are commercially available. Electrolyte solutions can also be made into ice cubes, which can be crushed and offered as ice chips.

Homemade ORS can be used (see Chapter 12), but it is always better to use commercially made ORS because homemade ORS may not have the correct concentration of salt. Homemade ORS should be used only in emergency situations when commercially made ORS is not available.

Most electrolyte solutions do not lessen the severity or duration of the diarrhea. They just prevent and treat dehydration. Giving solids may lessen the severity and shorten the duration of the diarrhea. Ceralyte may also lessen the severity and shorten the duration of diarrhea.

It is not necessary to use electrolyte solutions if your child has only mild diarrhea and is not dehydrated. See the section just below on other acceptable fluids.

Note: The younger the child and the more severe the diarrhea and dehydration, the more important it is to use electrolyte solutions.

Other Acceptable Fluids

Breast milk is an ideal fluid for most infants. If your infant vomits breast milk, offer the breast more often, but let your child feed for shorter periods.

Formula may be offered if your child is not vomiting and is well hydrated. Again, smaller amounts given more often may be better tolerated. Stop the formula if your infant is vomiting. Try to reintroduce the formula four to eight hours later.

Do not dilute milk or formula unless your child is vomiting, and even then dilute it only for short periods. When you dilute milk or formula, you also "dilute" the calories.

Some infants and children are unable to tolerate milk or formula because of temporary sugar (lactose) intolerance. Lactose intolerance may be present if your child passes a large watery stool after each milk feeding. These infants and children should be given a lactose-free preparation such as soy milk formula (Isomil, Isomil DF, and ProSobee, among many others) or lactose-free milk (Lactaid milk). Older children do *not* need milk at this time.

Vegetable juices such as carrot juice can be given.

For children with mild to moderate diarrhea, diluted fruit juices or sodas (one-third strength), half-strength strength Gatorade, or water may be used for short periods, especially if supplemented with starchy and salty foods such as rice cereal, oatmeal, mashed potatoes, and mashed bananas. Older children and adults should eat salted crackers or pretzels to increase the fluid and salt absorption.

Fluids to Avoid

- Do not give full-strength fruit juices, sodas, sports drinks, or Jell-O. They have a very high sugar content

and no or insufficient salts. They frequently make the diarrhea worse.
- Most commercial chicken broth has too much salt and no sugar, and so it is not suitable for rehydration.
- Do not give boiled skim milk.

ADDITIONAL INFORMATION ON APPROPRIATE SOLIDS FOR CHILDREN WITH DIARRHEA

If your child is vomiting or is dehydrated, you should stop his normal diet for a period of four to eight hours.

Once your child has stopped vomiting, and once she has been rehydrated, her usual foods should be introduced. Cooked cereal such as oatmeal or cream of wheat, mashed potatoes, rice, noodles, wheat (such as bread, crackers, and pretzels), and bananas will aid in water absorption, shorten the period of diarrhea, and decrease its severity. Lean meats, yogurt, vegetables, and fruit are usually well tolerated. Bananas are a good source of potassium, which is lost in diarrheal stools.

Avoid fried and fatty foods and foods that contain a lot of sugar, such as ice cream and Jell-O.

After the vomiting has stopped, the "BRATT" diet (bananas, rice, applesauce, tea, and toast) may be acceptable to use for short periods (one to two days) but does not supply enough calories, protein, and fat for long-term use.

OTHER CONCERNS

Stools

Note: Contact your child's physician if there is blood in the stool.

Stool color is not important. When your child has diarrhea, the stool color may vary from brown to yellow to bright green, but this should be of no concern. Many medications and fluids may change the color of the stools. Pepto-Bismol, for example, may turn your child's stools (as well as his tongue) black.

Do not be concerned if you see pieces of food in your child's stool.

The amount of fluid lost with each stool will depend on the age of the child, the size of the stool, and its consistency (see p. 343).

Weight Loss

Weight loss in a child with gastroenteritis is initially due to dehydration. However, a common cause of weight loss later in the illness, especially if your child is well hydrated, is not getting enough food—in other words, your child has not been given the essential nutrients to maintain and gain weight. Children usually regain their weight once they are eating normally.

Hygiene

Remember to wash your hands well after changing your child's diaper.

Dispose of diapers in a hygienic and environmentally friendly way.

When to Seek Medical Attention

For children with vomiting and diarrhea, seek medical care under the following circumstances:

- If your child is younger than six months old.
- If your child is limp and lethargic or appears very ill.
- If your child has any signs of dehydration. If you are traveling and can't contact a medical professional, follow the guidelines above, which should enable you to rehydrate your child on your own. Signs of severe dehydration, however, indicate a medical emergency.
- If your child has vomiting that persists despite the measures described above and the dehydration is worsening. In most children the vomiting settles on the second day of the illness.
- If your child consistently refuses to take liquids by mouth.
- If your child passes large amounts of watery stools and has increasing signs of dehydration—in other words, if your attempts to rehydrate your child are not sufficient to keep up with the volume of stool passed.

- If your child has a severe stomachache lasting longer than two hours. Note, however, that many children have recurrent bouts of abdominal pain or cramps, especially when passing gas or stools. Persisting pain (longer than one to two hours) or worsening pain indicates the need to seek medical attention to rule out more serious causes, such as appendicitis, bowel perforation, or obstruction.
- If the stool contains blood or a large amount of mucus, or if the stool is black and your child is *not* taking Pepto-Bismol.
- If the diarrhea is not improving after 2 to 3 days. It may take as long as 7 to 10 days before your child's stools are totally normal, but each day there should be improvement. Your child should be eating and drinking well and be active, alert, and interested in his or her surroundings.

IN SUMMARY

Vomiting

- Vomiting is *not* a contraindication to giving electrolyte solutions. Even infants and young children who are vomiting will usually be able to tolerate *small* amounts of electrolyte solutions. Give 1 teaspoon (5 ml) every one to two minutes. For older children, you can use a medicine cup. As the fluid is tolerated, increase the amounts and give less often.
- Children older than 18 months of age may suck on ice chips or Popsicles if vomiting is a problem. Electrolyte solutions may be made into Popsicle-type bars, which

Table 4. Summary of the Management of Diarrhea and Dehydration

Degree of Dehydration	Rehydration Therapy	Replacement of Losses	Nutrition
Minimal or none	Not applicable: Give usual fluids	*Less than 20–25 lbs weight:* 2–4 oz fluids for each diarrheal stool or large vomit *More than 20–25 lbs weight:* 4–8 oz of fluids for each diarrheal stool or large vomit	Continue usual diet
Mild to moderate	Give ORS, 1½ oz per pound of body weight over 4 hours	Replacement as above, but use ORS	Once rehydrated, resume age-appropriate diet
Severe	A medical emergency. Requires intravenous fluids.		

Note: Once the dehydration is corrected your child will need her usual maintenance fluids (see p. 344). ORS = oral rehydration solutions, or electrolytes.

your child can suck on, or into ice blocks, which can then be crushed and offered as ice chips.

- Breast-fed infants who vomit should be fed for shorter periods and more often.

Note: If your child continues to vomit despite these measures, medical care should be sought.

Diarrhea

- Assess your child's hydration status and refer to table 4 in this chapter for guidelines on how to proceed.
- Reassess your child's level of hydration frequently.
- Avoid fluids and foods that may make the diarrhea worse.
- Continue giving extra fluids until the diarrhea has resolved.
- Know when to seek medical care.

APPENDIX

Conversion of pounds to kilograms:
    Approx. 2 pounds = 1 kilogram (kg)
Conversion of ounces and quarts to milliliters and liters:
    Approx. 1 ounce = 30 milliliters (ml)
    Approx. 1 quart = 1 liter

32

Vomiting and Diarrhea with Causes Other Than Acute Gastroenteritis

Refer also to Chapter 31.

Although acute viral gastroenteritis is the most common cause of vomiting and diarrhea, these symptoms can have many other causes.

OTHER CAUSES OF VOMITING BESIDES ACUTE GASTROENTERITIS

There are many causes of vomiting in childhood. Some of these are serious, but most resolve on their own and are of no concern unless the vomiting is repetitive or accompanied by other symptoms. In addition, as discussed in Chapter 31, repetitive vomiting may lead to dehydration, especially if accompanied by diarrhea.

Below is a list of the more common causes of vomiting in different age groups.

Children Younger Than One Year of Age

- Many infants spit up or regurgitate small amounts of milk or food in the first year of life. In the true sense of the word this regurgitation, known as *gastroesophageal reflux* (GER), is not regarded as vomiting, which is forceful and unpleasant. GER is normal and is usually totally harmless. It may lead to a high laundry bill but does not usually lead to dehydration! If your child is not gaining weight adequately, is always fussy, or has breathing problems, he may need to be treated. Otherwise, you just need to wait until your child outgrows GER, which usually happens around one year of age.
- *Projectile vomiting* in the first three months of life often has a significant medical cause, and if it occurs repeatedly, you should seek medical care. With projectile vomiting, the vomited material "shoots out" many feet. An obstruction to the outlet of the stomach (*pyloric stenosis*) is an important cause of repeated projectile vomiting. This requires surgical correction.
- In the first few weeks of life, an infant who vomits green-colored fluid (bile) may have a bowel obstruction and needs to be seen by a physician immediately.
- Metabolic diseases and infection (*sepsis*) are other im-

portant causes of repeated vomiting in the first few weeks of life. If either of these are the cause, your infant will be very ill.

- Infections, especially urinary tract infections and meningitis, may cause vomiting.

Older Children and Adolescents

- Serious causes of vomiting requiring urgent surgical attention include appendicitis and bowel obstruction.
- Head injuries, both minor and severe, may also cause vomiting (see Chapter 47).
- A significant cause of vomiting in toddlers is the ingestion of poisons, toxins, or medicines.
- Infections, especially urinary tract infections, may cause vomiting. Meningitis is another important cause of vomiting. Less serious infections, such as ear infections and strep throat, may also cause vomiting.
- Migraine is another fairly frequent cause of vomiting in this age group as well as in younger children.
- Other causes of vomiting include peptic ulcer disease, irritating medications (aspirin, ibuprofen, certain antibiotics), and food poisoning.
- At any age, dietary indiscretion may lead to vomiting.
- Brain tumors or any other cause of raised pressure in the skull are *very rare* causes of recurrent or persistent vomiting at any age. The vomiting typically occurs in the early morning and is almost always associated with recurrent or persistent headaches.

Treatment

The treatment of vomiting varies depending on the cause. In all cases, you need to prevent dehydration. For more specific details, refer to "Management of Vomiting" in Chapter 31 and also see the section on when to seek medical care, below.

The following are some guidelines to help you prevent your child from becoming dehydrated.

- Stop all solids and milk products (apart from breast milk) for four to six hours. If your child is breast-fed, try feeding her for shorter periods but more often. If she continues to vomit, follow the steps below.
- Give *small* amounts of clear fluids to your child. If your child is *not* dehydrated, you may give sips of water, diluted Kool-Aid, diluted Gatorade, or a similar fluid. If your child is older than about 18 months, sucking on ice chips is a good way to get fluid into your child. If the vomiting continues past 6 to 12 hours, or if there are any signs of dehydration, it is preferable to give electrolyte solutions. This applies especially in the first year of life. Popsicles made from electrolyte solutions are a good option.

Note: I cannot stress enough that the secret to success is giving *small amounts of fluids* (as little as 1 teaspoon, or a medicine dropper full) *frequently* (every one to two minutes).

Once the smaller amounts of fluid are tolerated, increase the amount of fluid offered.

After four to six hours of clear fluids and with no vomiting, it is usually safe to reintroduce formula to a younger infant or a bland diet to the older child. This may consist of foods such as Saltine-type crackers, rice, mashed potatoes, and bananas. Start with small amounts.

It is important not to starve your child for prolonged periods. Get him back on a normal diet as quickly as possible.

Medications to Stop Vomiting

These frequently have unpleasant side effects in children and should be used only under the direction of your child's doctor.

When to Seek Medical Attention

- Vomiting that persists beyond 24 hours in a child younger than two years of age and beyond 48 hours in a child older than two years of age. You may, however, need to seek medical attention *earlier* than this, especially for young children, if the vomiting is severe or repetitive.
- If your child develops signs of mild or moderate dehydration (such as a dry mouth, sunken eyes, or listlessness) and the vomiting is persisting.
- If your child has signs of severe dehydration, seek medical care *immediately*.

- Your child is not dehydrated yet appears unduly ill or is very lethargic and apathetic—in other words, your child's condition appears to be worse than can be explained by the degree of vomiting or dehydration.
- Projectile vomiting in the first few months of life. Every child has an occasional projectile vomit, but if this happens repeatedly, medical care should be sought.
- Bile-stained vomit (yellow or green) in the first six months of life or persistent bile-stained vomit in older children.
- If there is a large amount of blood (more than a teaspoon) or blood clots in the vomit and your child has not just had a nosebleed. There may be streaks of blood in the vomit if your child retches repeatedly.
- If your child has severe abdominal pain. Children who vomit will be unhappy and uncomfortable, but they should not be in severe pain once each vomiting episode is over.
- If there is a swelling in the groin (this may be a hernia or a strangulated testicle).
- If your child has obvious abdominal distension (the abdomen appears very full).
- If your child has other worrisome symptoms, such as severe headache, neck stiffness, confusion, rapidly spreading rashes, or backache.
- If your child has recently had a head injury.
- If your child's condition is worsening.

OTHER CAUSES OF DIARRHEA BESIDES ACUTE VIRAL GASTROENTERITIS

There are many causes for diarrhea besides viral gastroenteritis. Among them are the following:

- Bacteria. Bacteria cause what is sometimes called "summer diarrhea." The stools in bacteria-caused diarrhea may contain mucus and blood. Sometimes antibiotics are needed to treat it. Bacteria also usually cause travelers' diarrhea (see Chapter 12).
- Excessive consumption of juice.
- A disease such as a urinary tract infection, meningitis, or appendicitis. If your child looks ill, is lethargic, or has severe pain, he should be seen by a physician, as one of these diseases (or others) may be causing his diarrhea.
- Antibiotics, which are an extremely common cause of diarrhea (see p. 295).

There are many other causes of diarrhea besides those mentioned above. Many of these causes result in chronic diarrhea lasting months to years. They may be associated with poor weight gain and abdominal pain. Your child needs to see a medical professional if this is the case.

The management of these other causes of diarrhea will vary depending on the cause. In all cases, your aim is to prevent dehydration. Maintaining adequate nutrition is another important goal, especially if the diarrhea is longer lasting.

See Chapter 31, "Management of Diarrhea," for guidelines on treating diarrhea.

Note: A breast-fed infant often has frequent loose to watery stools, but in the strict sense of the definition, this stool pattern should not be classified as diarrhea, as it is the infant's normal state. This is not a cause for concern if the infant is active and gaining weight. If you notice that your infant's stool pattern is changing (for example, larger amounts of more watery stools or a change in stool odor) or your infant's behavior is changing (for example, your infant is more irritable or more lethargic), or if your child develops a fever, you should contact your child's physician.

33

Abdominal Pain

There are many causes of abdominal pain ("bellyache" or "stomachache") in children, varying from simple causes such as indigestion or gas pains to serious causes such as appendicitis and obstruction of the bowel. Remember, children younger than two to three years of age have trouble pinpointing where their pain is. They may complain of abdominal pain when in fact they have a middle-ear infection or some other disease. Sometimes the pain may not even be due to an abdominal condition but may be referred pain from a chest condition such as pneumonia.

WHAT CAUSES IT?

- Constipation. This is probably the most common cause of abdominal pain in childhood (see Chapter 34).
- Strep throat. This is a particularly frequent cause of abdominal pain in the school-age child (see Chapter 24, p. 275).

- Dietary "indiscretion." This includes eating too fast, eating too much, and eating food that does not "agree" with you. Many children with lactose intolerance get stomach cramps and diarrhea when they eat dairy products. This condition often runs in families.
- Acute gastroenteritis. This often begins with abdominal pain. Vomiting, fever, and diarrhea usually follow soon afterward (see Chapter 31, p. 328).
- Infantile colic (see Chapter 19, p. 252).
- Emotional upset. Many children complain of stomachache when they are upset or worried. Anxiety related to problems at school or home is a common cause of stomachaches.

Abdominal pain or stomach upsets while traveling may be due to a combination of factors: constipation, dietary indiscretion, and the anxiety associated with travel. It may also be the first sign of travelers' diarrhea.

Other, more serious but less common causes of abdominal pain include urinary tract infections, kidney stones, appendicitis, intestinal obstruction, and poisoning, among many others.

 Treatment

Fortunately, most stomachaches disappear on their own.

The treatment of abdominal pain will depend on the cause. Initially the cause of the pain may not be obvious, and so parents usually try to comfort their child with a caring and commonsense approach. Below are some guidelines.

- Encourage your child to lie quietly and rest. During bouts of abdominal pain, reassure your child in a calm voice and tell him to take a few deep and slow breaths.
- If the pain persists, try a warm water bottle or a heating pad on your child's belly.
- Sucking on ice chips may help to distract your child as well as maintain hydration.
- Do not give your child medicines that may complicate the situation or make matters worse. Avoid aspirin- and ibuprofen-containing products. Unfortunately, acetaminophen (Tylenol) rarely helps a stomachache. Sometimes a dose of Pepto-Bismol or Maalox may provide some relief.

Before you call your child's doctor, consider the following:

- If the cause is constipation, follow the guidelines in Chapter 34. Encourage your child to sit on the toilet and to try to have a bowel movement. Once the acute episode is over, "tackle" the problem of constipation because unless it is dealt with properly and diligently, it is sure to recur.
- If the cause is lactose intolerance, avoid lactose-containing foods such as milk and cheese. Discuss this further with your child's doctor at your next routine visit.
- If you suspect strep throat, seek medical care (not usually an emergency).
- If it becomes obvious that the stomachache was the harbinger of acute gastroenteritis, follow the guidelines in Chapter 31.

- If the cause is some serious intra-abdominal condition, your child may be reluctant to walk or hop because such movement makes the pain worse. Ask your child to walk and hop and assess how she performs these actions.

When to Seek Medical Attention

- The pain increases in severity or lasts longer than three to six hours.
- Your child has repeated vomiting.
- Your child has signs of dehydration that do not respond to appropriate measures (see Chapter 31, p. 345).
- Your child is unable to walk or walks bent over. Many children with appendicitis or other serious abdominal conditions walk bent over, move very gingerly, and are reluctant to hop.
- Your child is persistently tender over the appendix area (lower right side).
- Your child vomits blood.
- Your child has blood in his bowel movements.
- Your child vomits bile (green or yellow fluid).
- Your child has a swelling in the groin or swollen and painful testicles.
- Your child has recently had an abdominal injury.
- Your child appears very ill, has a high fever (greater than 104°F, or 40°C), is very pale, has cold or mottled extremities, or is confused or is very lethargic.
- You suspect your child has strep throat. (Not a medical emergency!)

Happily, most children with a stomachache are not seriously ill. Your child will get better and you will have a few more gray hairs! Discuss stomach upset or abdominal pain with your child's doctor. Hopefully you can prevent a recurrence.

34

Constipation and Stooling Patterns

WHAT IS CONSTIPATION?

When defining constipation, one needs to take three things into account:

1. The consistency of the stools
2. The frequency of the stools
3. The difficulty in passing stools

There are many definitions of constipation, but a commonly accepted one is the passage of hard stools often accompanied by pain. Some definitions might include the word *infrequent* in reference to how often stools are passed, but passing stools infrequently is not always an indication of constipation. A person may pass a stool only once or twice a week, but if the stool is soft and its passage is not accompanied by discomfort, that person would not be considered constipated. This is often the case in breast-fed infants in the second and third months of life.

Also, a child's bowel habits commonly change with age and diet. Your child's stools at six months of age may not be the same as at six years of age. Use the discussions below to determine what you can expect as your child grows older.

Children Younger Than One Year of Age

Changes in a Child's Bowel Habits with Age and Diet

In the first few days of life infants pass meconium stools. These are black and tarry, but within two to five days the stools are usually yellow or green or various shades in between. Sometimes the stools have a seedy texture.

Typically, a breast-fed infant will have several (as many as 5 to 10) bowel movements a day, and the stools are often loose or even watery. Despite this, the infant is content, gaining weight, and thriving. Frequently, around the second or third month of life, breast-fed babies often pass only one to two stools per week. As long as the stools are soft and the infant is content and gaining weight, this is regarded as normal. This infant is not constipated and does not require any treatment.

Formula-fed infants usually have far fewer bowel movements a day, and the stools tend to be firmer and smellier. If the stools are hard and the infant appears to be in pain when passing them, the infant is considered constipated and should be treated accordingly. This is more likely to occur if the infant is on soy feeds.

Apparent Difficulty in Passing Stools

Many infants in the first few months of life appear to have great difficulty passing stools. They get red in the face, strain, grunt, cry, draw their legs up over the abdomen, and so on, but they eventually pass a totally normal, soft stool. This apparent difficulty is normal and is probably due to immature coordination of the muscles of the bowel. As long as the stool is soft and the infant is otherwise well and thriving, this is nothing to be concerned about. The problem usually resolves by three to four months of age. Such an infant is not considered constipated. (Imagine how difficult it must be to poop while lying on your back!) (See also Chapter 19, p. 248.)

 ### *Treatment*

First of all, try to determine whether your baby truly is constipated or whether she just has a bowel coordination problem. If the latter, no treatment may be the best treatment. If you feel your infant really does need help, try stimulating the rectum by inserting a well-lubricated (with Vaseline or KY Jelly) thermometer about one inch into your infant's rectum. Alternatively, insert an infant glycerine suppository into your infant's rectum. Usually within a few minutes a stool will be passed. Although effective, these techniques should not be overused. One to two ounces of water or diluted juice given once or twice a day may also help relieve this stooling difficulty.

If your infant has true constipation, there are a number of things you can try:

- Offer your infant 1 to 2 ounces of water once or twice a day.
- Give your infant an ounce of prune or pear juice diluted with an equal volume of water once or twice a day.
- Add 1 to 2 teaspoons of dark Karo syrup to your infant's formula once or twice a day.
- Consider using the infant glycerine suppositories described above.
- If your infant is already eating solids, add baby foods high in fiber such as apricots, pears, prunes, peaches, peas, and beans.

If these measures fail, consult your child's doctor. A medical examination and prescription stool softeners may be indicated.

Toddlers

Toddlers are especially prone to constipation and often do not pass a stool for many days. These problems often start around toilet training time. If your child passes stools infrequently, the stools become hard and cause pain when they are passed. Consequently your child may become afraid to pass stools and will hold them in as long as possible. This only worsens the problem, as the stools become harder and harder and larger and larger. This often leads to recurrent bouts of abdominal pain. Treatment of this problem should be discussed with your child's doctor and should consist of appropriate changes in diet, good toilet habits, and possibly the regular use of stool softeners and laxatives until the problem is resolved. Constipation tends to be a recurring problem, so be on the lookout for relapses.

Older Children

Constipation is very common at all ages. Have you watched TV lately and seen all the advertisements for laxatives?

Children with constipation may develop soiling and may even appear to have diarrhea! The sooner these problems are dealt with, the sooner they will resolve. They seldom go away on their own, and you will need expert help and guidelines on the appropriate diet, good toilet habits, and the use of stool softeners and laxatives.

CONSTIPATION WHILE TRAVELING

Constipation is an extremely common problem when traveling. It is probably even more common than travelers' diarrhea! The excitement and the stresses of travel, changes in diet, and erratic availability of toilet facilities all contribute to a tendency to constipation. Regular toilet habits are extremely important, and attention to these as well as an appropriate diet will go a long way to prevent constipation and bouts of abdominal pain. Make sure all the travelers in your party keep up their fluid intake, eat fiber-containing foods, and have regular bathroom breaks. It's a good idea to include a stool softener and laxative in your travel kit.

Note: Although fruit juices are helpful in the treatment of constipation, they are very poor sources of nutrition for an infant and young growing child. In the long term, fruit juice should not take the place of breast milk, formula, or ordinary milk in your child's diet. A common cause of poor weight gain in children in the United States is excessive consumption of fruit juices. This may also lead to chronic diarrhea.

35

Headaches

Refer also to the section "Children with Headaches" in Chapter 5.

Children fairly commonly complain of headaches, and this usually does not indicate a severe underlying disease such as a brain tumor. Many headaches occur in association with other illnesses such as infections—for example, strep throat. They may also occur with sinusitis, earaches, and other infectious diseases that have nothing to do with the head.

Very young children have trouble pinpointing where their pain is and may complain of a headache when, in fact, they have abdominal pain.

Headaches are often a manifestation of the psychological stresses of life. The stresses of travel, for instance, often cause headaches in the entire family.

Recurrent headaches are often due to migraine or tension, and these should be discussed with your child's physician.

Migraine headaches are frequently located in the front of the head, often behind one eye. They may be throbbing in nature and often are associated with visual symptoms, nausea, and vomiting. They are often relieved by sleep and an appropriate analgesic. Migraine headaches are common in childhood.

On occasion, there is a serious cause for a headache. If your child complains of a severe headache, has a fever or neck stiffness, or is confused, immediate medical attention should be sought. Your child is unlikely to have meningitis if she is alert and active and is happily watching TV and interacting with her environment.

 ### *Treatment*

Initial treatment of a headache, without other symptoms, should consist of an appropriate dose of acetaminophen or ibuprofen. Ibuprofen tends to be more effective than acetaminophen for treating migraine headaches. Having your child lie down in a dark room will also often help the headache. Headaches that do not respond to these simple measures should be discussed with your child's physician.

If your child complains of a headache but wants to watch TV or play Nintendo, he does not have a significant headache, and there may be an ulterior motive for complaining of a headache.

Children with recurrent headaches should see a physician who knows how to diagnose and treat headaches. Migraine headaches are aggravated by stress, caffeine, and a lack of sleep. Make sure your child has a headache action plan if she suffers from chronic headaches. This plan and an adequate supply of your child's headache medications are vital before setting out on your travels.

36

Seizures, or Convulsions

Three to four percent of children have seizures (also called convulsions) associated with fevers (see Chapter 20, p. 256). These seizures, which are known as *febrile seizures,* are usually short, lasting only a few minutes, and do not cause brain damage.

Some children have recurrent seizures unassociated with fever. When a child has recurrent seizures not triggered by fever, he is said to have epilepsy. A child with recurrent seizures should be seen by a neurologist and will probably be maintained on appropriate antiseizure medication.

Occasionally, a child who has never had seizures before will develop prolonged seizures. Such a child may have a serious disease such as meningitis, a brain hemorrhage, or poisoning and requires immediate medical care.

Treatment

First aid treatment for a seizure includes the following:

1. Try not to panic.
2. Lay your child down on his side and make sure that his head is lower than the rest of his body so that any mucus or vomit can drain out. Position your child's head so that it is slightly tilted back. This will help maintain an open airway.
3. Do not attempt to force hard objects, such as rulers or pencils, between your child's teeth. Do not attempt to give anything by mouth.
4. If your child has a fever, remove your child's clothing. If your child is prone to febrile seizures, insert an acetaminophen suppository if one is available.
5. If the seizure persists for longer than five minutes, seek immediate medical attention. Call 911.

Remember, most seizures are short and do not cause brain damage. There are, however, some very serious causes for seizures such as meningitis or clots on the brain. Therefore, medical attention should always be sought after your child has had a seizure. The exception to this is the child with known febrile seizures who shortly after the seizure is alert and running around and does not show any signs of illness. Even then, it is preferable to discuss the episode with your child's doctor, as the illness that caused the fever may need to be treated.

If your child has a recurrent seizure disorder (epilepsy) and you plan to travel, make sure you take sufficient antiseizure medication with you on your travels. Depending on the antiseizure medication your child is taking, it may be a good idea to have your child's blood level checked prior to your departure. Have a supply of rectal diazepam available to treat any prolonged seizures. You should know how to use the rectal diazepam. Ask your physician about this.

If your child is prone to febrile seizures, at the first sign of an illness such as an upper respiratory infection, keep your child lightly dressed and give your child an appropriate dose of a fever-reducing medication such as acetaminophen (Tylenol) or ibuprofen (Advil or Motrin). If your child has a fever and refuses to take medication by mouth or is confused, insert an acetaminophen suppository. Rectal diazepam may also be useful for a child with recurrent febrile seizures, especially if the seizures tend to be prolonged.

37

Rashes

Refer also to Chapter 14.

The skin is the largest organ of the body, and so it is not surprising that a lot can go wrong with it! Rashes may be an indication of a skin disease only, or they may be just the tip of the iceberg and reflect an underlying, more generalized disease. Many infectious diseases present with a rash and a fever. These may be relatively minor illnesses or very severe ones such as dengue fever or meningococcemia, both of which may be acquired while traveling.

> *Note:* If your child has a rash and is severely ill, medical care should be sought immediately.

Discussed below are a few of the more common skin ailments that your child is likely to get. Other skin problems are discussed elsewhere in the book.

DIAPER RASH

Most young children get a diaper rash (diaper dermatitis) at some time or another. This is not surprising, since diapers are essentially receptacles for urine and feces. Children who don't wear diapers don't get diaper rashes! Young children tend to have very sensitive and delicate skin, and diaper rashes can develop very rapidly, often overnight or after just one or two loose stools. Some children get diaper rashes very easily despite good hygiene. Diaper rashes are caused by irritants in the urine or stools and by infectious agents: bacteria, fungi (yeasts), and viruses. Diaper rashes may occur when new foods are introduced into the diet. Acidic foods such as citrus fruits or tomatoes are particularly likely to cause rashes when first introduced. Sometimes rashes are caused by irritation from the diaper itself. If you have recently changed diaper brands and your child develops a diaper rash, it may be prudent to go back to the old brand.

 Prevention

Most diaper rashes can be prevented by good hygiene and a few basic precautions:

- Change your child's diaper frequently, preferably as soon as he is wet or soiled.
- If your child has soiled, cleanse the area gently with wet wipes or with tap water and cotton balls. It is not

necessary to use soap to clean the diaper area after every bowel movement. Use soap only if the stool does not come off easily, and then use only a mild soap, such as Dove.

- Allow the diaper area to air frequently. Keep the diaper area uncovered as often and as long as possible. This is often easier said than done! Do not fasten the diaper so that it is airtight, especially overnight.
- Do not overuse wet wipes, as these may dry out the skin. Do not use scented wet wipes.
- Barrier creams and ointments may help to prevent diaper rashes and are useful as part of the treatment of diaper rashes. Most infants do not need to have one of these ointments or creams applied routinely—only if the skin is becoming irritated. It is often a good idea to apply these preventively overnight. Many of these contain zinc oxide or petrolatum or both. Some well-known brands are Desitin, A&D Ointment, and Triple Paste, the last being particularly effective. A very effective barrier agent is bentonite paste, but you will need to ask your pharmacist to make this up. You do not need a prescription for any of these agents.
- Disposable diapers, especially the more absorbent varieties, are more effective in preventing diaper rashes, so consider changing to these if your child is prone to diaper rashes.
- Get your child out of diapers as soon as possible.
- If your child is put on an antibiotic, follow these additional measures to prevent diaper rashes:

- Give him a probiotic, or yogurt that contains a live culture, while he is on the antibiotic.
- Change his diapers more frequently, especially if he develops diarrhea.
- Do not use plastic waterproof pants over cloth diapers.
- Use a barrier cream such as those mentioned above.
- If he develops a diaper rash, he may have a yeast infection, a common complication of antibiotic therapy. A yeast diaper rash is suggested by a bright red rash that is worse in the creases and has scattered red, satellite spots around it. Try an over-the-counter antifungal cream or ointment such as Lotrimin.

Treatment

- Follow the preventative measures outlined above.
- Expose the diaper area to the air more frequently.
- If your child's skin is too sensitive to touch, use a spray bottle of water to clean the skin after soiling. Fill a spray bottle with ½ teaspoon of baking soda dissolved in 16 ounces of warm water. Spray vigorously to remove stool and urine.
- Allow to air-dry or pat dry gently. It is not necessary to remove all the barrier cream at every change.
- Use one of the barrier creams described above. For severe diaper rashes consider using Triple Paste or bentonite ointment. If the diaper rash persists, or if it has

features of a yeast infection (see above), try an antifungal cream such as Lotrimin.

- If you have been using cloth diapers, try one of the newer, more absorptive disposable diapers.
- A weak steroid cream such as 0.5% or 1% hydrocortisone may help to decrease the inflammation in the diaper area but should be used in combination with other creams and ointments and only for short periods. Discuss the use of steroid creams with your child's physician. Unless directed by a physician, do not use potent steroid creams in the diaper area, as the steroid may be absorbed into the body and cause serious side effects.

 When to Seek Medical Attention

Consult a physician if

- the rash persists or gets worse;
- there are large blisters in the diaper area; or
- your child appears ill.

DRY SKIN

Many people have a tendency to develop dry skin. Children are no different and may be even more prone to dry skin and to eczema (see below), especially if they come from an allergic family.

When skin is dry, it tends to itch. An itch leads to scratching. Scratching, in turn, leads to rashes and often to secondary skin infections, the most common of which is impetigo.

  Prevention and Treatment

Follow these guidelines to prevent the skin from drying out and to decrease the discomfort caused by dry skin:

- Minimize washing and bathing.
- Use a mild soap or a soap-free cleanser. Soaps should be free of scents and dyes.
- Wash in warm rather than hot water.
- After bathing or showering, instead of rubbing your child dry with a towel, pat her dry.
- Apply a moisturizing cream or lotion immediately after bathing and while your child's skin is still damp. Moisturizing creams tend to be more effective than lotions. Use a cream free of dyes and as hypoallergenic as possible.
- Reapply these moisturizers liberally and often.
- Wear cool cotton clothes next to the skin. Many people react to wool next to their skin.
- If the dryness worsens or your child develops rough, dry patches over his body, apply an over-the-counter hydrocortisone cream to these dry patches. These patches suggest that your child has more than just dry skin. He probably has eczema.

ECZEMA
(ATOPIC DERMATITIS)

Eczema, also known as atopic dermatitis, is often described as "the itch that rashes" and is becoming increasingly more common. It usually starts in infancy or early childhood and is particularly common in allergic families.

Eczema in babies often shows up as very dry and red cheeks, a dry chin, and cracked and bleeding areas behind the ears. Later on, rough, dry patches appear on different parts of the body. These patches are frequently circular in shape and are often misdiagnosed as ringworm.

In older children, eczema is often worse in the flexures of the elbows and behind the knees. The skin is dry, thickened, and itchy.

Eczema is often worse during winter when the air is dry but may also worsen in hot weather. The skin tends to be more itchy after a hot bath or shower and after activity.

If you suspect that your child has eczema, you should meet with your child's doctor to draw up an eczema treatment plan. This will usually consist of moisturizing agents, steroid or other anti-inflammatory creams and ointments, and sometimes an anti-itch medicine to take by mouth. Benadryl, an antihistamine, is one anti-itch medication that you may have in your medical kit. If given in the evening, it may decrease itching during the night because of its sedative effect. Your doctor may prescribe more potent and longer-acting medications such as hydroxyzine (Atarax) to decrease itching.

Periodically eczema may flare up and make your child itch

even more. Causes of such flare-ups include new foods; new detergents, soaps, or medications; infections; stress; and allergies. A very common cause of an eczema flare-up is inadequate treatment, especially stopping moisturizer creams, which should be the mainstay of your child's eczema treatment. At these times you may need to intensify your child's treatment by applying creams and ointments more frequently, using stronger prescription steroid medications, increasing the dose of the oral anti-itch medications, and even trying a course of antibiotics. Superimposed infection is a common cause of worsening eczema and may be suggested by blisters, weeping, and oozing or by increased scabbing and crusting. These crusts are often honey-colored. Your child's doctor may prescribe an antibiotic to help take care of the secondary infection.

Before setting out on your travels, make sure your child's eczema is under control and that you know how to take care of eczema exacerbations (see Chapter 14, p. 188).

HIVES

Hives are raised, red, and itchy areas that tend to move from one area of the skin to another.

There are many causes of hives, including allergies (for example, to a drug, a food, or insect bites and stings) and infections. Factors such as changes in temperature or exercise bring out hives. Hives may last for days or weeks, and frequently a cause is never found.

Prevention and Treatment

- Try to identify the trigger and then avoid it. Ask yourself: Is my child on any medication? Has my child eaten a new food? Have I tried a new soap or detergent? Could my child have been stung or bitten by an insect?
- Give your child an antihistamine such as Benadryl or one of the newer nonsedating antihistamines.
- Keep your child as cool as possible. Hot baths or showers, excessive activity, sleeping in a warm bed at night, or being overdressed may all worsen hives.
- If your child is ill or has a fever that lasts more than three to four days, medical care should be sought.

CAUTION

Hives may be part of a more severe, generalized allergic reaction. If your child's lips swell or he has any breathing or swallowing difficulty, seek medical attention immediately. If you have an Epipen injector, use it immediately.

HEAT RASH, OR PRICKLY HEAT

See Chapter 14, p. 180.

FOLLICULITIS AND BOILS

See Chapter 14, p. 181.

IMPETIGO

See Chapter 14, p. 182.

FUNGAL INFECTIONS, INCLUDING RINGWORM AND ATHLETE'S FOOT

See Chapter 14, p. 185.

SUNBURN

See Chapter 38.

POISON IVY AND CONTACT DERMATITIS

See Chapter 42.

SCABIES

See Chapter 18, p. 229.

LICE, OR NITS

See Chapter 18, p. 230.

INSECT AND TICK BITES

See Chapter 39.

RASHES AFTER SWIMMING OR BEING IN CONTACT WITH WATER

See Chapter 41.

FOOT BLISTERS

See Chapter 45, p. 473.

PART THREE

Summer
Woes

38

Sunburn

WHAT IS IT?

We have probably all been sunburned at one time or another, and we know what causes it. Sunburn is due to overexposure to the ultraviolet rays of the sun. Mild sunburn is equivalent to a first-degree burn, and severe blistering sunburn is the equivalent of a second-degree burn.

WHY ALL THE FUSS?

Sunburn is probably the most common summer hazard most of us face. It is also one of the more common travel-related conditions. It is often stated that accidents, especially motor vehicle accidents, are the most common cause of travel-related deaths. However, some experts say that death from skin cancer attributed to serious sunburns acquired many years earlier while on vacation is an even more common cause of travel-related death.

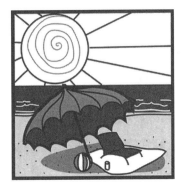

Sun causes not only sunburn but also aging of the skin and, most important, skin cancer. The incidence of skin cancer is increasing at a greater rate than that of any other cancer. One in five Americans can expect to develop skin cancer in his or her lifetime. The most serious type of skin cancer, melanoma, is often fatal and may lead to death in early adulthood. The death rate from melanoma has been increasing at a rate of 4 percent every year since 1973. Five or more blistering sunburns more than double the risk of getting melanoma later in life.

It has been estimated that up to 80 percent of a person's lifetime exposure to the sun has occurred by age 18. As a parent, you are in a position to ensure that your child's exposure to the sun is limited and safe. The damage caused by the sun is cumulative and often shows up only years later in the form of premature aging, wrinkles, sunspots, and cancer. Any tan is a sign of skin damage. Sun damage from sunlight builds up with continued exposure, whether sunburn occurs or not.

Young children are particularly sensitive to the effects of the sun. The skin of infants is thinner and more sensitive than that of adults. The younger the child, the less the protection against the sun and the worse the skin damage. Children also tend to spend more time outdoors than adults.

Sunburn in childhood is more likely to lead to skin cancer than sunburn in adulthood. The immature eyes of infants are also particularly vulnerable to the effects of the sun's rays.

What Is Ultraviolet Light?

Ultraviolet light (or ultraviolet radiation) is the light you can't see and is made up of UVA, UVB, and UVC rays. UVC is filtered out as it passes through the atmosphere and is not an important factor in sunburn. UVA and UVB have an additive effect on the skin and are responsible for the skin damage.

UVB is most responsible for sunburn and the later development of skin cancer and cataracts. UVB is most potent in the middle of the day. UVA is mainly responsible for skin aging (wrinkles, sagging, and brown sunspots) but also plays a part in the development of sunburn and skin cancer. UVA is present throughout the day and penetrates more deeply into the subcutaneous tissues. UVA is also harmful to the eyes and contributes to snow blindness and to the formation of cataracts. Unlike UVB, UVA is transmitted through window glass.

Heat, humidity, and wind can increase the effects of ultraviolet light. So does reflection of UV rays from snow and water. Moist skin reflects less ultraviolet light, allowing for greater absorption of ultraviolet rays.

The UV index is often published daily in the newspaper and will give you some idea of the amount of ultraviolet light that day. The scale is from 1 to 10. The higher the number, the greater the risk.

Prevention

As with all accidents and illnesses, prevention is the best medicine. Avoiding sun damage should involve a *total* program, not just the use of sunscreens.

Limit Sun Exposure

- Minimize the amount of time spent in the sun. This is especially important early on in the season when the skin is particularly sensitive. Increase sun exposure by a few minutes each day.
- Avoid deliberate sunbathing.
- Stay out of the sun at the hottest times of the day. UVB is most severe in the middle of the day (10 a.m. to 4 p.m.). "Only mad dogs and Englishmen go out in the noonday sun." A good rule of thumb is that if your shadow is shorter than you are, you should not be out in the sun. Plan your outdoor activities for early or late in the day.
- It is important to remember that you can still get severely sunburned on cloudy days, as 70–80 percent of the UVB can get through the clouds.
- The higher the elevation, the more severe the effects of the sun. Sun exposure increases by at least 4 percent for each 1,000 feet of elevation. In other words, at an eleva-

tion of 10,000 feet your body is exposed to 40 percent more UVB than at sea level. At higher elevations and during the winter there is less atmospheric ozone to protect you. You may get as much UVB exposure in snowy Vail, Colorado (elevation 8,500 feet), as you would get on a sunny day in Orlando, Florida! Skiers and mountain climbers are particularly prone to sunburn, not only because of the high elevation but also because of the reflected rays from the snow.

• You don't have to be in direct sunlight to get sunburned. Sun may be reflected from concrete, water, snow, and sand and burn you even though you wear a hat or are beneath a beach umbrella.

Wear Protective Clothing

• Wearing protective clothing is an essential part of sun protection.

   Not all clothing offers equal protection against the sun: Your child could still get sunburned through clothing! A thin, white cotton T-shirt has a sun protection factor (SPF) of only 5 to 7. If clothing becomes wet, the SPF is decreased. The tighter the weave and the darker the color, the greater the protection against UV rays. Before you buy, hold the garment up to a light source. If little light gets through, you have made a good choice.

• Long-sleeved shirts and long pants will give added protection.

- Clothing that is loose fitting is generally cooler and offers better protection against the sun than tight-fitting clothing.
- Your child should wear a wide-brimmed hat with a brim of at least 3 inches. Baseball caps provide very little sun protection for the face if worn backward!

Sun-protective clothes have a label listing the garment's UV protection factor (UPF) value. Blue denim has a very high SPF value.

You can purchase true, lightweight, sun-protective clothing from Sun Precautions (Solumbra clothing: 800-882-7860).

Use Sunscreen

The application of a sunscreen should *not* be the primary means of sun protection. It should only supplement sensible sun precautions and the wearing of appropriate clothing.

There are two main types of sunscreens: chemical sunscreens and physical sunblocks.

Chemical sunscreens absorb UV light before it penetrates your skin. They tend to be light and easy to apply but must be applied at least 30 minutes prior to sun exposure. They contain a variety of chemicals to block UVB. Some contain chemicals such as avobenzone (Parsol 1789) to block UVA as well. Most sunscreens are more effective in blocking UVB than UVA. The SPF rating applies only to UVB. Always buy a sunscreen that blocks both UVA and UVB.

Physical sunblocks are opaque and physically block, reflect, and scatter the sun's rays. They give immediate protection and do not have to be applied 30 minutes before sun exposure. Sunblocks block UVB and UVA.

Sunblocks usually contain titanium dioxide or zinc oxide (or both). They tend to be messy and uncomfortable, although newer micronized sunblocks that have very fine particles of titanium dioxide or zinc oxide are more user-friendly.

Sunblocks are especially useful on areas such as the nose, cheeks, lips, and tops of the ears. People allergic to chemical sunscreens can usually tolerate physical sunblocks.

Follow these guidelines when using sunscreens:

- Use a sunscreen with an SPF of at least 15. Very sensitive individuals (infants, fair people with blond or red hair, or people with many freckles or moles) should use a sunscreen with an SPF of at least 30.
    - A sunscreen with an SPF of 15 filters out 93 percent of UVB rays if applied correctly. A sunscreen with an SPF of 30 filters out 97 percent of UVB rays if applied correctly.
    - Sunscreens with SPFs greater than 30 are probably not necessary and are more expensive. It is better to buy a larger bottle of sunscreen with a lower SPF and apply it more liberally than to use a sunscreen with a higher SPF and not apply enough.
    - The SPF number gives you some idea of how long you can remain in the sun before burning. If, for ex-

ample, you would normally burn in 10 minutes, applying a sufficient amount of sunscreen with an SPF of 15 would provide you with about 150 minutes in the sun before burning. However, most people do not apply enough sunscreen to achieve the labeled SPF.

- The SPF number can be reduced by perspiration and swimming. A sunscreen is said to be *water resistant* if it lasts for 40 minutes in water and *waterproof* if it lasts 80 minutes or longer.

- Apply the sunscreen 30 minutes before being exposed to the sun to allow time for the lotion to penetrate the skin. Particularly sun-sensitive individuals should reapply the sunscreen just before going outside.

- Apply sufficient sunscreen. Most people use only a quarter to half of the recommended amount of sunscreen. An adult needs at least 1 ounce (one palmful) of lotion to cover the body completely. If the sunscreen is applied at least twice a day, an 8-ounce bottle of lotion will last only four days!

- Cover all parts of the body exposed to the sun. Apply an especially thick layer to the shoulders and to the nose. Do not forget the tips of the ears, the neck, the ankles, and the tops of the feet. Apply a sunblock or lip balm with sunscreen to the lips.

- Reapply the sunscreen frequently, at least every two hours. Reapply more frequently if sweating excessively or swimming. Reapply after toweling or when clothing rubs off the sunscreen—for example, when hiking. Waterproof sunscreens will last longer in water but should still be reapplied frequently. All sunscreens need to be reapplied.

Sunscreens may cause allergic or irritant rashes. Sunscreens containing PABA have a greater chance of causing allergic rashes. To avoid this, choose a sunscreen that contains PABA esters or other ingredients. You can do a patch test by applying a small amount to the inside of the forearm first and noting any redness or irritation. Sunblocks are less likely to cause allergic rashes.

Particularly suitable products for infants and young children are the range of Vanicream sun protection creams, which include sunscreens and sunblocks. Phone: (800) 325-8232. Web site: www.psico.com.

Delray dermatologicals manufacture a wide range of sun protection products under the label Blue Lizard Australian Suncream. Phone: (800) 877-8869. Web site: www.Delray derm.com.

Waterbabies, made by Coppertone, also seems to work well for many young children. Despite these recommendations, just about any product can cause skin rashes in infants, as they tend to have very sensitive skin. You may need to try several products before finding the right one for your child.

Sunscreen does *not* allow unlimited sun exposure. It merely helps to decrease sunburn. If you would normally get sunburned in 10 minutes and you have applied a sufficient amount of sunscreen with an SPF of 15, you may be able to spend 150 minutes in the sun. Once you have spent your 150 minutes in the sun, you need to cover up or get out of the sun. Reapplying the sunscreen does not allow you to spend another 150 minutes in the sun. In other words, sunscreens should *not* be used to prolong time spent in the sun.

We should all try to adopt the Australian slogan "Slip on a shirt, slop on sunscreen, and slap on a hat!"

SPECIAL SITUATIONS

Infants

Infants are especially prone to severe sunburn. Many sunscreen bottles state "not for use under 6 months of age." Most sunscreens, however, can be used on infants. It is far better to use a sunscreen than to let your infant get sunburned. It is better still *not* to expose young infants to the sun, especially in the middle of the day. If you have no option, use a sunscreen as well as clothing that covers the arms and legs. Shield your child with an umbrella and use a head covering as well. Remember, ultraviolet light is invisible and can be reflected onto an infant under an umbrella. It does not take much to burn an infant's skin.

Adolescents

Adolescents are especially fond of getting suntans. I don't know of any way to convince teenagers about the dangers of the sun, but you should try to teach them how to limit sun exposure and how to use sunscreens correctly.

Tanning Devices

Indoor tanning devices can be as harmful as direct sunlight. Most tanning salons use lamps that supposedly only emit UVA rays, but many lamps are not well calibrated and emit UVB rays as well.

Sunscreens with Insect Repellents

It is preferable not to use lotions that contain both a sunscreen and an insect repellent. You should use each separately. Apply the sunscreen first and allow time for it to penetrate the skin. Apply the insect repellent over the lotion just before exposure. Do not rub the repellent into the skin. The repellent will reduce the SPF of the sunscreen.

Medications and Sun Sensitivity

Some medications increase a person's sensitivity to the sun. This is especially true of some antibiotics, but some anti-inflammatory medications, oral contraceptives, and some diuretics also increase sensitivity.

Dark-Skinned People

It is a fallacy that dark-skinned people can't get sunburned or get skin cancer. They, too, should follow safe sun rules.

Treatment

Unfortunately, the symptoms of sunburn do not begin until two to four hours after the sun's damage has already been done. The peak reaction of redness, pain, and swelling does not occur for 24 hours. In other words, you will not realize your child has been sunburned until after the fact. Nothing can reverse the effects of sunburn that has already occurred. The damage is done! You can, however, treat the symptoms. The following measures may help:

- Cool baths or wet compresses are very effective in relieving pain and burning.
- Ibuprofen or acetaminophen may help relieve the sensation of pain and heat.
- Nonprescription 1% hydrocortisone cream and bland moisturizing creams can be applied two to three times a day and may help to decrease pain and swelling. Refrigerating creams and lotions prior to use gives added relief. Aloe vera gel or cream is soothing and may aid healing.
- Get your child to drink extra fluid to prevent dehydration.
- Peeling of the skin occurs some days after sunburn. The itching can be partly relieved by applying moisturizing creams and lotions frequently.

A variety of other topical remedies are often recommended. These include oatmeal or baking soda baths, vitamin E oil, and many other creams and lotions. Remember, the skin has already been damaged and can easily be further irritated. Probably very little else is as soothing as cool water soaks and compresses. Some physicians recommend high-dose ibuprofen or oral corticosteroids, but there is little scientific evidence to substantiate that they are effective once the sunburn has already occurred. They also may have unpleasant side effects.

Once your child has a sunburn, further damage and discomfort can be avoided by observing the following:

- Do not apply ointments, petroleum products, or butters to sunburn because they all prevent heat and sweat from escaping from the skin.
- Do not use first aid creams or sprays that contain benzocaine because they may cause allergic rashes.
- Do not apply DEET-containing insect repellents to sunburned skin. Damaged skin allows greater absorption of substances into the body.
- If your child has blisters, do not pop them. Once they are broken, cut away the dead skin and try to discourage your child from picking at the peeling edges until the skin has healed completely. Some physicians recommend applying a topical antibiotic such as Bacitracin to the exposed new skin, but this is seldom necessary, as secondary infection is uncommon.

The most important aspect of the treatment of sunburn is preventing further sun damage. Do not expose your child to the sun again until the skin is completely healed.

When to Seek Medical Attention

- If your child has extensive blistering.
- If your child appears ill or dizzy. A severe sunburn may be as serious as a severe burn from a hot liquid or other heat sources and may lead to fluid loss and shock.
- If your child has a temperature higher than 102°F.
- If the sunburn appears to have become infected. Fortunately, this rarely occurs.

EYE DAMAGE

Just as the sun's rays may cause damage to the skin, they may also cause damage to the eyes, increasing the chance that your child will develop cataracts later in life. Chronic sun exposure also increases the risk of macular degeneration, which is a significant cause of blindness in the elderly.

The acute effects of the sun on the eye are *photoconjunctivitis* (inflammation of the conjunctiva) and *photokeratitis* (inflammation of the cornea). These are the equivalent of sunburn of the eye. The eyes will be red and very painful, but these conditions do not usually lead to long-term eye damage. Snow blindness is a very severe form of photokeratitis.

Sunglasses

- Buy sunglasses with lenses that absorb 99–100 percent of UV rays. Look for labels that say "Photo, UV absorption up to 400 nm"; "Maximum or 99% UV protection or blockage"; "Special purpose"; or "Meets ANSI (American National Standard Institute) UV requirements."
- The larger the lenses and the closer they are to the eye, the better the protection.
- The darkness of the lenses does not correlate with the ability to block UV rays.
- Cheap toy sunglasses should be avoided. They give little or no protection and may harm your child's eyes further by encouraging him to look into the sun.

IN SUMMARY

Exposure to too much sunlight is dangerous to your child's health, both in the short term and the long term. Sunscreens alone will not provide sufficient protection, and there is no such thing as a healthy tan! The good news is that minimizing ultraviolet radiation during the first 20 years of life will decrease your child's risk of de-

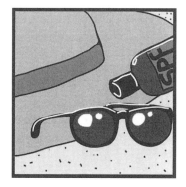

veloping melanoma and other types of skin cancer later on. Using the commonsense precautions suggested above will help prevent sun damage.

Children raised in households where putting on sunscreen is as routine as brushing teeth will find it easier to continue the habit even into adolescence. If you set a good example for your children when they are young, they are more likely to continue these habits into adolescence and adulthood.

Remember to protect your child's eyes from the sun.

Insect Bites and Stings

Refer also to Chapters 15, 16, 43, and 44.

The pleasures of the outdoors are often spoiled by the unwelcome attention of biting and stinging insects. Fortunately, in the United States, most bites and stings are harmless and cause only minor local irritation. In contrast, in many other parts of the world, diseases transmitted by insects are a major health hazard and cause severe illness and chronic ill health, as well as millions of deaths. It is important to remember, however, that even in the Unites States, insects and ticks may carry serious diseases. Mosquitoes may cause West Nile fever, and ticks may cause Lyme disease, Rocky Mountain spotted fever, and a number of other illnesses.

Stinging insects usually just inflict unpleasant and painful stings that get your attention immediately. A small number of people have severe reactions to bee stings that may be life-threatening. Others, especially children, have fairly significant local allergic skin reactions to bites from common insects such as gnats, mosquitoes, or fleas. Insect stings tend to cause immediate and noticeable pain; insect and tick bites, on the other hand, are usually painless and at first go unnoticed. Even spider bites may not cause much pain initially, but severe local pain, redness, and swelling may develop later along with more general symptoms such as headache, abdominal pain, and muscle cramps.

The measures you and your child should take to prevent insect and tick bites depend largely on the diseases you need to prevent, which in turn depends on the area you live in or intend to visit. It is extremely important to take preventative measures seriously if you are in an area where you might acquire serious diseases such as malaria, dengue fever, or yellow fever. Malaria causes up to 3 million deaths each year, mainly in children. Every 30 seconds, somewhere in the world, a child dies from malaria.

Just as the prevention of sunburn involves more than just one application of sunscreen, so the prevention of insect bites and stings involves more than just the use of repellents.

 Prevention

General Measures to Minimize the Chance of Insect and Tick Bites and Stings

- Choose your picnic or campsite carefully. Avoid places that attract insects such as fields of clover, orchards with fallen fruit, and areas near trash cans. Also avoid areas with dense vegetation. High and dry areas that have less vegetation are less likely to harbor insects and ticks. Breezes may deter flying insects.

- When camping, do not sleep or lie right on the ground but rather on a blanket or camping mattress.
- Avoid bright clothing and jewelry, perfumes, aftershave lotions, hair spray, and scented cosmetics and soaps, all of which tend to attract insects.
- Dress sensibly. Wear closed shoes, long-sleeved shirts, and long pants. Tuck the bottom of pants into socks or boots. Loose-fitting clothes are better, as mosquitoes and tsetse flies may bite right through tight-fitting clothing. Insects tend to be attracted more to dark-colored clothing than light clothing. It is also easier to spot ticks and other insects on light-colored clothing. Good colors are khaki, tan, and white. Wearing a hat, especially with permethrin sprayed on to it, will help greatly in preventing insect "attacks" on your head.
- When eating outside in the company of bees and other insects, eat and drink cautiously. Cover food and drinks tightly, and be careful when drinking directly from soda cans. Bees, especially yellow jackets, often crawl inside open cans to feed.
- Avoid rapid movements when in areas with many bees. If a bee lands on your child, do not slap or brush it away. Bees don't usually sting unless frightened or provoked.
- Keep insects out of your car. In areas with many insects, travel with your windows closed. Keep a cloth or towel handy to trap bees or other flying insects. Pull off the road before attempting to get rid of an intruder.

- Some insects, especially mosquitoes, feed only at certain times. The mosquito that carries malaria usually feeds between dusk and dawn, so try not to be outdoors at these times. The mosquito that transmits West Nile fever is most active in the early morning and at dusk.
- In your own backyard, get rid of standing water, where insects can breed.
- If you are in tick-infested areas, perform careful body inspections twice a day for ticks.

Insect Repellents and Insecticides

Insect repellents are usually applied directly to the skin and repel insects and ticks. Insecticides are usually applied to clothing or sprayed into confined spaces and often kill insects or ticks. The repellent you choose will vary depending on a number of factors:

- The "bug" you are trying to repel and the illness you are trying to prevent: if you need to prevent such severe diseases as malaria, yellow fever, Japanese encephalitis, and dengue fever, all of which can be fatal, you need to use an effective repellent, in other words DEET in a concentration of at least 20%.
- How long you need the repellent to be effective; the higher the DEET concentration, the longer the duration of action.
- Your location. For example, you will need a more potent repellent in a rain forest where the concentration of

"bugs" is high and where rain and sweat will tend to wash the repellent away.

- The age of the person using it. Some authorities feel that it is safer to use lower concentrations of DEET (less than 20%) in young children because of the widely held but possibly erroneous belief that DEET toxicity is related to concentration. The American Academy of Pediatrics recommends using preparations that contain less than 30% DEET. It also states that DEET should not be used for children in the first two months of life.
- Generally speaking, if it is important to prevent being bitten, you cannot beat the combination of DEET on the skin and permethrin on clothes.

The time of day that the repellent is applied will vary according to the disease you are trying to avoid. For example, when trying to avoid malaria or Japanese encephalitis, the repellent should be applied between dusk and dawn (the evening and nighttime hours). On the other hand, if you are trying to avoid being bitten by the mosquito that causes yellow fever or dengue fever, you will need to have repellent on during daylight hours as well.

DEET

There are many types of insect repellents, but the most reliable and effective by far are those that contain DEET (N,N-diethyl-3-methylbenzamide). However, these may be toxic in young children if not used correctly, as DEET is absorbed through the skin into the circulatory system.

It may be safer for children to use preparations that contain DEET at a concentration of 30% or less. The disadvantages of using lower concentrations of DEET are that they will not last as long and therefore may not give adequate protection and that, because they do not last as long, they will have to be reapplied frequently, which in and of itself may cause toxicity.

DEET preparations are available in many forms including sticks, sprays, creams, and lotions. The concentration of DEET in these preparations ranges from 5% to 100%. Lower concentrations of DEET are just as effective as higher concentrations when first applied but do not last as long. The duration of action generally correlates with the concentration up to 50%. There is not much point using preparations with concentrations in excess of 50%.

Some of the lotions containing DEET are available as extended-release formulations. Two excellent ones are listed here:

1. Ultrathon. This is one of the more effective preparations and is an excellent choice, especially when it is vital to prevent insect bites. This contains 33% DEET and can be purchased through Travel Medicine (800-872-8633; www.travmed.com). It is used by the military and is extremely effective, providing up to 12 hours of protection (the same as preparations containing 75% DEET).

2. Another very effective and long-lasting preparation of DEET for both children and adults is Sawyer Controlled Release Family Insect Repellent, which contains 20% DEET (Sawyer: 800-940-4464; www.sawyeronline.com). This lotion is easy to apply and minimizes the absorption of DEET. It lasts up to five hours and is probably one of the better choices, if not the best, for children.

Both these preparations (Ultrathon and Sawyer Controlled Release Family Insect Repellent) are now available at many camping stores and in the camping section of many large chain stores such as Wal-Mart.

To be effective, repellents must be applied to all exposed skin, as mosquitoes will readily bite unprotected skin just an inch or two away from the treated area. Ideally, especially when used on children, DEET should be applied only once a day to limit its potential toxicity. However, preparations with lower concentrations of DEET may need to be reapplied more often, particularly if your child is sweating or very active.

The following precautions should be taken when using DEET:

- Avoid applying DEET around the eyes or mouth.
- Do not apply DEET to the hands of small children, as they often put their hands and fingers in their mouth.
- Do not apply to cuts, wounds, or sunburned or irritated skin.

- When applying DEET, do not rub it in but apply it lightly.
- Do not let young children apply DEET themselves.
- Apply DEET only to exposed skin and not under clothing.
- Do not reapply DEET unless necessary.
- Do not spray DEET near food.
- Wash off the repellent with soap and water when it is no longer needed.
- DEET is combustible and is *highly toxic if ingested*, so keep any DEET-containing products in a safe place away from inquisitive children.

DEET can also be applied to clothing, although it may damage plastics and spandex. It may also damage wristwatch crystals and eyeglass frames. It is generally preferable to use DEET on skin and permethrin on clothing. DEET does not damage natural fibers such as wool or cotton.

Overall, DEET is extremely safe for children if used correctly. It is the best preparation to use when trying to prevent bites from insects that carry dangerous diseases such as malaria, dengue fever, and yellow fever.

Other Repellents

Many other insect repellents are available, some of which contain only "natural" substances. These include citronella, which is found in Avon's Skin So Soft. A testament to the fact that this preparation is not very effective is that Avon has recently introduced a new formulation of Skin So Soft that contains DEET. One of the more effective "green" formulations is Bite Blocker, which contains soybean oil, geranium oil, and coconut oil (www.biteblocker.com). Use this preparation if you feel you cannot use a DEET-containing preparation. If you use natural products that do not contain DEET, it is important to reapply them frequently because of their short duration of action. However, none of these natural preparations is as effective or lasts as long as DEET, which remains the gold standard.

Some newer insect repellents that contain picardin may be just as effective as DEET. Repellents that contain picardin include Cutter Advanced, Bayrepel, Autan Repel, and KBR3023. However, to be as effective as DEET, picardin-containing preparations should contain at least 20% picardin, which at present is not the case in the United States. More effective picardin-containing insect repellents are available in other parts of the world.

Insecticides: Permethrin-Containing Products

Permethrin is extremely effective in protecting against ticks and also against many biting insects, including mosquitoes. In fact, it is more effective against ticks than DEET. It should *not* be applied directly to the skin but should be applied to clothing, bedding, bed nets, and camping gear. It does not damage fabrics and will last through many washes. In areas with a high concentration of ticks and a high risk of Lyme disease, spray permethrin on socks, shoes, and trousers, and even consider ankle bands impregnated with permethrin. When spraying clothes, hold the can about 12 inches away and use enough spray to moisten the entire garment. Spray both sides and let the clothing dry before wearing. It is especially important to spray permethrin on bed nets when trying to prevent being bitten by the anopheles mosquito, which carries malaria.

Recommended permethrin-containing preparations to use on clothes and camping equipment include

1. Sawyer Permethrin Tick Repellent, which can be purchased by calling (800) 940-4464 or online at www .sawyeronline.com;
2. Duranon Tick Repellent;
3. Cutter Outdoorsman Gear Guard; and
4. Fite Bite Permethrin Solution, which can be purchased by calling (800) TRAV-MED.

Aerosol knock-down insecticides frequently contain permethrin-related substances. Examples of these include Doom and Raid. These types of insecticides are effective and can be sprayed in the bedroom before going to bed.

An ideal combination for preventing bites of insect *and* ticks is to use DEET on the skin and permethrin on clothing.

CAUTION
Neither DEET nor permethrin protects against stinging insects such as bees, wasps, hornets, or fire ants.

Folk Remedies

Vitamin B_1 and garlic are not effective repellents. The latter may have repellent effects on the human species! Sucking on lemons may prevent scurvy but not insect bites.

Simultaneous Use of Sunscreens and Insect Repellents

If your child requires both a sunscreen and an insect repellent, it is preferable to use each separately. Apply the sunscreen to your child's skin about 30 minutes prior to sun exposure, allowing time for it to be absorbed by the skin. Then apply the insect repellent. Do *not* rub the DEET in but apply it lightly. However, the DEET will lessen the protective effects of the sunscreen, so it is advisable to use a sunscreen with a higher SPF than you usually use. An alternative but less ideal approach is to use combination products that contain both DEET and a sunscreen with a SPF of greater than 15. Examples of such preparations are OFF! Skintastic with Sunscreen (SPF 30) and Cutter with Sunscreen. You will need to be cautious about reapplying these preparations to avoid DEET toxicity.

IN SUMMARY

It is better to use a combination of methods to prevent insect and tick bites and the diseases they transmit:

- Avoid infested habitats.
- Wear suitable clothing.

- Use an effective repellent.
- Apply an insecticide to your clothing, bedding, bed nets, and so on.

When to Seek Medical Attention

If you develop any unusual symptoms such as high fevers, severe headache, or unusual rashes after being in an infested area, seek medical attention. Be sure to tell your doctor about your travels.

TICK BITES AND TICK REMOVAL

Tick bites and tickborne illnesses are common throughout the world, including the United States. In fact, ticks cause almost as many human diseases worldwide as mosquitoes do. In the United States ticks are responsible for more disease than mosquitoes. Ticks transmit a variety of infectious illnesses, of which Lyme disease is by far the most common (see Chapter 44). Another important tickborne disease in the United States is Rocky Mountain spotted fever.

Prevention

The most important measures in preventing tick bites are listed below (see also the general measures to prevent insect and tick bites, p. 412).

- If possible, avoid tick-infested areas. Be especially vigilant when walking in long grass. Ticks do not jump, fly, or drop from trees. Ticks crawl onto you as you lie on the ground, stride through long grass, or brush against vegetation.
- Wear suitable clothing and enclosed shoes. Wear long pants and tuck them into socks or boots.
- Apply permethrin to clothing.
- Apply a repellent to exposed skin.
- Do twice-daily tick inspections. Remember, the tick stage that usually transmits Lyme disease is the nymph, which is very small—about the size of a sesame seed.

What to Do If You Find a Tick

If you detect the tick early, it may not be attached, and you may be able to pick it off very easily. If the tick is firmly attached, you will need to use tweezers or one of the instruments specifically designed to remove ticks. If using tweezers, grasp the tick as close to the skin as possible and pull upward 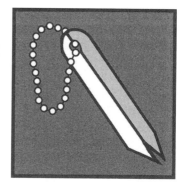 and backward with steady, even traction. Do not twist, jerk, squeeze, crush, or puncture the tick. You can purchase instruments specifically designed to remove ticks (Pro-Tick

Remedy: (800) PIX-TICK or (800) 749-8425; www.tickinfo .com). These instruments are particularly useful for removing very small ticks and also lessen the chances of crushing the tick.

Once the tick has been removed, disinfect the area with soap and water or an alcohol swab. You may also apply an antibacterial cream such as Triple Antibiotic or Bactroban. Discourage your child from scratching the area, as this may lead to secondary infection.

Occasionally the head of the tick may be left behind in the skin. It is not usually worth the extra trauma of digging it out. Apply an antibacterial cream for a few days, and the area will usually settle down and clear. Your child may develop a small, red inflamed area or nodule that will disappear over a week or two. This is *not* the rash of Lyme disease.

Although ticks can be disease carriers and the prevention of tick bites is important, keep in mind the following:

- By far the majority of tick bites in the United States are harmless and do *not* lead to any disease. At the most your child will develop a red area smaller than the size of a nickel.
- Except in certain high-risk areas, most deer ticks do *not* carry Lyme disease.
- Deer ticks need to be attached for at least 24 hours before they can transmit Lyme disease.

When to Seek Medical Attention

If the typical rash of Lyme disease develops in the ensuing days or weeks, seek medical attention. Also seek medical attention if your child becomes ill. Refer to Chapter 44 for further details on Lyme disease.

INSECT STINGS

For general measures on preventing insect bites and stings, see above, p. 412. As mentioned earlier, insect repellents do not protect against stinging insects, only against biting insects.

Treatment

- If the insect left a stinger in the skin, remove it immediately. The sooner the stinger is removed, the less time the poison has to be injected. Scrape the stinger off with a knife or credit card or fingernail. Avoid squeezing the stinger, as this will inject more poison. Yellow jackets and wasps do not leave a stinger and may sting repeatedly.
- Apply ice or a cold pack to the sting site. Cortisone cream will help soothe the sting and decrease itching.
- Diphenhydramine (Benadryl) by mouth will decrease the allergic reaction and itching. Newer nonsedating

antihistamines should be just as effective and do not need to be given as often.

- Give acetaminophen or ibuprofen for pain.

CAUTION

Signs of a severe allergic reaction include the following:

- **Difficulty swallowing, thick tongue, hoarseness.**
- **Chest tightness, wheezing, difficulty breathing.**
- **Confusion, fainting, and collapse.**

***Call 911* if your child has any of these symptoms. If you have an EpiPen injector, inject it *immediately*.**

Note: A person who has had a severe reaction to an insect sting should consult a physician to decide whether allergy injections (immunotherapy, or "shots") are indicated.

If your child has just had a severe reaction as outlined above and you used an epinephrine injector, your child should *still* be seen by a physician or taken to the nearest emergency room. Many people have a delayed second reaction that will require further treatment.

If your child has had a previous severe generalized reaction, you should *always* carry an emergency epinephrine kit (such as EpiPen or EpiPen Junior) wherever you go. This is especially important on trips outdoors, vacations, and so on. Learn how to use this kit. If your child has a severe reaction, **do not delay— use your kit.**

Most children who are stung by an insect will not have a severe reaction but may have an itchy, red swelling that can persist for as long as five to seven days. This swelling may extend far beyond the original sting and be tender, warm, and red. This is known as a "large local reaction" and does not usually indicate that the bite is infected. Continued use of cool compresses and appropriate doses of Benadryl or other antihistamines will help. Occasionally, with persistent scratching, children may develop a secondary infection at the site of the sting and may require antibiotics by mouth or application of an antibiotic cream.

FIRE ANTS

Fire ants, also known as imported fire ants, are becoming an increasing problem in the United States, particularly in the Gulf region, and are responsible for tens of thousands of stings each year. Originally natives of South America, these aggressive insects have taken up permanent residence in many of the southern states of the United States. They get their name from the intense burning sensation that follows after their sting.

The ants are small, only about 2 to 5 mm (less than a quarter of an inch) in length, and are red or black in color. They live in ant heaps but readily invade houses and other buildings.

Anyone can get stung. Children are frequent victims, especially in the summer months; feet, ankles, and legs are prime targets.

When the fire ant stings, it attaches to the skin of its victim by its jaw and stings with a stinger at the end of its abdomen. If the ant is not immediately removed, it will sting the victim in a circular pattern, holding on to the skin with its jaw as it pivots in a circular motion. An intense burning sensation follows immediately, and usually within 30 minutes the victim has a raised red itchy wheal. Over the next 24 hours this wheal evolves into a small, sterile pustule. The victim often scratches this, and secondary bacterial infection may follow. A large local reaction may also follow a sting: redness, swelling, and itching extending for inches around the original bite site.

CAUTION

A severe allergic reaction, anaphylaxis, may also follow the sting of a fire ant. Its signs include the following:

- **Swelling of the lips, tongue, and throat.**
- **Breathing difficulties.**
- **A drop in blood pressure.**
- **Collapse.**

Call 911 **if your child has any of these symptoms. If you have an EpiPen injector, inject it *immediately*.**

Prevention and Treatment

- As always, prevention is best. Avoid areas that fire ants are known to inhabit. Do not disturb their ant heaps. This is not always easy to do: in some areas in the South, their ant mounds cover fields, building sites, and playgrounds and may number up to 200 per acre!
- If attacked by fire ants, brush them off immediately.
- Once a sting has occurred, apply ice or cool compresses to relieve the burning and itch. Topical applications of lotions that contain camphor and menthol may also help, as may creams or gels containing benzocaine or steroids. All creams, lotions, and gels tend to be more soothing if refrigerated first. None of these remedies will halt the progression of the wheal into a pustule.
- Oral antihistamines may be needed for persisting or severe itching.
- Cleanse the area with soap and water frequently to avoid secondary infection.
- For those people who have severe large local reactions, elevation of the affected area and oral antihistamines and corticosteroids may be necessary.
- For those with anaphylaxis, immediate administration of epinephrine by injection (EpiPen) is the best treatment, followed by expert medical care. Call 911. After recovery from the event these people should see an allergist for possible immunotherapy. They should also

have immediate access to injectable epinephrine at all times.

For Your Reference

1. "Reactions to the Stings of the Imported Fire Ant," by R. D. deShazo, B. T. Butcher, and W. A. Banks, in the *New England Journal of Medicine* 323 (1990): 462–66.
2. "Imported Fire Ant Stings: Clinical Manifestations and Treatment," by P. R. Cohen, in *Pediatric Dermatology* 9 (1992): 44–48.

SPIDERS

There are more than 20,000 species of spiders in the United States and 34,000 worldwide. Many species produce venom, but few species are harmful to humans, either because the fangs are not strong enough to penetrate skin or because the venom is not toxic enough. In the United States, however, the black widow spider and the brown recluse spider can cause serious reactions or even death, especially in children. Fortunately, bites by these two spiders are relatively rare and often do not produce serious illness. Fatalities from spider bites are extremely rare, but arachnophobia (fear of spiders) is not!

Spider bites are far less common than insect bites or stings. Rarely is the bite witnessed, and so the diagnosis is often difficult. Spider bites often occur on parts of the body where clothing is constrictive, such as at the sites of cuffs, collars, and waistbands and at the groin.

 Treatment

If you suspect that your child has been bitten by a venomous spider, seek medical attention promptly. Spider bites may not cause much initial pain and may go unnoticed for some time. Young children suspected of having been bitten by a black widow spider or a brown recluse spider should be hospitalized for observation and treatment.

If you or your child have witnessed the bite, follow these treatment measures:

1. Clean the wound, immobilize the affected limb, and apply ice.
2. Administer a pain-relieving medicine such as acetaminophen (Tylenol) or ibuprofen (Advil, Motrin).
3. Keep your child still to minimize the spread of venom.
4. Seek medical care. Further treatment may be indicated, and your child may need a tetanus shot and antibiotics.

Black Widow Spiders

With its legs extended, the black widow spider is usually about the size of a quarter. It is usually shiny black in color and has a red, orange, or yellow hourglass-shaped marking on the underside of the abdomen. It may be found indoors or outdoors.

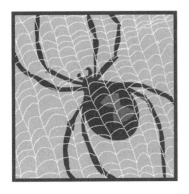

Immediately after being bitten by a black widow bite, a person may feel a pinprick or pinch sensation, but because the bite does not initially cause a lot of pain, it may go totally unnoticed. Usually within an hour or so, a dull burning or aching pain develops at the site of the bite. This pain may last for days. Redness, itching, and swelling develop, and two red puncture marks may be visible. These puncture marks are not usually visible at the time of the bite. In some people, other, more generalized symptoms develop later. These symptoms include muscle tremors and aches, cramps, flushing, excessive sweating, and salivation. Swelling of the face, rather like that seen with an allergic reaction, may occur. There may also be chest tightness, backache, severe abdominal pain, and fainting. Even more severe symptoms may develop later. By this stage, the victim is hopefully in the hospital. Infants may show none of the above symptoms but just cry inconsolably.

Brown Recluse Spiders

These spiders are smaller than black widow spiders. With their legs extended, they are usually between a nickel and a quarter in size. They are usually light or dark brown in color and have a violin-shaped mark on their back. They live both indoors and outdoors. They hibernate in the winter, so the most likely time for a bite from a brown recluse spider is between April and October. These spiders are more active at night.

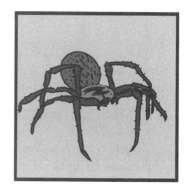

Again, the bite may hurt only a little or not at all. Over the next few hours, redness, swelling, and itching may develop, followed by blistering. Two tiny bite marks may be visible. The wound may have the appearance of a halo with a blue center surrounded by a white ring that in turn is surrounded by a red ring. The wound often develops a thick scab (eschar) that may last for weeks or even longer. When the scab falls off, a deep ulcer may be left that may take months to heal. There is usually no immediate danger from the bite of a brown recluse spider, as generalized symptoms are rare. However, generalized symptoms may occur in children, especially young children, and include fever, nausea, sweating, vomiting, and muscle spasms.

Other spiders whose bites may cause symptoms in humans include the hobo spider and the funnel-web spiders. The symptoms are more local and include pain and blistering at the bite site. Generalized symptoms rarely occur.

IN SUMMARY

- If you or your child is bitten by a spider, you will probably not witness the bite.
- Most spider bites are not dangerous and just require local treatment in the form of cleansing, ice, and possibly pain medication such as ibuprofen or Tylenol. Anti-itch medication such as Benadryl may also be useful.
- If you suspect that your child has been bitten by a black widow or a brown recluse spider, seek medical attention immediately. If there is any doubt, it is still wise to seek medical attention. Muscle aches or weakness, abdominal pain, excessive sweating, or salivation indicates a serious reaction.
- Infants, young children, and the elderly are more likely to have serious reactions to poisonous spider bites.
- If you have captured the spider, it is helpful to bring it along for identification. When trying to catch the spider, it is important to avoid being bitten yourself!

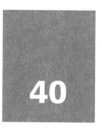

40

Snake Bites

Most snakes are not aggressive and will not bite unless disturbed or challenged. Despite all the horrific stories you hear, there are very few deaths from snake bites in the United States. There are approximately 45,000 snake bites a year in the United States and only about 10 deaths. Mexico has more poisonous species than the United States, and up to 150 people die each year from snake bites. Other parts of the world have a greater variety of snakes, many of which are very poisonous. Worldwide, there are probably more than 100,000 human deaths each year from snake bites, but still most snake bites do not lead to death, and many lead to very few symptoms other than extreme anxiety. Still, it is wise to have a healthy respect for snakes. A bite may lead to severe local tissue damage as well as collapse, cardiac arrest, and death.

Prevention

Remember, as always, prevention is better than cure:

- If you are planning a hiking or camping trip, learn beforehand about the type of snakes you are likely to encounter. Knowledge is power. There may not be any poisonous snakes in the area you plan to visit. If you have learned to recognize the poisonous species and you get bitten by one of them, you will know you need to get to medical care as soon as possible.
- Avoid areas that are known to be snake infested.
- Protect your feet and legs—wear closed shoes or boots and long pants. Tuck your pants into your socks or boots.
- Look where you put your feet and hands. The vine you are about to grab hold of may not be a vine!
- Be especially careful when disturbing rocks or piles of stones.
- If collecting firewood when it is dark, take a flashlight with you. Always use a flashlight when moving around your campsite at night.
- When camping outdoors, shake out bedding or sleeping bags before going to bed at night.
- Check shoes and boots before putting them on.
- If you come upon a snake, do not disturb it: many snake

bites occur when people (usually adolescent or young adult males) "mess around" with snakes.

The medically important species of snakes in North America fall into two families: the *pit vipers* (rattlesnakes, copperheads, cottonmouth water moccasins, and cantils), and the *elapids* (the coral snakes).

PIT VIPERS

Rattlesnakes, the most common of the pit vipers, are responsible for the majority of snake bites in the United States. Copperheads are the second most common cause of snake bites in the United States. Pit vipers are found throughout the continental United States. Most pit viper bites result in envenomation (release of venom), but less than one-third lead to severe poisoning. About 20 percent of bites are "dry," meaning that no venom is injected. Bites from pit vipers tend to cause immediate, severe pain and local tissue damage with discoloration and swelling at the site of the bite. Other symptoms and signs such as nausea and vomiting, weakness, and a metallic taste in the mouth may follow later.

Pit vipers have a triangular or spear-shaped head and vertical, elliptical pupils. They get their name from a facial pit between the eye and the nostril. Their top speed of travel is only 3 miles per hour.

CORAL SNAKES

Coral snakes belong to the elapids and are found in Arizona, the southeastern United States, and Texas. The bite of a coral snake may cause minimal local pain and swelling, and in fact the bite marks may be difficult to see. Many hours later (sometimes as much as 12 hours), the victim may have nausea and vomiting, headache, sweating, pallor, abdominal pain, and difficulty breathing. In contrast to pit viper bites, a much higher percentage of coral snake bites are dry, and enough venom to make a person ill is injected only about 40 percent of the time.

The coral snake is extremely colorful; it has red, yellow, and black bands encircling its body. The red and yellow bands touch each other. Some harmless species of snakes also have red, yellow, and black bands, with the red and yellow bands being separated by a black band. Which of these brightly colored snakes is poisonous may be remembered by the saying "Red on yellow, kill a fellow; red on black, venom lack." This rule does *not* necessarily apply to snakes found outside the United States. Coral snakes have an oval or round head and round pupils. They are shy and cause very few bites a year in the United States.

In other parts of the world, the elapid snakes include cobras, mambas, and kraits, all of which can be extremely dangerous and cause many deaths.

Treatment

The following measures should be taken if someone in your party is bitten:

- Back away, out of the snake's range. Try to stay calm. Reassure the victim. Remember, very few snake bites in the United States lead to severe poisoning or death.
- If you can identify the snake from a distance, this may help further management, but do *not* try to catch the snake. Dead snakes may bite reflexly for up to one hour after being killed.
- Keep the victim as quiet and as still as possible.
- Remove watches, jewelry and anything else that may become a tourniquet if the affected limb swells.
- If possible, keep the affected limb at the level of the heart to minimize absorption of the venom.
- If you know the bite was from a snake belonging to the elapid family, pressure immobilization of the affected limb may lead to less absorption of the poison into the circulation. This involves wrapping the entire extremity with an elastic or crepe bandage, starting at the bite site and working toward the heart. The bandage must be tight enough to collapse the superficial veins and lymphatics but *not* so tight as to occlude the blood flow in the arteries. Check the pulses in the victim's affected

limb frequently. The entire extremity is then immobilized in a splint.

- *Do no harm!* Do *not* incise into the skin and try to suck out the poison. Do *not* apply a tight tourniquet.
- *Get the victim to a medical facility that is equipped to deal with snake bites and their consequences as soon as possible.* If possible, carry the victim out. If this is not possible, walk the victim out slowly.
- Offer the victim sips of fluids frequently if he does not have nausea or vomiting and there will be delay in getting to a medical facility.

One expert has said that if you have been bitten by a really poisonous snake, the best first aid equipment to have is a set of car keys. In other words, you will need sophisticated medical care, which will be available only in a hospital!

 For Your Reference

Wilderness Medicine, by Paul. S. Auerbach, 4th ed. (2001).

Venomous and Stinging Marine Animals

Injuries from venomous marine animals have increased as more people visit tropical and subtropical waters to dive and snorkel in marine reefs.

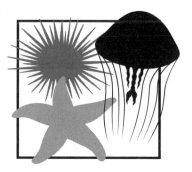

A variety of sea animals can cause extremely unpleasant stings, skin rashes, wounds, and more serious toxicity involving many organ systems. These animals include sponges, corals, sea anemones, sea urchins, starfish, jellyfish, Portuguese man-of-wars, stingrays, stonefish, sea snakes, and numerous others. Some, such as the box jellyfish, have such potent venom that their stings may be fatal. Tropical coral reefs in particular can harbor a multitude of venomous fish and other animals. The coastal waters of the United States harbor many of these venomous animals, so you do not have to travel far to be a victim! Toxic sponges occur all along the Atlantic coast from Cape Cod to Florida. Sea urchins, sea anemones, jellyfish and Portuguese man-of-wars are in the waters of the Atlantic and Pacific as well as the Gulf of Mexico. Sea nettles may be a major hazard in the Chesapeake Bay.

Fortunately, serious illness from contact with marine animals is rare. Most only cause unpleasant stings and irritating rashes, and if you are sensible, you should still be able to enjoy the wonders of the marine world. Pay attention to the preventive measures discussed below. Remember, the greatest risk around water is the risk of drowning. This is particularly true for adolescents and young children and for those who consume alcohol around water activities.

 Prevention

If you are planning a vacation around marine activities, especially those involving diving and snorkeling in tropical and subtropical marine reefs, some preparation is wise:

- Update the entire family's tetanus immunizations.
- Take along a medical kit and make sure it contains gloves, tweezers or forceps, an antiseptic solution, antibiotic cream or ointment, hydrocortisone cream, an antihistamine (e.g., Benadryl), painkillers, gauze, and bandages.

- If you plan to swim in an area where stings from marine animals are common, take along an antidote for the more common stings. Different antidotes are required for different stings: what works for one skin rash may worsen another. This is the main reason it is helpful to know what caused the sting or injury. Vinegar is useful for jellyfish and sponge stings. Baking soda pastes or solutions, rubbing alcohol, papain (papaya juice), and meat tenderizers may help others. A word of caution: many so-called remedies, such as urine or alcohol, may not only be useless but may make matters worse.
- Also take along cold packs (to treat tentacle stings), hot packs (for certain fish stings), and Safe Sea, a combined sunscreen and jellyfish block, which, if applied before swimming, may decrease the chance of tentacle stings.
- Do not forget hats, sunglasses, and large amounts of sunscreen. Sun-proof clothing is a good idea for very fair individuals (see Chapter 38, p. 399).
- If you are heading to isolated islands and remote locations where medical care is not readily available, it is a good idea to
  - take a first aid course and learn CPR;
  - visit your physician to discuss and request prescriptions for oral antibiotics, antibiotic eardrops (for swimmer's ear), a more potent painkiller than those sold over the counter, and medication to prevent and treat sea sickness; and
  - purchase and take along *All Stings Considered,* by Craig Thomas, M.D., and Susan Scott, to guide you

in case anyone in your party does suffer from a marine injury.

Once you are at your destination, take the following precautions, both before you enter the water and once you are in it:

- Be aware of the hazards where you plan to swim. Pay attention to warning notices on the beach. Ask the lifeguards about the surf conditions. There may be a reason that nobody is in the water!
- Never swim alone.
- Never consume alcohol around swimming and marine activities.
- Pay attention to changes in the weather, tides, and wind, which may rapidly transform a safe and peaceful haven into hazardous surf full of nasty stinging creatures. This is particularly likely to happen with the Portuguese man-of-war ("blue bottles"), as incoming tides and winds blowing onshore may bring an entire flotilla of blue bottles to the shore. Tentacles from jellyfish and Portuguese man-of-wars may extend for 80 feet or more from the body of the animal, so *stay out of the water* if these animals are sighted.
- Wear water shoes when wading in the water. These may not protect you from the sting of a stingray but may prevent other less toxic stings and coral cuts.
- Wear protective clothing (wetsuits) or a double layer of pantyhose if swimming in waters known to contain jellyfish.

- Do not handle sponges and coral with bare hands. Wear gloves when handling marine creatures, or do not handle them at all.
- Do not put your hands blindly into crevices and crannies and down dark holes when you are exploring reefs and rocks. You may get a very unwelcome bite or sting!
- Do not touch with bare hands jellyfish, Portuguese man-of-wars, sponges, and other creatures that have been washed up on the beach. They can inflict very serious stings for days after being beached.
- Shuffle when wading in water. In this way you will give fish warning of your approach and are also less likely to stand right on top of a stingray or other poisonous fish.
- Be cautious around tidal pools. Many of those beautiful looking "flowers" or stones in pools may be poisonous animals! Be especially cautious if you are with young children. They are often inquisitive and are prone to more severe reactions if stung. Sea urchins, anemones, and corals are often brightly colored and appealing but can cause very painful stings and nasty rashes.

SYMPTOMS

- Rashes or bite marks that have a characteristic pattern. These rashes often evolve over time: the skin may just be red initially; later, the rash often becomes raised; and even later, it may blister. Pigment changes in the skin may be evident weeks and months later.

Note: Anyone who collapses in the water should be suspected of having been stung by a venomous marine animal. Examine the person for the telltale skin rashes or bites.

- Swelling and discoloration occurring over hours to days.
- Pain and itching. These symptoms vary depending on the marine animal that caused the injury, whether venom was released; if so, how much; the location of the injury; and the response of the victim. Initially there may just be a prickling sensation and later more severe stinging. Pain is often excruciating and may last for hours or even days. The pain may extend into nearby joints, causing persistent and severe aching. Potent painkillers may be necessary. Inactivation of the venom by vinegar or heat may relieve the pain caused by some animals.
- Foreign bodies. Frequently the wound will contain stingers (nematocysts) or other particles of the offending animal. These may lead to further release of venom, secondary infection, and even more swelling and inflammation. Spines of some fish and coral may be deeply embedded. These spines often break off when you attempt to remove them. Consider the presence of a foreign body in any wound that is slow to heal or remains painful.
- Wound infection. Wounds often become infected and may take weeks or even longer to heal. Seawater is not sterile! Wounds on the hands and feet are particularly likely to become infected.

- Generalized symptoms. As well as the local damage or rash, there may be other symptoms such as pallor, sweating, nausea, vomiting and abdominal pain, dizziness, confusion and seizures, fainting, irregularities of the heart beat and a precipitous drop in blood pressure, breathing problems, chest pain, severe muscle aches and joint pain, kidney and liver failure, and death.

Note: The more serious manifestations in the preceding list are fortunately rare; they are more likely to occur in the very young and the very old. These require immediate treatment.

 ### *Treatment*

Although the management of specific injuries may differ depending on the type of stinging marine animal (see sections on various marine animals, below), there are general principles for treating all marine animal stings.

- Get the victim out of the water, as serious reactions may follow.
- Assess the person's general condition. Is he breathing normally? What is his color? Is he pale and sweaty? Is he confused? Immediate medical attention may be needed. The person may require CPR. Fortunately, in most cases, the victim will only be in pain and just be very frightened. If the victim is feeling faint, get him to lie down.
- Remove any visible tentacles using a stick, forceps, or

gloved hands. Do *not* touch the tentacles with your bare hands.

- In most cases the next step is to rinse the wound with *seawater.* (In many cases, washing the victim's skin with fresh water may aggravate the problem by causing more stingers to fire.)
- If you know the cause of the injury, applying a specific antidote may be the next step. For management of specific injuries, see the sections on various marine animals, below.
- Pain may be severe and in some cases can be alleviated to some extent by neutralizing the toxin (e.g., vinegar for jellyfish stings, hot water for scorpion fish stings). Potent painkillers will often be necessary. Applying ice packs is helpful with some stings, hot packs or non-scalding hot water with others (see the sections on various marine animals, below).
- Thorough and meticulous care of wounds is *essential,* as wounds are often contaminated by bacteria. The wound may need to be scrubbed and irrigated. If you do not have sterile solutions available, use tap water. Diluted povidone-iodine solution may be used (1 part povidone-iodine to 10 parts tap water).
- Marine injuries often contain foreign bodies (e.g., spines, stingers). These may be deeply embedded and require expert surgical removal. The more superficial stingers (nematocysts) are minute and may not be visible. Suggestions for removing these vary according to the cause of the sting and include applying adhesive

tape, a facial peel, or a thin layer of adhesive glue and then removing them. Other options are applying shaving cream or a paste of baking soda and shaving the area with a razor blade or similar object. As mentioned above, spines often break with attempted removal.

- Once the wound has been thoroughly cleaned, applications of steroid or anesthetic creams may help in alleviating the itch and pain.
- Tetanus prophylaxis is often indicated.
- Antibiotics are frequently needed both to prevent and to treat infection.
- Observation and care of the wound for weeks may be necessary.
- For stings involving the eyes, irrigate with copious amounts of tap water for at least 15 minutes. Seek medical care if the eyes remain painful and inflamed or if vision is affected.

Several types of marine animals and the types of injuries they cause are listed below, along with specific treatment measures.

Jellyfish

Jellyfish have tentacles that are lined by thousands to millions of stinging cells called nematocysts. These penetrate the skin and inject their venom. Reactions vary from unpleasant stings to life-threatening poisoning. The box jellyfish is the most notorious member of this group and is responsible for a number of fatalities each year in Australia.

- Soak the area in vinegar (acetic acid). If vinegar is not available, rinse the area with seawater. (Do *not* use fresh water.)
- Remove visible tentacles with a gloved hand, stick, flipper, or similar object. Do *not* rub the area with sand, a towel, or anything else.
- Remove the minute stingers remaining by applying shaving cream or a paste of baking soda and shaving with a razor or similar sharp-edged tool.
- Once the wound has been thoroughly decontaminated, applications of a steroid cream or anesthetic cream may be helpful.
- Further, nonspecific treatment includes pain control, tetanus prophylaxis, and antibiotics, as mentioned above.

Note: For severe stings, compression immobilization, resuscitation, intravenous fluids, and sophisticated medical care may be necessary, especially for children or the elderly.

For the Australian box jellyfish, specific antivenom may be indicated.

Portuguese Man-of-Wars ("Blue Bottles")

These are an extremely common cause of marine stings. Most stings are relatively minor, but severe reactions can occur.

- Remove all visible tentacles with a gloved hand, stick, or similar object.
- Rinse the area well with seawater or fresh water.

- Apply other general measures listed earlier in this "Treatment" section. Ice and oral painkillers will help the pain.

Sea Nettles

These are particularly common in the Chesapeake Bay area.

- Rinse immediately with seawater.
- Soak the area with a baking soda solution or cover with baking soda paste.

Fire Fern, or Fireweed

It is not unusual to brush up against fragments of these fern-like animals, which break up after storms and float in the water. A burning rash follows soon afterward.

- Wash the area immediately with seawater.
- Soak with vinegar or isopropyl (rubbing) alcohol.
- Apply a steroid cream after decontamination.

Fire Coral

This is not a true coral. It is often attached to rocks and resembles seaweed. It has a Christmas tree-like appearance and can cause severe pain.

- Treatment is similar to that of fireweed.

Sea Anemones

These are very common in tidal pools, are often brightly colored, and can cause painful and very unpleasant reactions, including dizziness, weakness, nausea, and vomiting.

- Wash the area thoroughly with seawater or fresh water.
- Apply ice for pain.
- Further, nonspecific treatment (pain control, tetanus prophylaxis, and antibiotics) is outlined above.

Sea Urchins

These are also found in tidal pools. They often have long spines that easily penetrate the skin and can cause a severe, burning pain. These spines frequently break off during attempted removal.

- Remove the larger, protruding spines carefully. Depending on the species, smaller spines may dissolve spontaneously.
- For large remaining spines, seek medical care.
- Some experts recommend applying heat to the wound to help relieve pain.

Starfish, Stonefish, and Scorpion Fish

These can cause very serious and extremely painful injuries. Fatalities have been reported with stonefish stings.

- Wash the area with nonscalding hot water (upper limit of 113°F, or 45°C).
- Remove foreign bodies with irrigation or forceps. Surgical removal may be required.
- Seek medical care if there are symptoms of generalized toxicity such as those mentioned on p. 447.

Cone Snails and Cone Snail Shells

Cone snails are often found in shallow waters. Their shells are often very beautiful, so you may be tempted to pick them up. Beware, especially if the snail's proboscis is protruding! Handle the shell with gloves, or leave them alone. Very nasty stings can result, and there is no specific antidote. Fatalities have been reported following cone snail stings.

- Scrub the wound.
- If symptoms of toxicity develop, seek medical care.

Sponges

Sponges may cause a variety of injuries. They often cause an irritant contact dermatitis with itching and blistering, similar to the skin reaction seen with poison ivy. There may also be spicules of silica or calcite embedded in the skin. Other symptoms include fever and chills, nausea, dizziness, muscle aches, and joint pains.

- Dry the area gently.
- Remove any spicules with adhesive tape or by applying a thin layer of rubber cement or a facial peel and then removing it.
- Soak the area with vinegar or rubbing alcohol three to four times a day.
- Later treatment may include application of a steroid cream and oral antihistamines to decrease the itch. Do *not* apply the steroid cream until the decontamination steps (earlier in this list) have been completed.
- Tetanus prophylaxis and antibiotics may be necessary.

Coral

The rash that develops after coral scrapes and cuts results from a combination of scraping across the coral, irritation from coral toxins, and fragments of coral particles penetrating the skin. Secondary infection often follows.

- Clean the cuts or scrapes well.
- Remove any coral fragments. Expert exploration and cleaning of the cut may be necessary.
- Secondary infection may occur and requires a course of antibiotics.

Stingrays

For prevention, see pp. 442–45.

Stingrays are not aggressive creatures and will usually attack you only if you step on them. The stingray's tail whips upward, and the spine at the base of the tail can cause a nasty, penetrating wound that is extremely painful.

- Immerse the wound in nonscalding hot water if possible. (Check the temperature of the water first to prevent a hot-water burn—the temperature of the water should not exceed 113°F, or 45°C.) If you do not have access to hot water, irrigate the wound with fresh water.
- Expert medical care is usually necessary to remove the spine, as fragments commonly remain embedded and will lead to secondary infection and delay healing of the wound.

Sea Snakes

These are usually very poisonous, and sea snake bites constitute a medical emergency. The bite wound is not always visible and may not be very painful.

- Try to keep the victim as calm as possible.
- Hold the bite site below the rest of the body.
- Apply a pressure immobilization bandage over the site of the bite.
- Get the victim to a hospital or other medical facility.

Table 5. Summary of Signs, Symptoms, and Treatment of Contact with Venomous and Stinging Marine Animals

Animal	Signs and Symptoms		Treatment
	Local	General/Systemic	
Anemone	Burning and itching. Redness and swelling	Yes (see text)	Wash with seawater or fresh water. Apply ice for pain. Appropriate treatment for severe reactions (see text).
Cone snails	Burning and stinging	Yes (see text)	Scrub the wound. Appropriate treatment for severe reactions (see text).
Coral	Abrasions and cuts	No	Clean well. Remove fragments. For deep cuts, seek medical care. May need antibiotics.
Fire fern/fireweed, fire coral	Patterned rash with burning and stinging	Rare	Wash with seawater. Apply vinegar or rubbing alcohol. Steroid creams *after* decontamination.
Jellyfish	Stinging and burning	Yes (see text)	Soak with vinegar. If not available, rinse with seawater. Remove tentacles (see text). Appropriate treatment for severe reactions (see text).
Portuguese man-of-war (blue bottle)	Stinging, burning	May occur	Remove tentacles. Wash with seawater or fresh water. Apply ice for pain. Appropriate treatment for severe reactions (see text).

Continued

Table 5. Summary of Signs, Symptoms, and Treatment of Contact with Venomous and Stinging Marine Animals *continued*

Animal	Signs and Symptoms		Treatment
	Local	General/ Systemic	
Sea nettle	Stinging and burning	May occur	Rinse with seawater. Soak with baking soda solution or apply baking soda paste.
Sea urchins	Spines cause severe, throbbing pain	May occur	Remove larger spines. Apply heat for pain. Medical help for deep spines.
Sponges	Itchy rash with blistering	No	Dry gently. Remove spicules with adhesive tape. Vinegar or rubbing alcohol 3 to 4 times a day. Steroid creams *after* decontamination.
Starfish, stonefish, scorpion fish	Severe pain	Yes	Immerse in nonscalding hot water.
Stingrays	Severe pain. May be a deep wound	May occur	Immerse in nonscalding hot water. Clean with soap and water. Medical care to remove spine.
Sea snakes	May be no visible bite	Severe	Calm victim. Immobilization. Get medical care.

For Your Reference

1. *Wilderness Medicine*, by Paul S. Auerbach, 4th ed. (2001).
2. *All Stings Considered*, by Craig Thomas, M.D., and Susan Scott (1997).

42

Poison Ivy, Poison Oak, and Poison Sumac Rashes

Poison ivy, poison oak, and poison sumac all have sap (resins) that can cause severe skin rashes. These plants are found throughout the continental United States but not in Hawaii or Alaska. These plants cause by far the majority of allergic skin rashes due to plants in the United States. About 50 percent of the adult population is sensitive to the resin (uroshiol) found in these plants. The intact plant does not cause rashes, but when it is damaged, the sap leaks out, and if it comes into contact with the skin, it can cause a severe rash. Contact with a damaged stem or root will have a similar effect.

Rashes may also result from contact with pets, articles of clothing, or tools that have been contaminated with the sap. Smoke from burning plants may also act as an irritant, causing severe breathing problems. The allergic skin reaction may start as soon as 6 hours after exposure but more typically occurs 24 to 72 hours later.

SYMPTOMS

Initially the affected skin is just itchy, but soon the area becomes red, raised, and rough. Blisters frequently follow, and later the skin tends to ooze. As the days go by, the skin dries out and crusts over. The blisters often occur in lines or streaks along the course of scratch marks. The rash is very, very itchy and may make your child very miserable for days.

The rash may continue to erupt for up to two weeks, giving the mistaken impression that the rash is being spread by the blister fluid or by reexposure to the resin. The delay in the appearance of the later eruptions is probably due to a number of factors, including the amount of sap that touches the skin at each location, the varying thickness of the skin, and differences in skin reactivity at various places.

Dermatitis caused by poison ivy, poison oak, and poison sumac is *not* contagious. *Once the initial sap has been washed off*, the dermatitis cannot be spread to other parts of the body or to other people. Not even the blisters are contagious.

 Prevention

Plant Identification

Knowing how to identify and then avoiding these plants is the mainstay of prevention. Learn how to recognize these plants:

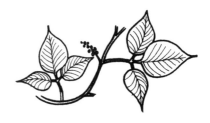

- *Poison ivy* usually has three leaves that are typically notched ("leaves of three, let them be"). However, there are numerous varieties of poison ivy, and some have five leaves! Poison ivy may occur as a vine or shrub. You may not need to go for a walk in the woods to come into contact with poison ivy. You will probably find it in your own backyard.

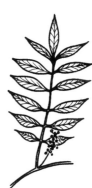

- *Poison sumac* usually has 7 to 13 smooth-edged leaflets. This plant grows in boggy areas in the East and South.
- *Poison oak* occurs in two forms, a low shrub (in the East and South) or a vine (Pacific coast). The leaves are often notched like those of the oak tree.

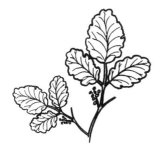

All three plants often have shiny black spots on damaged leaves, as the sap of the plant turns black when exposed to the air. The leaves of these plants tend to change color earlier than those of most other plants during the fall, often turning bright red.

Clothing

Your child should wear long-sleeved shirts and long pants when hiking through the woods. This may not be much fun, but the rash of poison ivy is a lot less fun! The poison ivy resin can penetrate clothing and even rubber gloves. Vinyl gloves offer better protection.

Ivy Block

You can apply Ivy Block to your child's skin before he ventures into poison ivy–infested woods. This will help to decrease the severity of the rash but not totally prevent it.

Eye and Skin Contact

Discourage your child from rubbing his eyes after coming into contact with these plants. Boys who may have come into contact with poison ivy outside and who want to "take a pee" in the woods should be careful when handling their genitals.

Washing

Take a shower or at least wash all exposed skin if you suspect you have been exposed to poison ivy. Once contact has occurred, the sooner the poison is washed off, the better. It should be washed off with soap and warm water, preferably *within 10 minutes*. It is very important to wash under nails, otherwise the resin may be spread to other parts of the body by scratching or rubbing. If there has been a long delay since contact, you stand a better chance of removing more resin if the skin is first washed with rubbing alcohol and then soap and water. Zanfel, a wash specially formulated to help remove the resin, has been shown to lessen the severity of the rash and decrease the itch (see "Treatment" section, below). When washing, avoid harsh soaps and do not scrub too vigorously, as you are likely to cause even more skin irritation.

Contaminated Objects and Animals

Remove contaminated clothing and wash these well. Handle these clothes with care to avoid coming into contact with the resin. Boots and boot laces may also become contaminated. It is a good idea to wash the bath towels as well, as they may have become contaminated with the resin. Bathe animals that may have come in contact with these plants. Clean tools that may be contaminated.

Allergy "Shots"

Desensitization (allergy "shots") for poison ivy dermatitis has been tried but is not very effective.

Treatment

- Keep your child as cool as possible. Heat and exercise make any itchy rash worse. Try to keep her in a cool environment and have her wear loose, cool cotton clothes.
- Wash the affected area with one of the recently marketed poison ivy washes such as Zanfel. Squeeze 1½ inches of the Zanfel paste onto one palm. Wet and rub both hands together for 10 seconds, working the Zanfel into a thinner paste. Rub both hands on the affected area and work the Zanfel into the skin. Rinse the area thoroughly. Repeat as necessary. (As discussed above, washing with soap and warm water is effective only if done within 10 minutes of exposure.)
- Cool baths, Aveeno compresses and soaks, bland creams, or lotions such as Calamine lotion will help to decrease the itch.
- Give your child an oral antihistamine such as diphenhydramine (Benadryl). This will help the itch and may even help your child sleep. Hydroxyzine (Atarax), especially if used in high doses, will have a similar effect. The newer, nonsedating antihistamines will also help to decrease the itch and should not sedate your child, although sometimes the sedation and drowsiness of the older drugs are an added bonus!
- If your child has an extensive reaction, and especially if it involves the face or genitalia (not an uncommon loca-

tion in little boys), consult your doctor, as oral steroids may be needed. It is often necessary to continue these oral steroids for 10 to 14 days. A common mistake made by many physicians is to prescribe too short a course of steroids. If this is done, the rash will often rebound. Shorter courses of steroids may be effective if started very early in the course of the illness.

- High-potency topical steroid creams may be effective *if used early* but should *not* be used on the face. These can be refrigerated before use: applying cool creams or gels is very soothing.
- These rashes are extremely itchy. Scratching may lead to bacterial infection of the skin known as impetigo, a skin infection usually due to "staph." or "strep." Keep your child's nails short and try to discourage scratching. If the area becomes painful and the area of inflammation continues to spread, you should seek medical attention, as your child may need an oral antibiotic or an antibiotic cream. A fever is a definite indication to seek medical care.

43

West Nile Fever

Refer also to Chapter 39.

WHAT IS IT?

West Nile fever is a viral illness that is transmitted by in-fected mosquitoes. Originally in the United States this dis-ease was transmitted by mosquitoes only to birds, but in the late 1990s the disease spread to humans and horses. In the United States, West Nile fever was first reported on the East Coast, but by 2004 it had spread to the West Coast. West Nile fever occurs as an epidemic every summer and fall.

SYMPTOMS

Symptoms typically develop 3 to 14 days after being bitten by an infected mosquito. Most people who are bitten by an in-fected mosquito have no symptoms at all. Some people have a mild flu-like illness with fever, headache, muscle aches, and gastrointestinal symptoms such as nausea and vomiting. Occasionally a rash or enlarged lymph glands may be present.

A very small percentage of people (less than 1 percent) become severely ill with neurological symptoms such as weakness, muscle tremors, and paralysis. Some of these people may even die.

The risk of catching West Nile fever is extremely low. Most mosquitoes do not carry the virus. Even if you are bitten by an infected mosquito, your chance of getting the severe form of the disease is less than 1 percent. The severe form of the illness tends to occur in middle-aged or elderly people. It is extremely rare for children to become severely ill from West Nile fever.

 Prevention

Even though the risk of acquiring West Nile fever is extremely low, it still makes sense to protect your children and yourself against the disease. This is particularly true for the elderly. You are more likely to get the illness if you spend a lot of time outdoors at the high-risk times.

- During the high-risk months, stay indoors at dusk, in the early evening, and dawn. These are the peak times for mosquito bites. This would deprive you, though, of being outside at a very pleasant time of the day, so it is more practical to follow the guidelines below.

- Wear long-sleeved shirts and long pants when you are outdoors, particularly at peak mosquito biting times.
- Use an effective insect repellent. At the present time this means a repellent containing DEET (see Chapter 39). Apply the repellent as recommended, and wash it off when no longer needed. If less effective repellents are used, reapply these frequently.
- Spray your clothes with permethrin.
- Make sure you have protective screens on windows and doors. Repair defective screens.
- Remove standing water around the house. Empty water from flowerpots, buckets, barrels, and so on. Change the water in bird baths and pet dishes at least once a week. Drill drainage holes in tire swings and keep children's play pools empty when not in use.

 Treatment

There is no specific treatment for West Nile fever. It is a viral illness. Antibiotics are not effective against viral infections. The treatment is supportive. Ill patients may require intravenous fluids, help with breathing, and specialized medical and nursing care.

44

Lyme Disease

Refer also to Chapter 39.

Lyme disease is caused by a type of bacterium known as a spirochete. It is transmitted to humans when they are bitten by certain types of ticks. In the United States, Lyme disease occurs in three distinct geographic regions:

1. The Northeast, extending from southern Maine to Virginia
2. The upper Midwest, especially Wisconsin and Minnesota
3. The West Coast, especially northern California

Lyme disease also occurs in other parts of the world, including Canada, Europe, and Asia.

In the Northeast, the deer tick is the usual culprit, whereas in the Pacific region the Western black-legged tick is usually

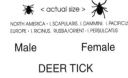

< actual size >

NORTH AMERICA · I. SCAPULARIS. I. DAMMINI. I. PACIFICUS.
EUROPE · I. RICINUS. RUSSIA/ORIENT · I. PERSULCATUS

Male   Female

DEER TICK

The nymph is usually much smaller, the size of a sesame seed.

responsible for transmitting the disease. The life cycle of the tick occurs in three stages. These are larva, nymph, and the adult. The nymph is usually responsible for transmitting the infection to humans; it is very small—about the size of a sesame seed.

SYMPTOMS

The symptoms of Lyme disease vary according to the stage of the disease. The three stages are as follows:

1. *Early localized disease.* Most people who get Lyme disease develop a typical rash called *erythema migrans.* This occurs 3 to 32 days (usually 7 to 14 days) after the initial tick bite. It starts as a red spot at the site of the tick bite and enlarges to form a circular lesion, usually with a clear center, often called a "bull's eye." This rash often reaches 2 to 5 inches in diameter or larger and may be mistaken for ringworm or eczema. At this time the person will often have flu-like symptoms—fever, chills, headache, and muscle aches.

2. *Early disseminated disease.* This stage occurs some weeks after the initial skin rash and again may include a flu-like illness as well as smaller but similar skin lesions scattered over the body. More significant symptoms include those of meningitis (severe headache and neck stiffness), paralysis of the facial muscles resulting in a

facial droop (Bell's palsy), and an irregular or slow heart rate.

3. *Late disseminated disease.* This stage may occur weeks to months after the initial tick bite. The main manifestation is joint pain (arthritis).

Note: Many people do not notice the initial tick bite.

Not all people develop the typical early rash (erythema migrans).

The tick needs to be attached for at least 24-hours or longer to transmit the disease.

DIAGNOSIS

The diagnosis of Lyme disease may be very difficult, especially if the typical early rash does not occur and there is no known history of a tick bite. Blood tests are not very helpful in the early stages and may also be confusing and inaccurate later on. The diagnosis is usually based on the typical symptoms occurring in a person who has been in an area where Lyme disease is known to occur.

 Prevention

To prevent Lyme disease you need to prevent tick bites:

• Wear long pants tucked into socks or boots when walking in long grass or the woods. It is easier to see the ticks if you wear light-colored clothing.

- Treat clothes with permethrin (see Chapter 39).
- Apply DEET repellents to exposed skin (see Chapter 39).
- After spending time outdoors, do a careful total body inspection for ticks. Look especially carefully in the hair. Remember, the ticks are very small, and you will need a good light source to see the ticks.

 Treatment

If you or your child develops the typical circular rash, seek medical attention. Lyme disease can be treated very effectively with antibiotics. A prolonged course of antibiotics may be needed.

Just because your child has been bitten by a deer tick, however, does not mean that she should start a course of antibiotics. Even in areas where Lyme disease is common, most ticks are not infected. As mentioned above, ticks need to be attached for at least 24 hours (and probably longer) before they transmit the spirochete that causes Lyme disease. A single dose of doxycycline may be indicated in very high risk areas and if the tick has been attached for longer than 24 hours.

HOW TO REMOVE AN ATTACHED TICK

See Chapter 39, p. 423.

Foot and Ankle Care

Whether you are hiking in the back country, sightseeing in Europe, or strolling around Disney World, having comfortable shoes and pain-free feet can make all the difference in whether or not you have an enjoyable trip.

BLISTERS

Blisters are common and frequently occur when hiking and sightseeing.

  Prevention and Treatment

- Before setting out on hiking expeditions or major sightseeing trips, purchase a blister prevention and repair kit. A well-known brand is Spenco. An extra supply of moleskin is also not a bad idea (see below).

- Make sure all footwear is comfortable. Wear shoes or boots that fit properly and have been broken in before your trip or hike starts.
- Wear comfortable socks. When undertaking prolonged hikes, wear two pairs of socks. Ideally wear the polypropylene socks next to the skin and the thicker wool or synthetic socks over the polypropylene ones. Check socks frequently to make sure they are not bunching up. Have spare pairs of clean socks readily available to change into if your socks become wet or damp.
- At rest stops take your socks and shoes off to allow your feet and socks to dry.
- Inspect feet frequently for "hot spots," which are the first sign of blisters. If you see any "hot spots," apply some moleskin or Spenco Second Skin over the area.
- If a blister develops, do not pop it. Fashion a piece of moleskin or mole foam in a doughnut shape and tape it so that it fits around the inflamed area. This should limit friction over the troubled area.

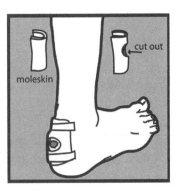

- If the blister does burst, apply an antibacterial ointment to the area and cover it with a nonadherent dressing. Change this dressing at least every day. If infection develops (the blister fluid becomes thick and cloudy or the surrounding area becomes very red), start warm soaks when you get back to your base camp or hotel. Continue using the antibacterial ointment. If the surrounding red area increases in size, seek medical care.

For Your Reference

For an excellent discussion on the prevention and treatment of blisters, refer to *A Comprehensive Guide to Wilderness and Travel Medicine,* by Eric A. Weis (2006).

ATHLETE'S FOOT

See Chapter 14, p. 186.

ANKLE SPRAINS

Ankle sprains are common and may ruin a vacation. They may even be dangerous if you are hiking in a remote area.

If planning a vacation that involves a lot of walking, especially if your travels will take you to areas where medical help is not readily available, prior to departure consider meeting with your local sports physiotherapist or orthopedic technician to learn how to put a compression bandage on a sprained ankle. Consider purchasing athletic tape or an ankle Aircast.

Make sure every member of your party has comfortable boots that provide adequate ankle support.

Injuries that cause sprains (tearing or stretching of liga-
ments) in adolescents and adults may cause fractures in
younger children. A fracture in the ankle region may be suggested by extreme tenderness over the bony prominence that
makes up the inner or outer aspect of the ankle (the malleoli).
Tenderness and swelling in front of or below the outer bony
prominence is more likely due to injury to the soft tissues (a
sprain).

 Treatment

Treatment for an ankle sprain may be remembered by the
mnemonic PRICE.

(Described below is the ideal treatment. Obviously if you
are in a remote area, you may not be able to do everything
listed.)

- Protection—from further injury. (Stop the activity that
  caused the injury!)
- Rest—this may last as little as a few minutes or as long
  as many weeks. Crutches may be necessary to make
  weight bearing less painful.
- Ice—applying ice not only decreases swelling but also
  helps to relieve pain. Ideally apply ice for 20 minutes
  four to five times a day and follow it by reapplying the
  compression bandage.
- Compression—by athletic tape or an elastic wrap helps
  to minimize swelling and also provides support. To ap-

ply adequate compression to a sprained ankle you will need to place some padding in the hollows on both sides of the ankle. This is *essential* to prevent soft tissue swelling. This padding may be a rolled-up bandage or sock or glove. Tape or a bandage is then wrapped tightly around the ankle to keep the padding in place. Periodically check the pulses in the feet and the color of the toes to make sure the wrap is not too tight.

- Elevation—keeping the foot elevated will decrease swelling.

When the acute pain and swelling have subsided (usually after two to seven days), the ankle needs to be rehabilitated with strengthening exercises. This is a vital part of the treatment, and if it is neglected, the person may be left with a chronically weak ankle that is prone to repeated sprains.

Accidents,
Injuries,
and
Emergencies

46

The Basics

Refer also to Chapter 2 and to the other chapters in Part Four.

Accidents are the leading cause of death in children from 1 to 15 years of age. We all worry about our children getting leukemia, brain tumors, West Nile fever, and other relatively uncommon illnesses. In fact, children are far more likely to die in a motor vehicle accident or as a result of some other preventable accident than from one of these illnesses.

It is important to remember that most accidents are *preventable*. This chapter discusses basic prevention and other safety concerns. Specific injuries and emergency situations (such as poisoning) are covered in subsequent Part Four chapters.

INJURIES CAUSED BY
MOTOR VEHICLE ACCIDENTS

Injuries sustained in motor vehicle accidents are by far the single greatest cause of death in childhood. You and your child are more likely to survive a motor vehicle accident if you use an appropriate restraint system, whether it is an infant car seat, a booster seat plus seat belt, or a seat belt. You should always set a good example for your child by wearing your seat belt.

All infants in the first year of life who travel in an automobile should be in a rear-facing car seat that is correctly fastened. Eighty percent of child safety seats are installed incorrectly! Find out how to install your child's car seat the correct way. You will reduce your child's chance of dying or being seriously injured by 70 percent if you use child safety seats correctly. In most communities you should be able to locate an organization that will be able to inspect the installation of your child's car seat to check that you have done this correctly. Often this service is available at your local police station or at a community hospital. Your pediatrician may also be able to advise you where to obtain assistance.

When your child is one year of age and weighs at least 20 pounds, you can switch her to a front-facing car seat. Again, check that it is properly installed. Once she is at least 40 inches tall and weighs about 40 pounds, she can progress to a booster seat used together with a seat belt. She should use a booster seat until she fits correctly into the car's combined lap and shoulder belt. The shoulder belt should not cross in front of her face or neck.

 For Your Reference

You can find more information about car seat safety from the following sources:

1. American Academy of Pediatrics. www.aap.org/parents.html
2. National Highway Transportation Safety. www.nhtsa.gov/
3. SeatCheck. www.seatcheck.org/

Remember, the back seat is almost always safer than the front seat!

Teen drivers. Teenagers are even more likely to be injured in car accidents. Driving at night is more dangerous, and the greater the number of occupants in the car, the greater the likelihood of an accident. If you add alcohol to the equation, you have a recipe for disaster!

DROWNING

In many parts of the United States drowning is the leading cause of death among children younger than five years of age. Infants and toddlers may drown in just a few inches of water

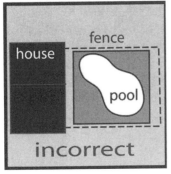 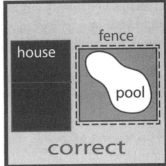

in a bathtub, bucket, toilet, or outside play pool. **Never** leave your young child in the bathtub alone, not even for a few seconds.

Sadly, drowning in swimming pools is also not a rare event. A swimming pool should be surrounded by an appropriate fence on *all four sides* and have a gate that locks securely.

Drowning is also a not uncommon cause of death among teenage males. In this group, alcohol consumption or swimming in unsafe waters often plays a role.

See Chapter 61 for a detailed discussion of drowning, including prevention.

FALLS

Falls often result in significant injury to young children and many visits to the emergency room. Falls may occur from changing tables, cribs, down stairs, or when an adventurous toddler climbs onto furniture. Do *not* place your child in a mobile baby walker. Accidents related to these have resulted in many deaths (see also Chapters 47 and 48).

BURNS

Burns are not only a cause of many childhood deaths but also often result in disfiguring injuries. See Chapter 51 for a detailed discussion of burns, including prevention and treatment.

OTHER SAFETY CONCERNS

Preventing injuries requires attention to many other aspects of safety, including the following:

- Crib safety.
- Firearm safety. Injuries caused by firearms lead to many tragic deaths among children in the United States. Suicide and homicide involving firearms are significant causes of death among adolescent males.
- Toy safety.
- Playground safety.
- Bicycle safety. Your child is more likely to wear a bicycle helmet if you set a good example by wearing yours. Make sure your helmets are fitted correctly.
- Safety around sports.

SIDS

SIDS (sudden infant death syndrome), or crib death, in no way can be classified as an "accident," but it does have a preventive aspect to it. SIDS is a significant cause of death in the first year of life.

Take the following measures to decrease the risk of SIDS:

- Place your infant on his back when you put him down to sleep.
- Do not let your infant sleep on soft surfaces.
- Do not put a pillow or blanket in your infant's crib.
- Do not smoke when you are pregnant and do not smoke around your baby.

47

Head Injuries

Note: The comments below do *not* apply to children who have multiple trauma, such as that seen in motor vehicle accidents, or who have fallen from a great height; nor do they apply to children with preexisting neurological problems or bleeding disorders. Children with any of these injuries or problems should be assessed by a medical expert.

Head injuries are extremely common in childhood. Fortunately, most injuries are minor. Infants and toddlers have a relatively large head as well as limbs that don't always do what they are supposed to do! Toddlers bump their head frequently as they learn to walk. Usually these bumps are of no consequence, and the parent is often more upset by the episode than the child. Your child will probably cry for a short while after banging his head and may develop a bump (an "egg"). Most of these bruises will be on the forehead. Over the next day or two, the bruise will darken and a black eye may appear. In fact, the injury often looks more impressive on day two or three than it did in the beginning! Bruises often take up to a week to fade.

The crying will usually cease in 10 minutes or less. Some children are a little sleepy after a mild head injury and may even vomit once or twice. This is a common reaction and usually does not indicate a more serious problem.

Prevention

Most head injuries can be prevented by taking the appropriate precautions.

Motor Vehicles

- Always wear your seat belt. Younger children should be in their child safety seat or a booster seat.
- *Never* drive under the influence of drugs or alcohol.

Helmets

- Use helmets when riding a bike, a snowmobile, and an all-terrain vehicle and when skateboarding, snowboarding, skiing, or riding a horse.
- Wear a helmet when playing contact sports such as football and ice hockey and also when playing baseball, softball, and lacrosse.

- Set a good example for your children by wearing a helmet when you ride a bicycle or partake in activities that may lead to head injuries.

Playgrounds

Playgrounds should have shock-absorbing surfaces such as mulch, sand, or rubber.

Firearms

Keep firearms away from children!

Falls from Heights

- Never leave your infant unattended on a changing table.
- Do not put your child in a mobile walker—these walkers have a tendency to make their way to the nearest staircase and descend rapidly!
- Keep house and apartment windows fastened.
- Do not let children play on balconies.

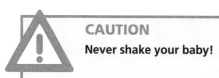

CAUTION
Never shake your baby!

Treatment

- If the skin is broken, clean the abrasion gently with soap and warm water. If your child has a laceration that is bleeding, apply firm pressure with a handkerchief, tissue, or gauze until the bleeding has stopped. The scalp is very vascular, and it may take some minutes and firm pressure to control the bleeding. If he has a *laceration with gaping wound edges,* however, he needs medical attention.
- An older child with a swelling on his head may be willing to hold an ice pack against the swelling. Wrap a plastic bag of ice (or a bag of frozen vegetables) in a cloth or towel and apply this to the wound. It is probably not worth trying to do this if you are dealing with an uncooperative toddler!
- Do *not* give your child ibuprofen (Advil or Motrin) or aspirin. You may administer a dose of acetaminophen (Tylenol) if you feel this is necessary.
- If your child is sleepy, let him sleep. You don't have to keep your child awake, but you do need to keep a close watch on him. If it is nighttime, wake him when you go to bed and then every four hours or so to determine whether he is behaving normally:
  - Does he make good eye contact and appear to be totally "with it?"

- If he has learned to walk, can he walk normally?
- If he is an older child who has learned to talk, is he talking normally? Ask him a few simple questions and assess his response.
- Are his pupils (the dark spot in the center of the eyes) the same size? If you shine a flashlight into his eyes, do the pupils constrict equally?

If you are unsure or concerned about any of the answers to these questions, call your physician. Usually, by the following day, your child will have recovered, but you will have a few more gray hairs! Occasionally it may be necessary to watch your child more closely for another day or night.

When to Seek Medical Attention

- If your child has a laceration with gaping wound edges.
- If your child is two years of age or younger *and* has *any* detectable abnormality of his skull, even if it is just a bruise or a localized swelling (an "egg").
- If your child vomits more than two times.
- If it is difficult to rouse your child, or if he becomes unconscious.
- If your child has a headache that lasts longer than just a few hours, or if he has a headache that is increasing in severity.
- If an older child is not behaving, walking, or talking

normally. If she seems confused or has slurred speech, persisting dizziness, clumsiness, or difficulty walking, seek immediate medical care.

- If your child's pupils are unequal in size.
- If your child has blurred vision, or if he sees double.
- If your child remains fussy, irritable, and inconsolable. These symptoms, as well as changes in eating or nursing, may be the only signs of a problem in a younger child. Most children do not cry for longer than 10 minutes after a minor head injury.
- If your child has blood or watery fluid coming out of one or both ears or his nose.
- If your child has a seizure.
- If, over the following days, your child loses balance easily, seems to regress, or loses interest in favorite toys or activities, or if his schoolwork deteriorates.
- If your child has a preexisting brain condition.
- If your child has any bleeding disorder or is on blood thinners.

RISK FACTORS FOR BRAIN INJURY

- Children two years of age and younger, especially those in the first year of life. The younger the child, the more vulnerable the brain.
- Falls from 3 feet and higher.
- The harder the surface, the more severe the injury. Falls onto a concrete floor are likely to be more traumatic than those onto a carpeted floor.

- Bumps over the temple or the back of the head have a higher chance of being associated with underlying damage. (Bumps on the forehead are the least likely to lead to underlying brain injury.)
- Children with blood clotting problems or who are on blood thinners.
- Children with preexisting neurological (brain) problems.

Remember, any child under two years of age who has had a fall and has signs of a skull injury (an abrasion, a bruise, a swelling, or a laceration) should be discussed with a physician.

48

Spine, Neck, and Back Injuries

Spinal injury should be suspected with any severe head injury from trauma—for example, severe head injuries sustained in a motor vehicle accident, a fall from a height, or similar accidents. Spine and spinal cord injuries are especially common in diving accidents and may also occur in sports such as football, cheerleading, horseback riding, mountaineering, and skiing. All-terrain vehicle accidents often cause multiple injuries, including those of the spine and spinal cord.

 Treatment

After an accident causing injury, if the person is conscious and cooperative, tell him not to move until his head, neck, and back have been stabilized. If the victim is unconscious, check that he is breathing adequately. If not, you should check his airway. You may need to gently straighten the head and neck to maintain an open airway.

Whenever a person has sustained an injury that may cause a neck or spinal cord injury, *assume that injury is present and take precautions to prevent damage to the spinal cord.* Do not move or elevate the head or neck unless the victim is in life-threatening danger. *Get help.* If you have to move the victim, roll the person like a log: roll the body as a single unit, taking care to keep the head, neck, and spine in a straight line. To safely roll an older child or adult in this manner requires the help of at least two other people. To transport the victim, you will need to use a litter or backboard. Place the litter alongside the victim and roll the victim like a log onto the litter. One person will need to cradle the head and neck and give commands to the other people assisting so that the all movements are coordinated. Pad and secure the victim with strips of cloth or tape.

Note: It is crucial to support the head during this rolling motion and keep the head, neck, back, and spine all in a straight line.

Remember, spinal cord injuries are common with head injuries, and one should always act as if they are present until they have been ruled out by X-rays.

49

Poisoning

U.S. poison control center: (800) 222-1222

As children acquire new skills, they expose themselves to new dangers. By six months of age, most infants can reach out and grasp objects. These objects go straight to their mouth! By nine months of age, babies have a pincer grip and can pick up small objects between their forefinger and thumb. Around this age they are also becoming more mobile and are starting to explore the world. The risk of accidental poisoning, as well as of choking, increases daily and persists throughout the toddler and early childhood years.

Children can ingest a variety of potentially toxic substances. These include both over-the-counter and prescription medications, household cleaning products, pesticides, plants, gasoline and kerosene, and paints and solvents, among many others. Medications that may seem innocuous in small doses, such as acetaminophen (Tylenol) and prenatal iron tablets, may be fatal in large doses!

When a parent discovers that his or her child has ingested a potentially dangerous substance, the parent's natural reaction is to want the child to vomit it out, but this may not always be wise. Substances such as strong acids (e.g., toilet bowl cleaner) or strong alkalis (e.g., drain cleaner and many detergents) are likely to cause just as much damage "coming up" as "going down." Gasoline and kerosene are more likely to cause a chemical pneumonia if vomiting is induced.

The United States has many superb poison centers. These collectively handle more than a million accidental ingestions and potential poisonings a year. Fortunately, death from poisoning is becoming increasingly rare in the United States. This is due to a combination of factors, the most important of which is the introduction of child-resistant containers and safer medications, as well as increasing public awareness of the dangers of poisoning.

 Prevention

Medications

- Keep all medications, including vitamins, out of sight and out of reach. Store them high up and in a locked closet.
- Always secure child-resistant caps in the locked position after use.
- Never transfer a medication from its original container to another one.
- Dispose of all unused or no-longer-needed medicines safely.

- Never refer to medications as candy.

Household Products

- Store potentially dangerous products in locked cabinets, preferably high up. Be particularly careful with bleach, drain cleaners, and similar extremely toxic materials.
- Never transfer these substances from their original containers to other ones.

In the Garage, Basement, or Garden Shed

- Store gasoline, kerosene, paint thinners, and varnishes in secure containers, locked up and out of reach.
- Never pour these substances into cups, soda bottles, or other containers. Even *you* may forget what that soda bottle contains!
- Store pesticides and fertilizers safely.

When Visiting

Children are often poisoned in someone else's home, so be especially vigilant when visiting relatives and friends. Grandmother's sleeping pills or blood pressure medicine may look particularly colorful and appealing to young children. People who are not accustomed to having young children around may not be quite as careful about keeping potentially toxic substances in a safe place.

CAUTION
Keep medicines and toxic substances in a safe place in a secure container.

Treatment

Note: Keep the poison center phone number close to the telephone. **The universal number for contacting the poison control center in the United States is (800) 222-1222.**

- Don't panic!
- Take the substance away from your child. If there is still some poison in your child's mouth, get her to spit it out or remove it with your fingers.
- Look for any obvious, immediate effects such as burns of the lips, redness around the mouth, or drooling.
- Contact the poison control center.
- Do *not* induce vomiting until you have discussed this with the poison control center.
- Watch out for side effects such as drowsiness, retching, stomach cramps, and behavior changes. *Call 911* if your child becomes excessively drowsy or unconscious or has breathing difficulties, jerking movements, or seizures. If your child does become unconscious or has a seizure before medical help can be reached, position your child on his side with his head lower than the rest of his body

so that should he vomit, he will not inhale what he threw up. Be alert for breathing difficulties.

• Take the poison, medicine container, or plant with you to the emergency room. If your child has vomited and you do not know what he ingested, take the vomited material with you to the hospital.

Ipecac

Ipecac syrup is a liquid that induces vomiting. Your pediatrician or family practitioner may have recommended that you purchase ipecac syrup and keep it in the home so that you can administer it to your child in the event that she ingests a poisonous substance or a potentially dangerous medication. In 2003, the American Academy of Pediatrics changed its recommendation to keep ipecac in the home and use it routinely as a poison treatment intervention. This was done for a number of reasons: (1) ipecac is not always very effective; (2) it is sometimes inappropriate to administer it; (3) it is frequently not necessary to induce vomiting.

There may be circumstances in which it is advisable to have ipecac available for the treatment of poisoning. Such a circumstance would be the traveling family that does not have easy access to a poison control center. Families traveling to malarial areas may be carrying chloroquine with them to prevent malaria. If an inappropriately large amount of chloroquine is ingested by a young child, the consequences may be fatal! *Prompt administration of ipecac in this situation may be life-saving.*

There may be other occasions when you do not have access to a poison center or medical care. In this case check the container that contained the substance. There may be instructions on how to take care of the ingestion. Remember, sometimes these guidelines are out of date, so it is always better to contact a poison center if possible. If you have ipecac with you, you may decide to use it. Give 3 teaspoons, or 1 tablespoon (15 ml), followed by a glass of juice or water.

CAUTION

Do not administer ipecac if
— the ingested substance is a strong acid or a strong alkali;
— the ingested substance is gasoline, kerosene, or similar volatile material;
— the victim is very drowsy or unconscious.

Remember, no matter where you are, it is always better to prevent these sorts of accidents.

50

Cuts, Scrapes, and Bruises

All children have falls and minor accidents from time to time. Many of the injuries caused by these minor accidents can be handled at home and do not require professional medical attention.

Treatment

- Remain calm—your child will pick up cues from your behavior. The more upset you act, the more frightened he will become. Often, the louder your child cries, the less severe the injury! The wound often looks worse than it is, especially if there is brisk bleeding. Sometimes, relatively minor injuries are associated with a lot of bleeding. This is likely to happen if the injury is on the scalp, where there is a large supply of blood vessels close to the surface. Abrasions or superficial (first-degree) burns are very painful but usually not very serious.

- Clean the wound properly. If possible, hold the affected area under running water and clean the wound thoroughly. If this is not possible, clean the area with soap and water. In the case of animal or human bites, hold the affected area under running water for at least 5 to 10 minutes. A small amount of bleeding will do no harm.

- When the wound is thoroughly cleaned, apply an antiseptic or antibacterial ointment and cover it with clean gauze and fasten it with tape. At times, all that is needed is a bandage.

- If the wound is still bleeding after you have cleaned it, place clean gauze directly over the area and apply firm pressure to the wound. If you do not have clean gauze, use a clean handkerchief or clean cloth. Elevating the affected part, for example, the foot or the hand, will also help to control the bleeding. If the bleeding continues, medical care should be sought.

- If the wound is deep and gaping, your child will probably need stitches—seek medical attention. If you are traveling and away from home and medical help is not easily accessible, you can try to pull the edges of the wound together using Steri-strip or a butterfly bandage. You can make your own butterfly bandage from adhesive tape.

- Your child may need a tetanus shot, especially if he is not fully immunized or the wound is contaminated with

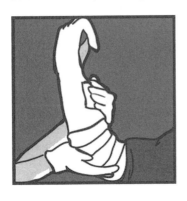

debris. Most children get tetanus immunizations as part of their routine childhood immunizations.

- In the case of an animal bite, your child might need protection against rabies. Contact your physician for guidance. In certain parts of the world, especially Asia, animal bites have a much higher risk of rabies (see Chapter 56).

- It is important to keep the wound clean and dry as it heals. Many wounds will become infected if a bandage or other dressing is left on for too long. Replace the bandage or dressing on a daily basis. Clean the wound every day and allow it to aerate and dry.

- Watch out for signs of infection, which include redness and swelling that spreads outward from the wound, red streaks spreading up the limb from the wound site, worsening pain, or a fever. Wounds of the hands and feet may be deeper than they appear, and infection can spread rapidly in these sites. Many puncture wounds are deep and

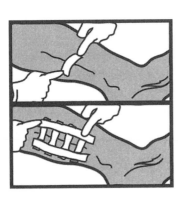

often become infected. Puncture wounds of the hands or feet should be assessed by a medical professional.

When to Seek Medical Attention

- If a wound continues to bleed.
- If the wound is deep and gaping.
- If your child has a puncture wound of the hands or feet.
- If a wound appears to be infected.
- If your child is not fully immunized against tetanus or the wound is contaminated with debris.
- If your child is bitten by an animal that may have rabies (contact your physician for guidance).

51

Burns

Each year, more than 2 million people in the United States suffer from burn injuries. Children, especially boys, make up the majority of these burn victims. The most common burn encountered is a scald caused by hot liquids or steam. Scalds usually occur in the kitchen or bathroom. Burns may also be caused by flames, chemicals, electricity, or radiation. Sunburn is the most frequent cause of a radiation burn. If your child has been sunburned, refer to Chapter 38.

The skin is the largest organ in the body, and its thickness varies greatly according to the location. The skin of the palms and soles may be up to 10 times thicker than that of the eyelids. The thinner the skin, the greater the sensitivity to heat.

Burns may also be associated with other injuries, including smoke inhalation damage to the lungs.

CAUTION
If your child has suffered a severe burn injury, seek medical care immediately.

CLASSIFICATION

The severity of a burn—and its consequences—depend on its size, depth, and location.

Size

The larger the burned area, the more severe the consequences. Even a superficial (first-degree) burn covering 10 percent of a child's body can have serious consequences. (The palm of a person's hand is equal to about 1 percent of his or her entire skin surface area.)

Depth

Heat burns can be classified into three degrees according to the depth of the burn. The degree of a burn is not always easy to determine, and the classification often has to be revised a day or two after the burn occurred.

First-Degree Burns

These are fortunately the most common and are characterized by superficial redness and pain. The skin will turn white when you press on it. The skin often peels within the next two to three days and is totally healed by one week. Sunburn is usually a first-degree burn.

Second-Degree, or Partial-Thickness, Burns

Second-degree burns are characterized by deeper redness, more severe pain, and swelling and blistering. Depending on their depth, these burns may take up to four weeks to heal. If these burns become infected, their classification may be revised to a third-degree, or full-thickness, injury. Less severe scalds are usually second-degree burns and usually take 7 to 14 days to heal.

Third-Degree Burns

In third-degree burns, the burned area is leathery and either white or charred. The burned skin itself is not painful, but the surrounding area may be. These burns will require skin grafting.

Note: Second- and third-degree burns readily become infected by bacteria.

Location

Burns of the face, hands, feet, and genital area have complications out of proportion to their size and should always be assessed by a medical professional.

Prevention

Most burns can be prevented by taking appropriate precautions, including the following:

- For the prevention of sunburn, refer to Chapter 38.
- Make sure your home has a number of functioning smoke detectors and *use them.* Newer photoelectric models cause fewer false alarms than the older smoke detectors, so consider switching to these newer models if you are tempted to disconnect your smoke detectors because of frequent false alarms. Replace the batteries in your smoke detectors every six months (some people do this in the spring and in the fall at the same time they adjust their clocks for the beginning and the end of daylight saving time).
- Keep matches and cigarette lighters in a safe place. Do not leave lighted cigarettes and pipes around. Better still, give up smoking!
- Be careful in the kitchen. Turn pot handles to the side or back of the stove. Preferably use the back burners of the stove.
- Do not hold your child on your lap when drinking hot beverages.
- Keep your hot water temperature between 120° and 125°F.

- Check the water temperature before putting your child in the bath.
- Be especially careful when using curling irons. These are extremely hot and cause deep burns very quickly.
- Don't leave a hot iron on the ironing board. Both the iron and the board are too unstable.
- Don't leave burning candles within your toddler's reach.
- Keep caustic chemicals (strong alkalis and acids) in a safe place and in secure containers.
- Put covers on electrical outlets.
- If your car has been standing in the sun, check the temperature of your child's car seat before putting her in it. Hot buckles can burn an infant's sensitive skin.
- Do not purchase your own fireworks. Attend public displays instead. Fireworks not only result in serious burns but are also a frequent cause of blindness (see Chapter 59).

 Treatment

The following treatment measures apply only to minor burns.

- Remove your child from the heat source.
- Remain calm.
- Immerse the area in cold water. If this is not possible, cover the area with a cloth soaked in cold water. This will not only limit the burn size but also provide some pain relief.

- Do *not* apply butter, oil, salves, or sprays to the burn. Benzocaine and other local anesthetic sprays may lead to sensitization, leading to allergic or irritant reactions.
- Give your child an analgesic such as ibuprofen (Advil or Motrin) or acetaminophen (Tylenol).
- After the initial cool water soaks, for first-degree burns apply a skin care product such as aloe vera cream. For second-degree burns apply either aloe vera or an antibiotic ointment, and cover the burn with a nonstick dressing such as Telfa if you have it. Keep it in place with gauze and tape. An ideal cream for preventing infection is Silvadene, which is available only by prescription.
- Do *not* pop the blisters.

When to Seek Medical Attention

- If the burn covers an area larger than the palm of your child's hand.
- For any burn of the face, hands, feet, or genital area.
- If the burn is anything other than a first-degree burn. The degree of the burn may be difficult to assess. If you are unsure, seek medical care.
- If the burn becomes infected. Signs of infection include the following:
  - Wound discharge that is green or yellow
  - Increasing pain at the burn site after a day or two

- Increased swelling or redness of the skin surrounding the burn
- A fever
- If your child gets an electrical burn.
- If your child has a second- or third-degree burn, he may require a tetanus shot.

FOLLOW-UP CARE

- Burns other than first-degree burns will require dressing changes once a day. Soak the burned area in cool water for 15 minutes, allow to air dry, and then apply an antibiotic ointment. Cover with a nonstick dressing such as Telfa, and keep it in place with gauze and tape. It is a good idea to give your child a suitable analgesic one hour *before* you change the dressing.
- Be on the lookout for secondary infection (described above).
- Once the burn has healed, soften the area by rubbing in vitamin E cream.
- Be extra careful to avoid sunburn to the area for at least one year.

ELECTRICAL BURNS

Electrical burns may appear to be very minor at the surface, but serious deep tissue injury may have occurred. Internal injuries may also be present.

1. Do not touch the victim until the current has been turned off or the source of the current has been removed with an implement that does not conduct electricity, such as a wooden broomstick.
2. If the victim is unconscious, call 911 and begin CPR if necessary.
3. If the victim is otherwise "OK," treat the burn like other heat burns by immersing the burned part in cold water, if possible.
4. Use pain medicine as necessary.
5. Seek medical care.

52

Foreign Bodies in the Ear

Occasionally while camping or being outdoors, an insect may fly or crawl into your child's ear. This is extremely distressing to the child (as it would be to anyone). Treatment consists of reassuring your child and gently pouring lukewarm water into the affected ear. The insect will often float out. If the insect does not come out, medical attention should be sought. Mineral oil can also be gently poured into the ear to drown the insect. It will then need to be removed by a physician. Do not pour liquids into the ear if your child has "tubes."

Children often put other objects into their ears, favorites being beads and popcorn kernels! Do not attempt to get these foreign bodies out. Seek medical attention instead. Do *not* put sharp objects into the ear or try to remove the foreign body with a paper clip or similar "instrument."

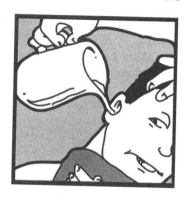

It can be risky to assume that ear pain is always due to an infection. Early one morning, my wife and I were awakened by our seven-year-old son, who came to our bedroom clutching at his right ear and crying in pain. Not having an otoscope (an instrument to look into the ear canal) at home to check on his ear, I assumed the pain was due to a middle-ear infection. I gave him a dose of ibuprofen and propped him up in his bed, and after about 30 minutes he settled down and went back to sleep.

The next day, our son seemed fine, and since it was the weekend, I did not take him to my office to check on his ear. The following night the scenario was repeated. I repeated the treatment I had tried the night before, but this time I started him on an antibiotic.

Three days later, David was still complaining of an earache, so I took him to the office and looked into his ear. Several pairs of hairy and spiky legs faced me down the otoscope. I removed the offending insect, a Japanese beetle, dead but still very much intact!

Lessons to be learned:

1. Do not treat your own family.
2. Cooperate when your child's doctor suggests that you bring your child into the office to be examined. You may be surprised by what he finds.
3. It is seldom a good idea to start a patient on an antibiotic for earache without examining the patient first.

53

Foreign Bodies in the Nose

It is not unusual for children to put things other than their fingers up their nose. Objects that commonly find their way into the nose are popcorn kernels, buttons, beads, eraser tips, and candy! More potentially dangerous objects that are put in the nose are small batteries such as camera or watch batteries. These can cause erosions of the nasal septum (the part of the nose that separates the two nostrils). If batteries find their way into the bowel, they can perforate the bowel.

If your child confesses that he has put something up his nose, it is wise to seek medical help immediately. Your doctor may be able to remove it fairly easily, but occasionally this may have to be done by an ENT (ear, nose, and throat) surgeon under anesthesia.

You may be able to see the object in the nose, and if it is protruding, you may be able to remove it yourself. However, do *not* try to remove it yourself if you cannot easily get hold of it, as you may push it in deeper. Do *not* try to push it in deeper hoping it will end up in your child's throat and be coughed out or spat out. If you do this, it may be aspirated into the windpipe or lungs. Rarely, a cooperative older child may be able to force the object out his nose by blowing his nose or by sneezing.

Sometimes a child does not tell the parent what she has done, and the parent gradually becomes aware over time that the child has bad breath and a nasty discharge from one nostril.

Rarely, a child who has put an object up his nose will swallow it, in which case there is usually nothing to be concerned about unless it is a battery or a sharp object. The major concern with a foreign body up the nose is that it will be aspirated into the airway or lungs. If your child has a choking episode, medical care should be sought immediately. If your child is in severe distress, you may have to perform the Heimlich maneuver or some similar age-appropriate maneuver (see Chapter 63).

When to Seek Medical Attention

- A foreign body in the nose that cannot be easily and immediately removed.
- A persistent foul-smelling discharge from one nostril.
- A choking episode or breathing difficulty in a child who was known to be playing with small objects.
- If you suspect your child may have swallowed a potentially dangerous object such as a camera battery, watch battery, or sharp object.

54

Knocked-Out Tooth

Dental injuries are common in childhood, and one of the more common ones is a knocked-out tooth.

 Treatment

- If a young child knocks out a "baby" or milk tooth, do not attempt to replace it in the gum socket.
- If your child knocks out a permanent (adult) tooth, this should be replaced as soon as possible. Do *not* touch the root end. Rinse the tooth gently under running water and replace it. Do not scrub or attempt to clean the tooth too vigorously. If you are unable to replace the tooth, put it in a glass of water or milk and seek dental attention right away. The sooner the tooth is replaced in the gum socket, the more likely it is to take hold and survive. Even if you have successfully replaced the tooth,

consult your dentist, as the tooth may need to be splinted. Your child may also need an antibiotic.

- If the tooth is only partially dislodged and is just sticking out of its socket farther than normal, push it back in until it is in its normal position and seek medical or dental attention.
- After dental trauma, your child should be on a liquid or soft diet until the tooth has healed.
- If the tooth cannot be found, your child may need to be checked because the tooth may have been inhaled. If this is the case, your child will probably be coughing or in respiratory distress. A chest X-ray may be needed. If the tooth has been swallowed, apart from the fact that your child has lost a tooth, there is no need to be concerned.
- To control bleeding from the gum apply pressure with clean gauze or a clean cloth. Bleeding will usually stop if pressure is applied for long enough. As with bleeding in other locations, you may need to apply constant pressure for 5 to 10 minutes.

55

Mammal Bites

Bites not only cause immediate tissue damage but also carry the risk of infection and rabies. Human bites are the bites most likely to become infected, followed by cat bites and then dog bites. Cat bites may look very minor, but infected material is often injected deeply into the tissues.

Treatment

The most important treatment of any bite is vigorous cleaning of the wound as soon as possible. This is best done by holding the affected area under running water for at least 5 to 10 minutes. Contact your doctor for further treatment such as tetanus shots, rabies prevention, antibiotics, and/or suturing if needed. This will depend on the size and location of the bite and the likelihood of infection.

For crush injuries, splinting and elevation of the affected extremity is recommended.

When to Seek Medical Attention

It is especially important to seek medical care for bites involving the face and puncture wounds of the hands and feet.

If your child has been bitten by a wild animal or a domestic animal that you don't know, rabies prophylaxis may be needed (see Chapter 56).

INFECTION

Signs that the bite wound is infected include the following:

- Increasing redness
- Increasing swelling
- Increasing pain
- Pus discharging from the wound
- Red streaks extending from the bite site toward the heart
- Fever

56

Rabies

Rabies and rabies prevention are still a significant public health issue in the United States. Rabies in humans fortunately is rare because of prophylactic measures after animal bites and because of control of rabies in domestic animals. It is a major medical issue in developing countries, with up to 100,000 human deaths worldwide annually.

In the United States, the animals that usually spread rabies are raccoons, skunks, foxes, and bats. Raccoons are the number one cause. In developing countries the most frequent cause of rabies is dog bites.

 Prevention

- Immunize your pets against rabies.
- Use caution around animals you do not know, even domestic ones.

- Avoid physical contact with strays and wild animals, whether dead or alive.
- Do not attempt to domesticate wild animals, especially raccoons.
- Tightly secure garbage can lids and make them less accessible to prowling dogs, raccoons, and skunks.
- If you have young children and you plan an extended stay in a country where rabies is common, consider getting them immunized against rabies.

Remember, in developing countries, dogs are the number one cause of rabies. Caution your children about petting dogs in third-world countries, especially in Asia.

Domestic pets such as white rats, hamsters, and mice do not carry rabies. Squirrel bites would be very unlikely to lead to rabies. If there is any doubt, contact your doctor or local state public health authorities. Be especially wary of bats: your child does not have to be bitten by a bat to get rabies. Rabies may be transmitted via bat urine or other bat secretions entering through mucous membranes such as the eye or mouth. If there is any doubt about your child's exposure to a bat while sleeping, contact your doctor or local health authorities.

 ### Treatment

Initial treatment of any animal bite includes extensive cleansing, as described in Chapter 55, followed by further wound care as necessary. Your child may also need tetanus prevention as well as antibiotics. Your doctor will then determine whether a course of rabies shots is necessary.

> *Note:* If you are planning an extended stay in an area where there is a high incidence of rabies, consider immunizing your children against rabies before you depart. This may be important if you are planning a long stay in a lesser-developed country where rabies is common. Discuss this with your doctor prior to your travels.

57

Heat-Related Illness

There are other causes for elevated temperatures besides the fever that occurs with infections. Heat-related illnesses include heat syncope, heat cramps, heat exhaustion, and heat stroke. Unlike the fever that occurs with infections (which is the body's normal way of fighting infections), heat-related illnesses are abnormal and may be very serious. Each year, heat stroke is responsible for more than 400 deaths in the United States.

- *Heat syncope* refers to symptoms of lightheadedness and fainting that may occur when a person is standing for a long time in a hot environment.
- *Heat cramps* usually follow strenuous exercise such as cycling on a hot day when the body has been depleted of salts and water. The muscles most commonly involved are the calves, the thighs, and the abdominal muscles. People with heat cramps are generally alert, have a nor-

mal temperature, and complain of muscle cramps. Treatment is to rehydrate with salt-containing fluids such as sports drinks or electrolyte solutions. Muscle cramps may also occur with heat exhaustion and heat stroke, in which case more aggressive treatment will be needed.

- *Heat exhaustion* is a more serious condition. A child with heat exhaustion will be very fatigued and complain of headache, dizziness, and nausea. He may be mildly confused and may vomit. He will sweat excessively. The skin is often cool and clammy. His temperature is usually elevated, but it may be normal. If he remains in the hot environment and without fluids, heat exhaustion may progress to heat stroke.
- *Heat stroke* is the most severe type of heat illness. It is extremely dangerous and a life-threatening emergency requiring immediate treatment. People with heat stroke are usually very confused, and their body temperature is usually markedly elevated, often to 105°F or higher. The skin is often dry. As heat stroke worsens, the level of consciousness deteriorates; the person may have a seizure or lapse into coma. Shock frequently develops. Heat stroke is extremely dangerous and is a medical emergency.

People of all ages can get heat-related illnesses, but certain groups are particularly prone to developing them. These groups are discussed below.

INFANTS AND YOUNG CHILDREN

Infants and young children do not sweat as readily as adults and have greater fluid requirements relative to their size. They are more prone to dehydration and heat-related illness. Young children also tend to be more active than adults and are often "too busy" to stop to drink. Infants have an immature temperature-regulating system, which contributes to the problem. Infants may develop heat exhaustion or heat stroke when they are overbundled or overswaddled, especially if they have infections associated with a fever. A very serious and preventable cause of heat-related illness in infants and young children is being left in a closed car. Temperatures in the car on hot days may exceed 150°F. Even a few minutes at these temperatures may be fatal!

OLDER CHILDREN

Older children are prone to heat illness when they exercise on very hot days, especially if it is humid and they have not yet acclimatized to the heat. Young athletes are especially likely to develop heat stroke if they do not drink sufficient fluid or if they are overweight. This type of heat illness may occur even in very fit adults who are dehydrated and exercising on hot days.

THE ELDERLY

The elderly may develop heat exhaustion or heat stroke without exercising if they are exposed to high environmental temperatures for several days, as occurs during heat waves.

 Prevention

- Infants and young children should not be overdressed, particularly if they have a fever or infection. The fever associated with an infection does not cause brain damage and is seldom cause for worry. However, if an infant who is ill and has a fever is overdressed or is in a warm environment, his temperature may reach dangerous levels. This may lead to severe medical problems, including brain damage.
- Never leave children in hot cars, even for short periods.
- Prevention of exercise-related heat injury:
  - Gradual acclimatization to hot weather is important. Expose your child to hotter temperatures for a few minutes longer each day. Increase activity intensity and duration a little each day. Do not let your child exercise vigorously in hot and humid weather until this acclimatization has taken place.
  - Do not let your child exercise at the hottest times of the day. At the beginning of the sports season, plan activities for the early morning or evening when temperatures are cooler. As your child becomes acclima-

tized to the warmer weather and is fitter, activities can take place in hotter and more humid weather, and exercise periods can last longer.

− Dress children in lightweight and light-colored clothing, which allows their skin to breathe and allows them to sweat adequately.

− Drink extra fluids before beginning exercise. Children should stop frequently (every 20 minutes) for drinks of water or sports drinks. Children should *not* wait until they are thirsty to drink. If your child waits until he is thirsty to drink, he is far more likely to become dehydrated and develop heat-related illness. Adolescents at football practice may want to appear "macho" and say they do not need to drink. Everyone at the practice must drink! Avoid caffeine-containing drinks, as these increase urine output.

− Children also need to have frequent breaks in the shade to cool off. This is especially important for overweight children. Any child who appears to be very fatigued, flushed, or dizzy or who seems less alert than usual should be called off the field immediately, be taken to a cooler location, and given fluids. Such a child should be closely watched.

− All children should try to get fit before the sports season starts. This is especially important for overweight children, as they are particularly prone to heat exhaustion and heat stroke.

Prevention while Traveling

Travelers are particularly prone to heat illness. It is not unusual to be at subzero temperatures in the Northeast on one day and be in a hot and humid climate the next. These measures may help you avoid heat-related illness and ruining your vacation.

- Schedule activities for early and late in the day when it is cooler.
- Increase your sun exposure gradually.
- Wear a hat and apply sunscreen if out in the sun.
- Wear loose-fitting, cool cotton clothes.
- Drink plenty of fluids.
- Limit your caffeine and alcohol intake.

 Treatment

The treatment of the *less severe* forms of heat-related illness includes moving to a cooler environment (such as the shade), removing excess clothing, and taking plenty of fluids. Wetting the person with cool water or fanning is very beneficial. If a person has heat cramps, give salt-containing fluids such as Pedialyte or sports drinks. If these are not available, drinking water to which a small amount of salt has been added (¼ teaspoon of salt to 1 quart of water) is a good alternative. Do *not* give the victim salt tablets. If the person is confused or vomiting, *immediate medical care* should be sought. Do *not*

administer aspirin, ibuprofen, or acetaminophen because they do not help this condition and may be harmful.

As mentioned above, *heat stroke is a medical emergency* and may be fatal. Call 911. While waiting for medical help to arrive, you should do the following:

- Move the person to a cooler area.
- Remove all the clothing down to the underwear. Young children and infants should have all their clothing removed.
- Sprinkle or spray the person with cool water or repeatedly apply wet towels or cloths.
- Fan the person.
- Place ice packs, cold compresses, or chemical ice packs around the neck, the armpits, the groin, and the scalp.
- Do not force the person to drink if he is confused or comatose.
- Do not give him aspirin, ibuprofen, or acetaminophen.

58

Cold-Related Illness
and Injuries

Just as children are more prone to heat illness than adults, so are they more likely to suffer from cold illness and cold-related injuries. The younger and smaller the child, the greater the risk. Children have a large surface area relative to their body weight, as well as a relatively large head from which they lose heat. They also have thinner skin, which loses heat more easily; less subcutaneous fat; and fewer energy reserves. All this is compounded by immaturity and poor judgment. The elderly are also prone to the development of hypothermia.

If the body temperature drops to 95°F (or 35°C) or lower, this is known as *hypothermia*. If a part of the body freezes, this is known as *frostbite*. Hypothermia and frostbite often occur together.

HYPOTHERMIA

This occurs when the body temperature drops. It is classified as mild, moderate, or severe (deep) hypothermia. The more severe forms are extremely serious and may be fatal. The signs of mild hypothermia may be very subtle; this form frequently "sneaks up" gradually and insidiously.

Signs of *mild* hypothermia include the following:

- Shivering
- Cold, blue, and mottled extremities
- Numb hands and feet; stiff muscles that lead to clumsy and uncoordinated movements and stumbling
- Lethargy, apathy, weakness, confusion, and poor judgment
- Slurred speech

As the hypothermia becomes more severe, the person will become more and more confused and irrational. With severe hypothermia, shivering ceases, the heart rate slows, and the person lapses into unconsciousness. This is a *medical emergency.*

FROSTNIP AND FROSTBITE

The areas most likely to be affected by both frostnip and frostbite are the fingers, toes, cheeks, and the tips of the ears and nose. All but the most minor degrees of cold injury require medical attention.

Frostnip is the mildest form of cold injury and involves only the superficial layers of the skin. The affected area is cold and white. Initially it may be painful, but later it becomes slightly numb but still has some sensation. As the area is warmed, it turns red, and the person may feel a tingling sensation ("pins and needles"). Frostnip is associated with the constriction of the blood vessels and is totally reversible and is cured by warming. There is no permanent damage, but if not treated early and adequately, it will progress to frostbite.

Frostbite is more severe than frostnip, as ice crystals actually form in the tissues and cause damage.

Frostbite is classified into superficial frostbite and deep frostbite depending on the depth of the freezing injury. Early on, it may be extremely difficult to differentiate between the different degrees of frostbite.

Superficial frostbite affects the skin and the tissues immediately below the skin. The affected area usually has a pale and waxy appearance, but there may be surrounding redness. The area will feel doughy and thickened. It will be numb. With thawing, blisters that contain a clear fluid may form. If the injury is slightly deeper, the fluid may be milky.

Deep frostbite is an extremely serious injury extending into the underlying tissues and may involve tendons, muscles, and sometimes bone. The entire area will have a woody feel and have no sensation. If blisters form, they are filled with a purple fluid.

As frostbite is warmed and thawed, the affected area often becomes red, blotchy, and very swollen. Thawing is often accompanied by extreme pain. The deeper degrees of frostbite may lead to death of the tissues, and amputation may be necessary.

 Prevention

Most cold injuries and incidences of hypothermia are preventable. It is important to remember that hypothermia can occur in all seasons and not only in the winter months.

When planning outdoor activities where cold illness or injury is possible, consider the following.

Clothing

- Dress your child in layers. Air gets trapped between layers and provides extra insulation. Layering also allows you to remove clothing as you get warmer and add a layer as you get colder. Ideally, the layer closest to the skin should be made of a synthetic fiber such as polypropylene or polyester, which wicks perspiration away from the skin. The middle layer provides insulation and some protection from the outside and may be made of wool, fleece, or cotton. This layer also absorbs some of the moisture from the inner layer. The outer layer should provide insulation as well as be wind- and water-resistant. This layer should also allow some ventilation so that sweat may evaporate.
- Children should wear hats. The younger the child, the

greater the heat loss from the head. A person may lose up to 80 percent of her body heat from the head and neck. A warm hat, a warm scarf, and ear muffs are essential.

- Wear gloves or mittens. Mittens provide greater protection from the cold but with loss of dexterity. On very cold days it is a good idea to use silk or polypropylene glove linings.

- Foot protection and boots are also important. Boots should fit well so as not to restrict the circulation. Just as having two layers on the hands is a good idea, so wearing two pairs of socks will help keep the toes and feet warm. Always have spare dry pairs of socks available. Change socks frequently so that the feet remain dry. Cold feet lead to frostbite, clumsiness, and misery.

- Remove underlying layers of clothes as your child heats up with activity. Being too warm leads to sweating. Clothing gets damp, and this leads to chilling as your child cools down. Add these layers back on as your child cools down again.

Fluids and Nutrition

A person is more susceptible to cold injury if he is dehydrated. Encourage your child to drink even if he is not thirsty. Avoid caffeine-containing drinks. Adults *must* avoid alcohol. Urine color, usually a good indication of the state of hydration, should be a light yellow.

Calories are also needed to help ward off the cold.

Frequent high-carbohydrate snacks provide instant energy. If camping outdoors at night, eat foods that contain fat and protein as well to provide your body with energy all night.

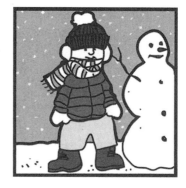

Environmental Conditions

Use common sense:

- Do not allow your child to go outside on extremely cold days. Make sure your child is adequately and appropriately dressed even on days that are not that cold but when wind chill is possible.
- Wind and wetness make cold injury much more likely. Your child should not be outside if the wind chill index is below 10°F, or −12°C.
- Limit time spent outdoors on cold days. Do not wait until your child is chilled before getting him indoors.
- Suspect hypothermia if a child who has been playing outside in the cold is irritable or lethargic or behaving strangely!
- Plan hiking, climbing, or camping trips carefully, paying attention to the weather conditions and location.
- Plan ahead. Anticipate changes in the weather and temperature, and even on sunny days include a water-resistant and wind-resistant shell, a warm hat, mittens, extra

pairs of socks, food, and adequate fluids. A space blanket is lightweight and packs easily.

- Hunger, exhaustion, and demoralization all make hypothermia more likely. Plan excursions carefully and sensibly. Don't try to do too much. Activities should be set at the level of the weakest and slowest participant. Eat snacks regularly.

- Periodically "windmill" your arms. This involves swinging arms around vigorously in a rotary fashion. This movement dilates the blood vessels to the fingers and hands, increasing the blood supply to them and so warming them.

- Keep an eye on your companions. Use the "buddy system" to check each other's faces (the nose, ears, and cheeks) for the telltale signs of frostbite (redness or white or yellow plaques). Repeatedly assess your companions:
  - Are they drinking enough?
  - Are they becoming irritable, lethargic, irrational, or confused?
  - Do they just want to be left alone?
  - Are they becoming less coordinated?

These signs may all indicate hypothermia. Take action!

Driving in the Winter

- Put blankets, gloves, extra clothes, and some food and water in the car when setting out on winter travel. A cell phone, a flashlight, flares, and a shovel may also turn out to be very useful.

- If you become stranded:
  - Stay inside your car for shelter if it is cold outside.
  - Make sure the snow does not block your car's exhaust pipe.
  - Turn off the engine and anything that consumes energy (lighter, heater, and radio).
  - Run the engine and heater for 10 minutes every hour.
  - Open the window a little now and then. Snuggle together but exercise a little to keep awake and keep warm.
  - If snow starts to bury your car, it is a good idea to make an air hole with an umbrella, a ski, or similar object.
  - Do not drink alcohol.

Treatment

The treatment will depend not only on the severity of the hypothermia or the type or severity of the injury but also on where you are and your proximity to medical help. If you are at home and your child is getting cold, get him to come inside.

If hypothermia and frostbite occur together, which is the often the case, treat the hypothermia first, as it is more likely to be fatal.

Hypothermia

> ### ⚠ CAUTION
>
> Severe hypothermia (as described on p. 533) is a medical emergency. Although the basic principles of treatment apply to all degrees of hypothermia, the in-hospital treatment needed for more severe cases of hypothermia is beyond the scope of this book. If you are in a situation where you can call 911, do this immediately. Prevent further heat loss by *gently* removing wet clothing and covering the person with layers of dry clothing, blankets, and/or sleeping bags. Handle the person very gently.

For the *milder degrees of hypothermia,* do the following:

1. Get the person out of the cold and wind if possible.
2. Remove all wet clothing. Put on dry clothing in layers.
3. Cover the person with warm, dry blankets or put her into a sleeping bag. Two sleeping bags are better than one.
4. Offer the person a warm, sweet drink.

Once the person is out of the cold and you have followed the directions listed above, shivering will generate heat and raise the body temperature. If at all possible, do *not* leave a hypothermic person alone.

Frostbite

Always try to detect and treat frostnip and frostbite early—as soon as the part turns numb and white.

- Get out of the cold.
- Windmilling, as described on p. 538, may prevent and limit the extent of frostnip and frostbite.
- For *mild* frostbite, remove wet clothing (gloves, mittens, boots, and socks) and warm the affected body part by skin-to-skin contact. Place hands in the armpits and place cold feet under clothing on somebody else's belly or in an armpit.
- Remove rings, watches, and tight or constrictive clothing that may compromise the circulation as swelling occurs.
- Put on dry gloves or mittens, dry socks, dry boots, and warm clothing.

More severe frostbite will require more intensive treatment. Get medical help if possible. The ideal treatment is rapid thawing accomplished by soaking the affected part in warm water (100° to 108°F). If you are "in the field" and this treatment measure isn't possible, you will have to allow slow and spontaneous warming. Once thawing has occurred, it is essential to prevent refreezing of the affected area. If this occurs, more damage will result. If you cannot prevent refreezing, it is better *not* to allow thawing in the first place.

If you are out on the trail or in the mountains and a member of your party gets frostbite of the feet, it is OK to let that person walk out with frozen feet. Thawing may take place spontaneously. Again, prevent refreezing. If boots are taken off out on the trail, you stand the risk of not being able to put them back on again.

Remember, frostbite is often associated with hypothermia. Treat this first!

Important Don'ts

- Don't rub frostbitten tissues. This may lead to further damage. Especially do not rub with snow.
- Don't allow the thawed body part to refreeze.
- Don't heat the frostbitten area in front of the fire or heater. Don't try to warm the frozen area with a blow dryer. You may complicate the injury with a burn.
- Don't break blisters.
- Don't touch cold metal with bare hands.
- Don't handle fuel and supercooled liquids with bare hands.

SOME FACTS ABOUT COLD-RELATED INJURIES

- Dehydration predisposes a person to hypothermia and frostbite. Keep well hydrated.
- Wetness often leads to hypothermia. This wetness may come from the outside—rain, snow, or water. It may also come from the inside—sweating leads to damp clothes, conduction of heat away from the body, and

chilling. Heat is lost 25 times faster in water. If you are out boating and your boat capsizes, you are more likely to survive by clinging to the overturned hull than by trying to swim to a distant shore through cold waters. This applies even if your clothes are soaked and you are exposed to the rain and wind.

• Hypothermia can occur in all seasons, not only in winter. A person may get dangerous hypothermia even when the outside temperature is 50° to 60°F if there is wind chill or clothing is damp or inadequate. A person who sets off on a hike on a sunny day in shorts and a T-shirt and gets caught in the rain is more likely to get hypothermia than the well-prepared skier in the middle of winter.

 For Your Reference

If you are undertaking more adventurous activities, it is strongly recommended that you read more to learn about cold- and heat-related injuries, first aid in the wilderness, and similar topics. *Wilderness and Travel Medicine,* by Eric Weiss, and *Wilderness First Aid,* a collaboration between the National Safety Council and the Wilderness Medical Society and published by Jones and Bartlett publishers, are excellent sources for further information. The truly adventurous are advised to take one of the survival courses offered by the Wilderness Medical Society.

59

Fireworks Injuries

Every year, particularly around the Fourth of July, children are injured by fireworks. Almost 10,000 people visit the emergency room each year with injuries caused by fireworks. More than 1,000 of these injuries involve the eye. In fact, fireworks are a significant cause of blindness.

- Burns are the most common injury due to fireworks.
- Bottle rockets cause the greatest number of eye injuries.
- Sparklers frequently cause eye injuries. They can reach temperatures of 1,800°F, hot enough to melt gold!
- Bystanders are more often injured than those who operate the fireworks.

Prevention

Leave fireworks to the professionals. Do not set off fireworks yourself. Don't be around amateurs setting off fireworks. That is all you need to know!

Treatment

For *burns,* see Chapter 51. Fireworks can cause deep burns. Hold burned hands and fingers in cold water. Give painkillers such as ibuprofen (Advil, Motrin). Seek medical attention.

For *eye injuries,* seek medical attention *immediately.* In the meantime:

- Don't panic. Stay calm.
- Don't rub the eye.
- Don't rinse out the eye.
- Don't apply any ointment.
- To prevent a child from rubbing the eye, shield it with the bottom half of a styrofoam cup taped to the brow, bridge of nose and cheek bone.
- Don't give ibuprofen or aspirin. These might increase bleeding.

CAUTION

If an eye injury has occurred, don't delay. Seek expert medical attention immediately.

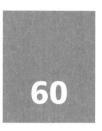

60

Lightning Injuries

It is often said that you are more likely to be struck by lightning than win the lottery! Sadly, this may be true. Lightning causes more deaths each year than tornadoes. In some years it has caused more deaths in the United States than any other natural disaster. The good news is that most people who are struck by lightning do not die, but many are left with severe injuries.

Lightning occurs most commonly in the summer months, typically in the afternoon. Lightning injuries are especially prevalent in mountainous areas and around large bodies of water, such as river basins and lakes. A significant proportion of injuries occur in persons who are inside their homes or places of employment. These injuries are fortunately much less likely to be fatal.

One of the most dangerous times for a fatal strike is *before* a storm. Lightning may travel nearly horizontally as far as 10 miles in front of a storm and may seem to come "out of the clear blue sky" and when there is still some sunshine. Violent and fast-moving storms are particularly likely to produce lightning. Lightning strikes may occur up to 30 minutes after the storm is over. The potential for lightning strikes before and after a storm, as well as during it, has given rise to the *30/30 rule*: if the interval between seeing the lightning and hearing the thunder is less than 30 seconds, you are close enough to be struck. The second "30" is to warn you to wait 30 minutes after the storm has ended before venturing out.

Lightning may strike you directly, but more frequently you will be harmed by a lightning "splash," which takes place when lightning that has struck a nearby object, such as a tree or fence, "splashes" onto you. This also may happen if you wait out the storm in small shelters, such as you may find on a golf course or on a hiking path, or if you take shelter under a tall tree. The lightning strikes the shelter or the tree and then splashes onto you. You are more likely to be struck by lightning *directly* if you are out in the open. It is a myth that lightning "never strikes in the same place twice."

Objects that contain metal or that are taller than you, such as golf clubs or umbrellas, may act as conductors and significantly increase the chances of a direct lightning strike.

 Prevention

- Be aware of weather conditions and weather predictions before going on excursions, playing sports outside, or working out in the open. Watch out for darkening skies and increasing wind. Remember that lightning may strike before the storm starts and after it is over. If you can hear the thunder, you are close enough to be struck. Seek shelter.

- Tips for finding adequate shelter:
  - Shelter in a substantial building or in an all-metal vehicle, such as a car. Roll up the windows and don't touch metal surfaces inside or outside the vehicle. Lightning can strike automobiles, but the metal surfaces will conduct the current to the ground.
  - Avoid convertibles or cloth-top jeeps.
  - Do not seek shelter in small sheds, gazebos, or picnic or golfing shelters, especially if these are isolated or exposed.
  - Do not take shelter under tall trees.
  - Tents offer very little protection, and the metal support pole actually may act as a lightning rod. Occupants of a tent should stay away from the poles and from the wet cloth.
  - In the forest, seek shelter in a low area among smaller trees.
- If you are unable to find shelter, do not stand near tall, isolated trees; on hilltops; or on exposed areas. If you are totally in the open, stay away from single trees to avoid lightning splashes. Stay away from metal objects such as flagpoles, motorcycles, tractors, fences, and bicycles. Put down metal objects such as ice picks, axes, hunting knives, umbrellas, and golf clubs.
- You do not want to be the tallest object around! De-

crease your height by crouching down, kneeling, squatting, or sitting cross-legged on the ground. Do not hold an umbrella above your head, and if your backpack projects above you, put it down.

- Try to minimize how much of your body comes into contact with the ground. Keep your feet as close together as possible. Do not lie down.
- Hold your hands over your ears to minimize ear damage from the thunderclap.
- If you are with a group of people, spread out and stay several yards apart. In the event of a strike, fewer people will be injured by ground currents or by side flashes between people.
- Avoid swimming, boating, or being the tallest object near a large, open body of water. If you are on the water, head for the shore.
- If indoors during a thunderstorm, avoid being near open doors and windows; fireplaces; metal objects such as pipes, sinks, and radiators; and plug-in electrical appliances. Do not use the telephone or the computer. Do not use a cell phone, as you can get ear damage from the static.

Lightning more frequently causes injury than death. If death occurs, it is most likely due to immediate cardiac or cardiorespiratory arrest. Starting CPR may be lifesaving. The sooner you start it, the more likely it is to be successful.

It is a myth that a person retains the charge once he or she has been struck by lightning. It is totally safe to touch a person who has just been struck by lightning.

Lightning injuries may cause severe brain damage, burns, eye and ear injuries, and many other types of injuries. Anyone struck by lightning, even if he or she appears well, should be taken to the nearest emergency room for assessment and therapy.

61

Drowning Prevention

Drowning is one of the most common causes of death in childhood in the United States. In some states it is *the* leading cause of death in childhood. On average, one child drowns every day in a backyard swimming pool. Drowning is also one of the more common causes of death while on vacation.

In the home setting, drowning may occur in the bathtub, the toilet, a bucket, a water barrel, a children's play pool, or the backyard swimming pool. Drowning also frequently happens during water recreational activities such as sailing, canoeing, or swimming.

Although people of any age can drown, there are two age groups in which drownings are more common. The first is the toddler age group; toddlers can drown in the bathtub or in as little as 1 inch of water in a bucket. Water holds an endless fascination for many of us, but especially for young children. They are naturally inquisitive and seem to be instinctively drawn to water. The second age group is adolescence, and in this group males are much more likely to drown than females. Boys tend to be risk takers, and some also seem to be especially lacking in common sense at this age. Among older adolescents, alcohol frequently plays a role in drowning incidents.

 Prevention

Prevention, prevention, prevention! You may be lucky enough to arrive in time to resuscitate your child, but this is not the way to prevent death by drowning.

- *Never* leave your child alone in the bathtub, not even to answer the front doorbell or the telephone.
- Do not leave buckets of water around.
- Empty your child's play pool once your child has finished swimming.
- Teach your child how to swim at a young age.
- No one should swim alone.
- *Never* leave young children alone around water. *Responsible adult supervision is the most important aspect in the prevention of drowning.*
- Teach your child safe water behavior.
- Do not allow diving into shallow water.
- When boating, everyone should wear an approved life vest or life jacket that is able to support the wearer so that the head is above water even if the person is uncon-

scious. A responsible and capable adult should be present during all boating activities.

- Respect the sea! Dangerous back currents and side washes can get the better of even the most powerful swimmer. Swim where there are lifeguards. Obey their instructions. If they tell you to get out of the water, get out!

- Counsel adolescents about the dangers of drinking and swimming. This combination is just as dangerous as drinking and driving.

CAUTION
Begin CPR immediately if your child is found unconscious in the water. Call 911.

If You Have a Swimming Pool

- Swimming pools should be fenced on all four sides with a fence that is at least 4 feet high. The gate should be self-closing and self-latching. Keep the gate locked. Keep a telephone close so that you do not need to leave the pool area to answer it. In the event of an accident the telephone will be close by should you need to call 911.

I grew up in sunny South Africa in a home with a swimming pool. It did not have a fence around it. (In those days very few pools did.) One day my younger brother went missing. We all raced to the swimming pool to see if he was there. It was midwinter, and we had not bothered to keep the water clean. The water was murky, so we all jumped in to look for his body. Fortunately he was not in the pool. We found him later asleep behind the sofa, but I still shudder each time I think of the incident!

- Keep the pool water clean.
- If your child goes missing, look in the pool first.
- Learn how to do CPR and keep your certification up to date.

62

Breathing Difficulties

There are many reasons why an infant or child may have trouble breathing. The causes of breathing difficulty range from a seemingly minor illness such as a stuffy nose (especially in an infant) to more serious causes such as severe asthma and pneumonia. Other chapters in this book contain discussions on bronchiolitis, asthma, croup, and coughs. Refer to these chapters where indicated.

This chapter contains guidelines on how to assess your child if he is having significant breathing problems and is seriously ill.

OVERALL APPEARANCE AND ACTIVITY LEVEL

The following questions are very sensitive guides to determining the severity of childhood illness including the degree of breathing difficulty.

- Does she really look ill? Does she appear anxious?
- What is she doing? Is she playing actively and happily, or does she just want to sit quietly on your lap?
- Does she show any interest in her surroundings?
- Is she interacting normally with you? Will she make eye contact? Will she smile?

How your child is behaving and acting may be more important than any one of the individual signs discussed below. If your child is active and running about, she probably does not have severe pneumonia or breathing difficulties even though she may have noisy breathing and a loud cough. On the other hand, a child who is quiet, inactive, and anxious may be in severe respiratory distress but have no cough or apparent breathing difficulty. Observe your child closely.

BREATHING PATTERN

- Is your child breathing in her usual way, or is she struggling to breathe?
- Is her breathing smooth and regular?
- Are there periods of breath holding?
  - Most newborns and babies in the first few months of life have very irregular breathing patterns. At times they breathe quickly, and then a few seconds later, they slow down and sometimes hold their breath for 10 to 15 seconds. Just when you are convinced they have totally stopped breathing, they start up again! This

breathing pattern is known as *periodic respiration*, and although it is very disconcerting, it is normal at this age.

– Older children with *sleep apnea* often have struggling respirations interspersed with periods of breath holding. You may hear loud snoring, then periods of gasping, and then silence. This condition is often due to enlarged tonsils or adenoids.

Note: Deep, sighing respiration may indicate dehydration or out-of-control diabetes.

BREATHING RATE

Newborn infants breathe around 40 times a minute and at times much faster. After feeding or crying, the respiratory rate may get as high as 80 times a minute or faster. After a minute or two, this rapid breathing should settle back to normal. A very good time to count your infant's respirations is when she is asleep. Count the number of breaths over a two-minute period and divide the number by two. Older children and adults usually breathe about 15 to 20 times a minute. A persistently high respiratory rate (above 60 times a minute in a child younger than one year of age or above 40 times a minute in an older child) is often an indication that your child has a problem This may just be a blocked nose (typically in a young infant), or it may be a sign of a more serious condition such as asthma, bronchiolitis, or pneumonia. Many other diseases such as heart disease or dehydration may also cause your child to breathe rapidly. If your child has a high fever, she may also breathe faster than normal.

NOISES WHEN BREATHING

- If your child has *croup,* you may hear a high-pitched, raspy sound as she breathes in, which is called *stridor.* This is often accompanied by the typical croupy cough, which is "barky" and "seal-like." When your child talks, you will usually notice hoarseness. Croup often comes on suddenly in the evening (see Chapter 26, p. 287).
- *Wheezing* usually is more marked when your child breathes out and is present in many childhood diseases including asthma and bronchiolitis (see Chapter 26, p. 285, and Chapter 28, p. 304).
- Your child may generate a variety of strange and disturbing sounds when she breathes through mucus in her nose or throat. These include "snuffly" sounds, whistling sounds, wheezing sounds, and coughs that may be loose, "junky," "fruity," or "mucousy." You may think that your child is really ill and may be convinced the "mucus is in her chest," but on closer inspection your child is often unperturbed by all the noise and not in any distress.

Blocked Nose

A blocked nose may be a serious problem in a baby. Try blocking your own nose and see how it affects you! If you don't open your mouth, you will soon be in serious trouble. Infants don't automatically open their mouth to breathe. A few drops of saline (salt water) instilled in the nose followed by suctioning may cure a blocked nose and the breathing difficulties!

"Rattly" Chest

Often, when you hold your child, you will feel a rattle in his chest and be convinced that he has mucus or fluid in his chest. This rattle is seldom due to mucus in his chest or pneumonia. It is more commonly due to the transmission of the *vibration* of mucus in the throat down to the chest cage. If your child is happy and has no signs of respiratory distress, he almost certainly does not have pneumonia but just has mucus in his throat.

OTHER SIGNS OF RESPIRATORY DISTRESS

Retractions

Retractions are also known as *recessing*. Each time your child breathes, you will notice "sucking in" of the tissues above the collarbones and between and below the ribs. The abdomen may also suck in with each respiration.

Flaring

If your child's nostrils flare in and out (like a horse's) with each respiration, she is said to have flaring.

> *Note:* Flaring and retractions are both signs of significant respiratory distress. They also may be present in dehydration and shock.

Color Changes

- *Pallor.* Does your child look pale? Children may occasionally look pale even when they are not ill, but paleness may also be a sign of many different illnesses, including breathing problems. Serious infections (sepsis) often cause marked pallor.
- *Bluish discoloration of the lips or fingertips.* This is known as *cyanosis.*

Note: Cyanosis develops only late in respiratory disease and should be taken seriously. Infants with serious infections may also be pale and cyanosed. Seek medical care.

At times, young infants have very blue hands and feet and may have a dusky tinge to their upper lip. This is usually a sign of poor circulation, which is normal in infants and seldom indicates any serious underlying disease. Older children who are cold also may have blue lips, hands, and feet. They should "pink up" with warming. These children will appear otherwise well and don't have any other signs of respiratory distress.

- *Red or blue in the face with coughing.* Many children become red in the face with coughing. If the coughing bouts are prolonged, they may even become blue in the face. Their normal pink color should return once the coughing bout is over.

COMPLAINING OF SYMPTOMS

An older child may complain of chest tightness, difficulty breathing, or chest pain. Keep in mind, however, that some children and adults with long-standing breathing problems such as chronic asthma may not complain of any symptoms despite having severe lung disease. (If your child has a cough in addition to breathing difficulties, refer to Chapter 28.)

When to Seek Medical Care

Seek medical care if your child

- appears ill;
- is struggling to breathe;
- has cyanosis (bluish discoloration) that is not just due to poor circulation (see above);
- has a persistently elevated respiratory rate;
- has retractions and nasal flaring;
- is very pale;
- has severe croup or wheezing;
- complains of chest tightness or chest pain;
- has a persistent cough; or
- has symptoms of sleep apnea.

Sometimes your child may have none of these symptoms or signs, but your parental intuition tells you there is something seriously wrong. If in doubt, seek medical care.

Choking

People of any age can choke, but children younger than four years of age are particularly prone to choking. As always, your goal should be prevention.

 Prevention

- Foods that easily lead to choking in young children include peanuts and other nuts, popcorn, hard candy, pieces of hot dog, and raw carrots. Do not give nuts and hard candy to young children. Cut food into small pieces before feeding it to young children.
- Do not let your child eat while running around. Supervise eating and mealtimes.
- Keep small toys and other small objects away from your children. Select toys appropriate for your child's age.

Latex balloons are particularly dangerous, as are eraser tips, buttons, and button batteries.

- Instruct the older children in your house not to give infants and younger children pieces of food and small objects.
- Learn CPR. Take a course at your local hospital, Red Cross, or similar organization. Update and practice your skills frequently. Renew your certification regularly, at least every two years.

 First Aid

Most choking episodes in children occur while they are eating or playing and are often witnessed by adults who can intervene while the child is still conscious and responsive. If your child appears to be choking, assess the situation before you intervene:

- *Do not* start first aid for choking if your child can cry or talk, has a strong cough, or is breathing adequately.
- Do start first aid for choking if your child cannot cough, talk, or emit normal sounds; is changing color (turning blue or pale); or cannot breathe; or if an older child uses the universal sign for choking (hands clutching the neck). If a child is found unconscious, you should always suspect upper airway obstruction as a possible cause and initiate appropriate first aid. See below for appropriate first aid measures by age group.

Call 911 after starting rescue efforts.

Infants Younger Than One Year of Age

If your baby appears to be choking, his breathing is obstructed, or he is turning blue and trying to cry but just making weak sounds, you will need to intervene:

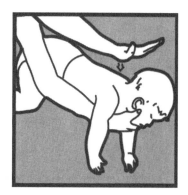

- Lay your baby face down with his head low along your forearm. His legs will straddle your forearm. Give five sharp *back blows* between his shoulder blades.
- If this fails to clear the blockage, turn your baby over and give five *chest thrusts* using two fingers on the lower half of the breastbone.
- Look in the mouth to see if this has dislodged anything.
- If the blockage does not clear, ***call 911.***
- Repeat the above steps until the blockage has cleared or until help arrives.
- If your child stops breath-

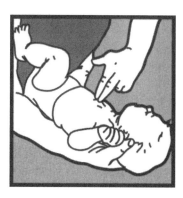

ing or remains blue, ***start cardiopulmonary resuscitation (CPR).***

- See below for management of the unconscious infant.

Older Children

Conscious Child

If your child appears to be choking but is coughing or crying or is able to talk, encourage her to cough forcefully and try to expel the foreign body.

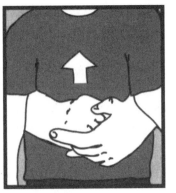

If your child cannot breathe or make a sound, you need to intervene with the Heimlich maneuver. If this does not dislodge the object and she loses consciousness, try abdominal thrusts.

If your child becomes blue or stops breathing, ***start CPR. Call 911.***

Unconscious Child

If you come across an unconscious child, you should always consider a foreign body or upper airway obstruction as a reason for the unconsciousness. This is more likely to be the case if the child is not breathing normally or is blue.

- Make sure the child is unresponsive.
- Shout for help.
- Open the airway and check for breathing. If the child is not breathing, attempt rescue breathing.
- If the child's chest does not rise, reposition the head and try the rescue breathing again. If you still are unable to give effective breaths (the chest does not rise), perform abdominal thrusts in a child or back blows in an infant.
- After each set of five abdominal thrusts (child) or five back blows (infant), open the child's mouth and look for a foreign body. If you see a foreign body, try to hook it out with your finger. If you cannot see a foreign body, do not put a finger in the mouth, as it may push an object in deeper. If you do not see a foreign body, repeat the cycle.
- ***Call 911.***
- If the child is not breathing, give rescue breaths until help arrives. Assess the pulse/circulation and if necessary ***begin CPR.***

64

CPR and Basic Life Support

It is strongly recommended that all parents learn cardio-pulmonary resuscitation (CPR) and basic life support. These skills cannot be learned from books or texts, but classes are often provided by your local hospital and by the local chapter of the American Red Cross.

Contact your local hospital or local chapter of the American Red Cross for CPR classes in your area.

Don't put this off! Phone today to reserve your place.

Renew your certification at least every two years.

PART FIVE

A Medical Kit for Children

This section of the book discusses the items suitable for a medical kit for children. Although this section is titled "A Medical Kit for Children," with just a few modifications the contents of the kit would also work for the entire family. You can create your own kit, or you can purchase one from one of the sources listed at the end of this section. Your kit should contain all the essential items and medications that you will need at home and while traveling. Even if you purchase a ready-made kit, you will need to purchase additional items to complete the kit or modify it to make it suitable for your family. I am not aware of any prepackaged kit that is totally suitable for children, especially young children. The specific contents of your kit will depend on

- the ages of your children;
- how many children are in your family;
- your destination; and
- your type of travel: adventure/"roughing it," or more sophisticated with ready access to medical care.

This section provides details about the components of a comprehensive medical kit you may want to assemble and take along with you during prolonged travel to lesser-developed countries. However, most families will require only a more basic kit for use at home or for travel in the United States. Below are the recommended contents for such a basic kit for infants and young children.

This section also includes suggestions for additional items and medications that you might like to take with you when traveling. There may be essential items you will need to get through a physician if you are traveling to countries where more exotic diseases, such as malaria, may be present. Please discuss your travel plans with your child's physician *several weeks before* you are due to depart. When traveling, do not forget to take your child's *routine medications* along—for example, allergy and asthma medications.

All medications have an expiration date. Check the medications in your kit and replace and update them as necessary. This check should take place routinely before any trip and periodically between trips. This will ensure that you always have unexpired medications to use in the event of an emergency. Just as it is a good idea to change the smoke detector batteries in your house when you adjust your clocks for daylight saving time in the spring and fall, it would also be a good idea to check your medical kit at these times. As your child grows, you may also need to change the formulation of the different medicines—for example, Tylenol syrup instead of Tylenol drops.

All the medications in your medical kit are over-the-counter medications, and most can be purchased from your local drugstore. You may have difficulty finding these medications outside the United States, especially in developing countries. Additionally, many medications in developing countries do not have expiration dates printed on their containers. Moreover, many of these medications may have different names outside the United States—for example, paracetamol instead of acetaminophen (Tylenol). For all these reasons, it is suggested that you go through each item in your kit before you leave home and replenish the supplies as needed.

For further details on how to use these medications, consult the appropriate chapter in this book.

Basic Medical Kit for Infants and Young Children

- Pain and fever medication
  - Acetaminophen (e.g., Tylenol drops *and* acetaminophen suppositories, either Feverall or Acephen)
  - Ibuprofen (e.g., Advil children's suspension)
- Allergy, cough, and cold medication
  - Saline nose drops
  - Diphenhydramine (Benadryl liquid, Benadryl chewable tablets, or Benadryl Fastmelt tablets)
- Medication for constipation, diarrhea, and stomachache
  - Electrolyte salts such as Liquilyte solution or Kaolectrolyte powder
  - Glycerine infant suppositories, Milk of Magnesia
  - Chewable antacids such as Tums, Maalox, Mylanta, or Pepto-Bismol
- Ointments and creams
  - Barrier cream or ointment for diaper rashes (Desitin, A&D Ointment, or Triple Paste)
  - 1% hydrocortisone cream or ointment (e.g., Cortaid)
  - Antifungal cream to treat yeast diaper rashes (e.g., clotrimazole cream, Lotrimin)
  - Antibacterial cream for cuts and scrapes (e.g., Triple Antibiotic, Neosporin, or Bactroban cream)
  - Aloe vera gel for burns

Continued

Basic Medical Kit for Infants and Young Children
continued

- Basic wound care supplies. These should include bandages, gauze swabs, a roll of adhesive tape, an Ace bandage, and an antiseptic cleaning solution.
- Hygiene aids. These should include an alcohol-based hand sanitizer or towelettes such as Purell.
- Instruments and supplies
  - Flexible digital thermometer
  - Pair of scissors
  - A 5-ml medication dropper
  - Disposable gloves
  - Tweezers to remove splinters and ticks
- Sunscreen
- Insect repellent

For correct dosage and how to use medications and supplies, refer to the appropriate subsections and tables later in this part of the book.

MEDICATIONS

Most children's medications are dosed according to weight. It is advisable to know your child's approximate weight so that you can calculate the correct dose of a medication.

It is easier to carry tablets than liquids when you travel, but your child should be able to chew or swallow them. Most children can chew tablets soon after their first molars erupt, which is usually around 15 to 18 months of age. The medication does have to taste good! Many medications are marketed as pleasant-tasting chewable tablets that are suitable for children as young as 18 months to 2 years. Beware of choking. For younger children, tablets can be crushed between two spoons and mixed with food. Be sure you have the correct dose. Some tablets do not even require chewing and are marketed as readily dissolving formulations that dissolve on contact with saliva.

Keep your kit and all medications in a safe place.

Keep your kit and all medications in a cool place away from direct sunlight.

Medications for Pain and Fever

Refer also to Chapter 20 for more information on the use of these medications.

Acetaminophen

Also known as paracetamol in many countries, acetaminophen is the best-known medication used to control fever and mild to moderate pain in children. It is sold in different forms (infant drops, children's elixir or syrup, chewable tablets, tablets, and suppositories) and marketed under a variety of trade names, the most recognized one in the United States being Tylenol.

- Acetaminophen infant drops (trade name: Tylenol infant drops). This medication is deal for treating fever and pain in the first year of life but may also be used in older children. Consult a physician before using in the first two to three months of life. Any fever or illness in the first two to three months of life should be discussed with a physician.

Dosing: The bottle contains a dropper with two marks—at 0.4 ml (half a dropper) and at 0.8 ml (full dropper). There are 80 mg of acetaminophen in 0.8 ml. Use only the dropper supplied with the bottle. Not all medication droppers are the same size!

- Acetaminophen elixir, syrup, suspension liquid. These forms contain 160 mg of acetaminophen per 5 ml (1 teaspoon) and are suitable for older infants and pre-school children. This form is less concentrated than the infant drops.

- Acetaminophen chewable tablets. These are pleasant-tasting tablets that come in two strengths: 80 mg and 160 mg. Chewable tablets are ideal for children two years and older and are easier to carry and administer than the liquid.

- Acetaminophen tablets and caplets. These come in a variety of strengths (80 mg to 500 mg) and are suitable for adults and older children who can swallow tablets.

- Acetaminophen suppositories (trade names: Feverall and Acephen). These are inserted rectally and come in a variety of strengths from 80 to 600 mg. For easy administration, coat with Vaseline or KY Jelly before insertion. Hold your child's buttocks together for one to two minutes after inserting the suppository.

Table 6. Acetaminophen Dosing

Child's Weight	Infant Drops*	Children's Suspension†	80-mg Chew Tabs	120-mg Suppository
6–8 lbs	0.4 ml			
9–11 lbs	0.6 ml			½
12–18 lbs	0.8 ml	½ tsp (2.5 ml)		¾
19–24 lbs	1.2 ml	¾ tsp (3.75 ml)	1	1
25–29 lbs	1.6 ml	1 tsp (5 ml)	2	1¼–1½
30–35 lbs	2.0 ml	1¼ tsp (6.75 ml)	2	1½–2
36–48 lbs		1½ tsp (7.5 ml)	3	2
49–64 lbs		2 tsp (10 ml)	4	2½
65–70 lbs		2½ tsp (12.5 ml)	5	3
71–87 lbs		3 tsp (15 ml)	6	4
More than 87 lbs	Because of the large amounts needed, it would be more practical to use a higher-strength formulation			

Note: See Caution on p. 578.

* 80 mg/0.8 ml.

† 100 mg/5 ml.

The suppository will melt and be rapidly absorbed. If the suppository has been kept in a warm environment, it may have softened. Place in the refrigerator to firm. A solid suppository is easier to insert.

Occasionally your child may eject the suppository. Reinsert and hold your child's buttocks together.

CAUTION

- Do not use acetominophen in the first two to three months of life without consulting a physician.
- Can be given every 4 hours, but do not exceed five doses per 24 hours.
- Not all teaspoons are equivalent to 5 ml. Use the medicine dropper supplied with the infant drops when using the infant drops. When using the suspension, use the measuring cup supplied with the suspension or an appropriate, accurately calibrated medicine dropper.
- Beware! Some cold medications contain acetaminophen. Always check the ingredients of other medications you are administering to your child so that you do not give too large a dose of acetaminophen.
- Acetaminophen is extremely safe when used correctly, but if overdosed or used for prolonged periods at usual doses, it can cause severe liver damage and even be fatal.
- Do not use for longer than three to four days without consulting a physician. Consult a physician earlier if you feel your child's condition is deteriorating. See Chapter 20.
- Acetaminophen is dosed according to body weight. The recommended dose is approximately 4–7 mg per pound of body weight (10–15 mg per kg body weight). The doses listed here are the *maximum* dose and may differ from the recommended dose on the medicine box or bottle.

Ibuprofen

Ibuprofen is also extremely effective for treating fever and pain in children and adults. It has the advantage over acetaminophen because its fever-reducing and pain-relieving effects last six to eight hours. It also has an anti-inflammatory effect. Its main disadvantage is that it may cause stomach irritation and bleeding problems. It is extremely safe if used correctly. Ibuprofen is *not* recommended for infants younger than six months of age.

- Ibuprofen infant concentrated drops (50 mg / 1.25 ml). This is a concentrated form of ibuprofen and comes with a dropper or syringe.

Note: These drops should *not* be administered with a teaspoon or larger medicine dropper.

- Ibuprofen children's suspension (100 mg / 5 ml). This form is ideal for older infants and young children. It comes in a pleasant-tasting liquid and is usually very easy to administer. The two best-known ibuprofen suspensions are Motrin Children's Suspension and Advil Children's Suspension.
- Ibuprofen chewable tablets. These come as 50-mg and 100-mg chewable tablets. Both the Advil and the Motrin brands are pleasant tasting.
- Ibuprofen tablets (200 mg of ibuprofen per tablet). These are suitable for adults and older children who can swallow tablets.

Table 7. Ibuprofen Dosing

Child's Weight	Infant Drops*	Children's Suspension†	100-mg Chewables
12–16 lbs	1.25 ml	½ tsp (2.5 ml)	
17–21 lbs	1.87 ml	¾ tsp (3.75 ml)	
22–32 lbs	2.5 ml	1 tsp (5 ml)	1
33–43 lbs		1½ tsp (7.5 ml)	1½
44–65 lbs		2 tsp (10 ml)	2
66–78 lbs		3 tsp (15 ml)	3
79–87 lbs		3½ tsp (17.5 ml)	3½
More than 87 lbs		4 tsp (20 ml)	4
		Because of the large amounts needed, it may be more practical to use a higher-strength formulation	

* 80 mg/0.8 ml.
† 100 mg/5 ml.

Note: Neither acetaminophen nor ibuprofen will be effective in reducing fever if the child is too warmly clothed or is in a very warm environment. Neither medication may return your child's temperature to normal and will often lower the temperature by only two or three degrees.

As mentioned in Chapter 20, the height of your child's fever is less important than how your child is acting.

Even though acetaminophen and ibuprofen are over-the-counter medications, both may be extremely toxic if overdosed or if used for too long a period. Always check other medications you are administering to your child to make sure that they do not contain these ingredients.

CAUTION

- Ibuprofen is not recommended for children younger than six months of age.
- Give every 6–8 hours but not more than three doses in 24 hours.
- Do not use for longer than three to four days without consulting a physician.
- If your child's condition is deteriorating, consult a physician.
- Ibuprofen can cause severe gastric irritation, bleeding, and kidney and liver damage. As with all other medication, it is essential to dose accurately.
- Ibuprofen is dosed according to body weight. The dosage range is 2–4 mg per pound of body weight (5–10 mg per kg body weight). The doses listed here are the *maximum* dose and may differ from the recommended dose on the medicine box or bottle.

If in any doubt, consult a physician.

Keep these and all other medications out of the reach of children.

Medications for Allergies, Coughs, and Colds

Diphenhydramine Allergy Liquid and Chewable Tablets

Diphenhydramine is a very effective medication for allergies and is often marketed under the trade name Benadryl. It comes in many forms:

- Benadryl Allergy Liquid (12.5 mg / 5 ml). This form is suitable for younger children.
- Benadryl Allergy Chewable Tablets (12.5 mg per tablet). This form is suitable for younger children.
- Benadryl Allergy Fastmelt Tablets (12.5 mg per tablet). This form is suitable for younger children.
- Benadryl Allergy tablets (25 mg per tablet). This form is suitable for older children who can swallow tablets.

This medication is very effective for treating the itch associated with hives, insect stings, food allergies, and many other allergic reactions. Diphenhydramine also has a beneficial effect on coughs and the runny nose and sneezing associated with the common cold. For dosing, see table 8 in this chapter.

Note: Some Benadryl formulations contain pseudoephedrine as well as diphenhydramine (e.g., Benadryl Allergy/Cold Fastmelt Tablets). The pseudoephedrine may make these preparations more effective for treating colds but less suitable for treating allergies. They also tend to have far more side effects (irritability, sleeplessness, fast heart rate) and are usually best avoided, especially in young children. When buying Benadryl or other diphenhydramine medications, read the label carefully to make certain you are getting the correct medication.

Table 8. Diphenhydramine (Benadryl) Dosing

Approximate Weight	Age	Liquid*	Benadryl Allergy Chewable Tablet or Benadryl Allergy Fastmelt Tablet (12.5 mg)	Tablets (25 mg)
12–20 lbs	6–12 months	¼–½ tsp	½	
21–26 lbs	12–24 months	½–1 tsp	½–1	½
27–36 lbs	2–4 years	1–1¼ tsp	1–1¼	½–¾
37–44 lbs	4–6 years	1¼–1½ tsp	1–1½	¾
45–90 lbs	6–12 years	1½–2 tsp	1½–2	1–1½
More than 90 lbs	Older than 12 years	2–4 tsp	2–4	1–2

Note: Dosed every 6 hours. Usual dose: 0.5 mg per pound of body weight every 6 hours. Do not exceed 24 teaspoons or 12 tablets in 24 hours. See Caution on p. 584.

* 12.5 mg/5 ml.

CAUTION

- **Benadryl is not recommended for children younger than six months of age.**
- Benadryl tends to cause drowsiness and should not be taken by adolescents and adults who intend to drive a motor vehicle or operate machinery.
- Occasionally, Benadryl may cause excitability, difficulty falling asleep, and extreme irritability.
- Do not use with any other product containing diphenhydramine.
- When purchasing Benadryl or similar preparations, check the label carefully to ensure that the medication does not contain pseudoephedrine (see *"Note"* above).
- Individuals with severe food and insect allergies should not rely totally on Benadryl but also must carry with them an injectable antianaphylaxis medication such as EpiPen.

Nonsedating Antihistamines

Nonsedating antihistamines are now available both over the counter and by prescription. Examples of these include loratadine (Claritin, Alavert), desloratadine (Clarinex), cetirizine (Zyrtec), and fexofenadine (Allegra). They have the advantage of lasting 12–24 hours and have fewer side effects. They are definitely less sedating than Benadryl. Zyrtec may cause sedation in some people. Many are available as syrups, chewable tablets, or fast-dissolving tablets that young children will have no trouble taking. If you see a "D" after the antihistamine's name, it usually means the medication contains a decongestant as well, and the comments above and below about pseudoephedrine apply. The medication may be more effective, but at the cost of increased side effects. Ask your physician or pharmacist for help in deciding which medication is right for you and your child.

Pseudoephedrine Nasal Decongestant Medication
This comes in many forms. Examples are:

- Sudafed Children's Nasal Decongestant Liquid
- Sudafed Chewable Tablets

These medications provide temporary relief from a stuffy nose due to a cold or allergy. They promote nasal and sinus drainage and may temporarily relieve sinus congestion and pressure, but they often have unpleasant side effects.

There are a variety of cough and cold medications that may help the nasal congestion due to colds and allergies. Most of these medications, like Sudafed mentioned above, have the potential for unpleasant side effects and have only limited benefit in alleviating the symptoms of the common cold. In contrast, allergy medications are far more effective in alleviating allergies. For further details on the management of colds and congestion, see Chapter 23.

Table 9. Sudafed Dosing

Age	Sudafed Liquid (15 mg/5 ml)	Sudafed Chewable Tablets (15 mg)
6–12 months	Consult your physician.	
1–2 years	Consult your physician (an appropriate dose for a child heavier than 32 pounds is ½ tsp of liquid or ½ tablet every 6 hours).	
2–6 years	1 tsp	1 tablet
6–12 years	2 tsp	2 tablets
12 years and older	3–4 tsp	3–4 tablets

Note: Can be administered every 6–8 hours.

Topical Nasal Sprays

A variety of topical nasal sprays are available for treating colds, stuffy noses, and allergies.

- Nasal saline (salt water). This is ideal for clearing infants' noses and for moisturizing dry noses—for example, when flying. Nasal saline can be purchased commercially (Nasal, Ocean Drops, Little Noses, Simply Saline, Entsol), or you can make up your own saline solution (dissolve ½ level teaspoon of salt in 8 ounces of clean water).
- Nasal decongestant drops or sprays. Examples of these are oxymetazoline (Afrin) and pseudoephedrine nose

CAUTION

- Pseudoephedrine tends to make children and adults feel anxious and restless and may result in difficulty falling asleep.
- Pseudoephedrine may also cause palpitations, cardiac arrhythmias (irregularities of the heart beat), high blood pressure, and glaucoma.
- Use of Sudafed for children younger than two years of age is usually at the discretion of your physician. However, recommended doses for children 1 to 2 years of age are given in table 9. Be careful: you may end up with a restless, nervous, and irritable child who will not or cannot settle down.
- Despite all the warnings discussed above, Sudafed may be useful in preventing earache during air travel, especially in a child or adult who is traveling with nasal congestion, a cold, or allergies. The medication should be given just prior to air travel and during prolonged journeys may be repeated every six hours as necessary.

drops (0.25% or 0.5%) (¼% or ½%). These should *not* be used for longer than five days.

- Steroid nose sprays. These are very effective for treating nasal allergies and are available by prescription only, although some may soon be available over the counter. They may also have a place in the prevention of recurrent sinusitis. Steroid nose sprays are mentioned here for completeness sake and to remind you to take them along on your travels if your child suffers from nasal allergies.

Epinephrine

This is an *essential* medication to have at home and on your travels if anyone in your family is severely allergic to bees or has severe food allergies. This medication is often supplied in a kit, the best known being EpiPen, and is an injectable medication.

Medications for Motion Sickness

Dimenhydrinate

Dimenhydrinate comes as a liquid, chewable tablet, and tablet. A well-known preparation is Dramamine chewable tablets. These are fairly effective in the prevention and treatment of travel and motion sickness (see Chapter 10). To prevent motion sickness, the first dose should be taken one-half to one hour *before* starting the activity that may induce motion sickness. For dosing, see table 10 in this chapter.

CAUTION
- **Dimenhydrinate may cause drowsiness and interact with other sedatives, antihistamines, and alcohol.**
- **Should not be used for children younger than two years of age unless directed by a doctor.**

Table 10. Dimenhydrinate (Dramamine) Dosing

Age	Tablets*
2–6 years	¼–½ tablet
6–12 years	½–1 tablet
12 years or older	1–2 tablets

Note: Repeat every 6–8 hours, as necessary.

* 50 mg per tablet.

Scopolamine Patches

Scopolamine patches, such as Transderm Scop, are very effective in preventing motion sickness, but their use is *not* approved for children younger than 12 years of age. A prescription is required for these patches. Side effects include dry mouth, drowsiness, blurred vision, and difficulty with urination.

Homeopathic Preparations

Ginger is a homeopathic preparation that may be effective for some people and is very safe.

Medications for Diarrhea

Oral Rehydration Salts

- Many commercially available powders can be mixed with drinkable water to make ideal solutions to prevent and treat dehydration associated with vomiting and diarrhea. Examples of these are Kaolectrolyte, Ceralyte, IAMAT oral rehydration solutions, and Jianas Brothers

Rehydration Powder. Packets of oral rehydration powders can often be purchased at stores that sell camping and outdoor recreation supplies. Other preparations can be purchased as ready-made solutions—for example, Pedialyte and Liquilyte. However, the ready-made liquid preparations are bulky and heavy. They are ideal for home use but may weigh too much to take with you on your travels.

- These solutions can be used safely at any age.
- See Chapter 31, p. 347, for guidelines on the administration of electrolyte solutions.

> **⚠ CAUTION**
> - It is essential to mix the solution accurately, adding the correct amount of liquid to the powder (e.g., 1 packet of Kaolectrolyte powder is added to 8 ounces of water).
> - It is essential to use safe drinkable water (see Chapter 13).

Imodium AD

Imodium chewable tablets may be used for treating diarrhea in older children and adults. Most episodes of diarrhea and diarrheal disease in children are *not* treated with any medication. Pay attention to maintaining hydration and preventing dehydration by the regular and appropriate use of suitable fluids and electrolyte solutions as mentioned in Chapter 31.

Table 11. Imodium Advanced Chewable Tablets Dosing*

Age	1st Dose	Next Dose	Maximum Number of Tablets per Day
6–8 years	1	½	2
9–11 years	1	½	3
12 years and older	2	1	4

Note: Take the first dose after the first loose bowel movement. Take subsequent doses (½ of the first dose) after each subsequent loose stool. Do not exceed the maximum recommended number of tablets per day.
* 2 mg per tablet.

Imodium, in combination with certain antibiotics, may be very effective in treating travelers' diarrhea in older children and adults.

CAUTION
- Imodium should *not* be used if your child has a high fever or blood or mucus in the stool.
- If the diarrhea persists, consult a physician.
- Not recommended for children younger than six years of age.
- May cause bowel obstruction in young children.
- As mentioned above, the mainstay in treating diarrhea is fluid therapy and *not* medication. This particularly applies to the treatment of diarrhea in young children.

Bismuth Subsalicylate (Pepto-Bismol)

Pepto-Bismol may be used for both the prevention and treatment of travelers' diarrhea (see Chapter 12).

Note: Pepto-Bismol may color the tongue and stools black.

Table 12. Bismuth Subsalicylate (Pepto-Bismol) Dosing

Age	Pepto-Bismol Liquid	Pepto-Bismol Chewable Tablets
Under 3 years	2.5–5 ml	Not recommended
3–6 years	5 ml	⅓ tablet
6–9 years	10 ml	⅔ tablet
9–12 years	15 ml	1 tablet
Older than 12 years	15–30 ml	2 tablets

Note: May repeat every 30–60 minutes to a maximum of 8 doses in 24 hours. Pepto-Bismol may color the tongue and stools black.

Medications for Indigestion and Heartburn

Examples of these are Mylanta, Maalox, and Pepto-Bismol.

Mylanta Chewable Tablets

Table 13. Mylanta Chewable Tablets Dosing

Weight	Age	Tablets
Under 24 lbs	Under 2 years	Not indicated
24–47 lbs	2–5 years	1
48–95 lbs	6–11	2
More than 95 lbs	12 years and older	3

Note: Maximum of three doses per 24 hours. Maximum of three tablets under 6 years of age or six tablets from 6 to 11 years of age during a 24-hour period.

CAUTION
- **Consult a physician if indigestion persists.**
- **Do not use Mylanta for longer than two weeks without consulting a physician.**
- See Chapter 33.

Pepto-Bismol

See table 12 in this chapter.

Medications for Constipation

A variety of agents may be used to prevent and treat constipation. These include simple measures such as increasing water and juice intake as well as using over-the-counter or prescription medications. Convenient medications to take along on your travels are listed below.

Milk of Magnesia

Table 14. Milk of Magnesia Dosing

Age	Dosage
Under 2 years	Consult a physician
2–5 years	1–3 tsp once a day
6–11 years	1–2 tbsp once a day
12 years and older	2–4 tbsp once a day

Note: Follow each dosage with a full glass (8 oz) of liquid.

Senokot Liquid

A bowel action generally follows 6 to 12 hours after taking Senokot.

Table 15. Senokot Liquid Dosing

Age	Dosage
Under 2 years	Not indicated
2–6 years	½–¾ tsp
6–12 years	1–1½ tsp

Note: May give once or twice a day. If constipation persists, consult a physician.

Glycerine Suppositories

These are especially useful for infants. Keep suppositories in a cool location. One infant suppository is inserted into the rectum and the buttocks held together for one to two minutes. A bowel movement will usually follow shortly thereafter. Larger glycerine suppositories may be used for older children.

For easier administration, coat the glycerine suppository with Vaseline or KY Jelly. If the suppository has softened or melted due to warm temperatures, put it in the refrigerator prior to use to solidify it.

Bisacodyl (Dulcolax Suppositories)

The suppository is inserted into the rectum and the buttocks held together for one to two minutes. The suppository may be coated with Vaseline or KY Jelly to facilitate insertion. If the suppository has softened, place it in a refrigerator prior to use to solidify it. These suppositories are usually effective within 60 minutes.

Table 16. Dulcolax Suppository Dosing (5 mg/suppository)

Age	Number of Suppositories (once a day)
Under 2 years	Not indicated. Preferably use a glycerine suppository.
2–11 years	1 suppository
12 years and older	2 suppositories

CAUTION

- **Dulcolax may cause abdominal cramps and rectal irritation.**
- **If constipation persists, consult a physician.**

Prescription Stool Softeners and Laxatives

A variety of very effective and gentle medications are available to prevent and treat constipation. Examples of these are Miralax, Kristalose, and lactulose. These are available only by prescription. Ask your physician about these medications if your child is prone to constipation.

> *Note:* You should *not* rely on medication alone to treat constipation. Management of constipation should consist of the administration of appropriate fluids, a suitable diet, correct toilet habits, and stool softeners and laxatives if necessary. If constipation persists despite these measures, medical care should be sought.

Constipation tends to be a recurring problem, and vigilance is necessary to prevent its recurrence.

Constipation is a common problem while traveling. Plan ahead. Take stool softeners or laxatives with you on your travels. Drink plenty of fluids. Take regular bathroom breaks.

OINTMENTS AND CREAMS

1% Hydrocortisone Cream or Ointment

This is used for the treatment of itchy rashes such as eczema (atopic dermatitis), insect stings and bites, and contact dermatitis.

CAUTION

- **Hydrocortisone (or any steroid cream) may make certain skin conditions worse, especially fungal infections such as ringworm and bacterial skin infections such as impetigo. If the rash does not improve, consult a physician.**
- **Do not use on the eyelids.**
- **Do not use for prolonged periods in the diaper area.**

Clotrimazole Cream or Ointment

This is used in the treatment of fungal infections of the skin such as ringworm, athlete's foot, and diaper rashes caused by yeasts. A well-known brand is Lotrimin AF.

CAUTION

If the rash does not clear, consult a physician.

Topical Antibiotic Cream or Ointment

Examples of these are Triple Antibiotic ointment, Neosporin ointment (all over the counter), and Bactroban ointment or cream, which is only available by prescription.

Diaper Rash Cream or Ointment

Essential if you have a child in diapers! Examples are Desitin ointment, A&D Ointment, and Triple Paste (especially effective).

Calamine Lotion

This is useful for insect bites and other rashes.

Vaseline

Vaseline is ideal for the treatment of dry cracked lips, raw noses, and facial eczema. It is also used for the lubrication of thermometers and suppositories.

Aloe Vera Gel

This gel is useful for the treatment of burns.

EYE CARE

The following items may be useful:

- Artificial tears or eyedrops.
- Contact lens solution (if appropriate).
- Prescription antibiotic eyedrops or eye ointments.
- Saline solution. This may be made up by dissolving ½ teaspoon of table salt in 8 ounces of clean water. Commercial saline eyedrops may also be purchased. This is an ideal solution for irrigating irritated eyes and for removing foreign bodies from the eye.
- An extra pair of eyeglasses or contact lenses. If your child wears eyeglasses or contact lenses, do not forget to take an extra pair along on your travels.
- Sunglasses.

SUN PROTECTION

- Sunscreen. This is essential for the prevention of sunburn. Ideally use sunscreen with a SPF of 15 or greater. Apply at least 30 minutes before exposure to the sun. Reapply often. See Chapter 38.
- Lip balm with a sun protection factor of 8 or greater.
- Sunglasses.
- A hat. Not part of a medical kit, but essential when traveling to sunny areas.

INSECT PROTECTION

Insect Repellents

Preparations containing DEET are by far the most effective. The following preparations are recommended:

- Sawyer Controlled Release Insect Repellent (20% DEET). This is probably the best preparation to use on children.
- Ultrathon (33% DEET). This is probably the most effective preparation overall (see Chapter 39).
- Newer picardin-containing insect repellents may soon be suitable alternatives to DEET. (However, picardin-containing insect repellents available in the United States are *not* of sufficiently high concentration to be equivalent to DEET.)

CAUTION

- **DEET-containing preparations are extremely safe if used as directed.**
- **Do not apply to the fingers or hands of young children.**
- **Do not apply on cuts, wounds, or irritated skin. Do not put in eyes or mouth.**
- **See Chapter 39.**

Insecticidal Sprays and Liquids

Sprays and liquids containing permethrin are used on clothing and mosquito nets (see Chapter 39). Knock-down insect sprays that contain pyrethroids are also available. Examples of these are Doom and Raid. Although too bulky for your medical kit, these are very useful to rid a room of insects. These aerosol cans should *not* be transported by air.

DRESSINGS, BANDAGES, AND WOUND CARE

- Alcohol swabs for cleansing wounds.
- Antibacterial towelettes for cleaning fingers, hands, and wounds.
- Betadine or povidone lotion for sterilizing wounds.
- Topical antibiotic ointment such as Triple Antibiotic ointment, Neosporin, or Bactroban (also listed under Ointments and Creams).
- Bandages.
- Liquid bandages.
- Sterile gauze swabs, 2 × 2 inches, and 4 × 4 inches.
- Telfa dressing to apply directly to burns and other wounds. This will not stick to the wound.
- Steri-Strips for repairing lacerations.
- Butterfly bandages for repairing lacerations.
- Compound Benzoin Tincture USP. This can be applied directly to the wound prior to applying the Steri-Strip. Allow the Benzoin to dry and then apply the Steri-

Strip. This allows the Steri-Strip to attach to the skin more securely.
- Gauze bandage to secure dressings.
- Roll of adhesive tape to secure dressings, repair mosquito nets, fasten diapers, and so on.
- Ace (elastic) bandage.
- Cold pack.

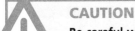

CAUTION
Be careful when applying bandages to the fingers and hands of young children. They may suck the bandages off and choke on them.

INSTRUMENTS AND OTHER MEDICAL EQUIPMENT

- Flexible digital thermometer (for oral and rectal use).
- Metal tweezers.
- Scissors.
- Tick remover.
- 5-ml medication dropper.
- Large and small safety pins.
- Latex-free protective gloves.
- Bulb aspirator for sucking mucus from noses and for irrigating ears and wounds.
- Ziploc-type plastic bags. Useful for transporting dirty diapers, wet bathing suits, and so on. The smaller ones

are useful for transporting a knocked-out tooth, ticks, and so on.

OPTIONAL ADDITIONS TO YOUR MEDICAL KIT

These may be needed on hiking and camping expeditions or if traveling to tropical and underdeveloped countries.

- Wet wipes.
- Hand sanitizer gel.
- Zanfel cleanser to help treat allergic skin reactions to poison ivy, poison oak, and poison sumac.
- Toilet paper and facial tissues.
- A knock-down insect spray such as Doom.
- Moleskin to prevent and treat blisters.
- Athlete's foot powder.
- Water disinfection equipment or water purification tablets.
- Prescription antibiotics to be obtained from your child's physician. These may include antibiotics for treating ear infections, travelers' diarrhea, skin infections, and so on. Antibiotic eyedrops or eye ointment and antibiotic eardrops for swimmer's ear may also be a good idea.
- Antimalarial medication if traveling to a malarial area.
- Survival wrap or thermal blanket.
- Dental emergency kit.
- Sterile needle syringe kit—recommended if traveling to countries where medical care and medical supplies are

limited and the risk of transmission of AIDS and hepa-
titis is high.
- Mosquito net.
- Large collapsible plastic water bottle for storing water
and making up oral rehydration solution.
- N-95 face masks (if traveling to areas with outbreaks of
SARS or similar contagious illnesses).
- Compression stockings for adults, especially those at
risk for traveler's thrombosis.
- Athletic tape for taping ankle injuries, or ankle Aircasts
for sprained ankles. Consider these if hiking or back-
packing in a remote area.

 For Your Reference

Supplies:

1. Travel Medicine Incorporated. Phone: (800) TRAV-
MED. Web site: www.travmed.com. A great source for
a variety of travel, first aid, and outdoor recreational
supplies. This company has a good selection of medical
kits, mainly appropriate for older children and adults.
2. Chinook Medical Gear. Phone: (800) 766-1365. Web
site: www.chinookmed.com.
3. SCS Ltd. Phone: (800) 749-8425. Web site: www
.scs-mall.com.
4. Adventure Medical Kits. www.adventuremedicalkits
.com.

Rehydration Salts for Treating Diarrhea and Vomiting:

1. Jianas Brothers Packaging Company. (816) 421-2880.
2. Cera Products. (301) 490-4941 or (888) 237-2598.
3. Most stores that sell outdoor recreation and camping supplies.

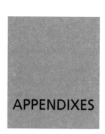

APPENDIXES

Appendix A. Average Weight of U.S. Children

Age	Weight (lbs.)
Birth	8
6 months	17
1 year	23
2 years	28
3 years	32
4 years	36
5 years	40
6 years	46
7 years	50
8 years	56
9 years	64
10 years	70
11 years	80
12 years	90

Note: To convert to kilograms, divide by 2.2.

Appendix B. Converting Degrees Fahrenheit to Degrees Centigrade

Degrees Fahrenheit	Degrees Centigrade
98	36.6
98.4	36.9
99	37.2
100	37.7
*100.4	38
101	38.3
102	38.9
103	39.4
104	40
105	40.5

Note: A temperature of 100.4°F (38°C) or higher is the definition of a fever.

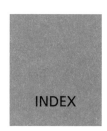

INDEX